I C 924449 3

Imperial College London

2407240797

AF759757

IMPERIAL COLLEGE, LONDON

AUTHOR/HEADING

LATHAM , R.V.

TITLE

High voltage vacuum insulation .

CLASS No. 537.222.3

ACCESSION No. 2726939 01

Books should be returned by the last date stamped.

We reserve the right to recall 2 weeks after issue.

28 APR 1989

30 JUN 1989

-5 OCT 1990

19 OCT 1992

18 JAN 1993

29 APR 1996

1-7-09.

30 APR 2012

K
6/11/81
PR

HIGH VOLTAGE VACUUM INSULATION:
The Physical Basis

HIGH VOLTAGE VACUUM INSULATION: The Physical Basis

R. V. LATHAM

Department of Physics
University of Aston, Birmingham
England

1981

ACADEMIC PRESS

A Subsidiary of Harcourt Brace Jovanovich, Publishers

London New York Toronto Sydney San Francisco

ACADEMIC PRESS INC. (LONDON) LTD.
24/28 Oval Road,
London NW1

United States Edition published by
ACADEMIC PRESS INC.
111 Fifth Avenue
New York, New York 10003

Copyright © 1981 by
ACADEMIC PRESS INC. (LONDON) LTD.

All Rights Reserved
No part of this book may be reproduced in any form by photostat, microfilm, or any other means, without written permission from the publishers

British Library Cataloguing in Publication Data
Latham, R. V.
High Voltage Vacuum Insulation.
1. Electric insulators and insulation
2. High voltages
I. Title
621.319'37 TK3401 80-41602

ISBN 0-12-437180-9

537.222.3
27269390l

Printed in Great Britain by
Whitstable Litho Ltd., Whitstable, Kent

Preface

The aim of this book is to provide a contemporary "introduction" to the physics and technology of high-voltage vacuum insulation; to this end, it gives a concise account of the basic physical concepts, together with a detailed source for further specialised reading. Each chapter deals with a specific aspect of the subject and, as far as possible, has been written as a self-contained entity with inclusive referencing. Whilst the book is chiefly directed towards the research worker or development engineer, its format makes the text equally suitable for use as a basis for "special topic" lecture courses at either under-or postgraduate level within Electrical Engineering or Applied Physics departments of universities or polytechnics.

In the opening chapter, the reader is given a general perspective of the electrical insulating properties of the vacuum gap, together with a brief historical survey of the main developments in the identification of the fundamental physical processes that ultimately determine its performance. This is followed in chapter 2 by a detailed account of the design criteria for practical high voltage electrode pairs and how their operational characteristics are influenced by such basic parameters as their material, geometry,separation and surface preparation. The central chapters (3 to 6) of the book are devoted firstly to an analysis of the theoretical models that have been evolved to explain how the electrical breakdown of a gap is initiated, and secondly, to a review of the corroborative experimental evidence that has been obtained from controlled laboratory simulation studies. Attention is then directed in the penultimate chapter(7) towards a very important series of experimental investigations that have used diagnostic techniques to identify the physical processes that actually occur in normal operational gaps; in particular, it highlights a number of sophisticated systems that have recently been developed for making in situ dynamic studies of phenomena. The final chapter opens with a discussion of the practical implications of some exciting new findings that have emerged from these latter studies,and concludes with an objective assessment of the "present state of the art" that integrates the well established concepts presented in the earlier chapters of the book with some new but relatively undeveloped ideas. It should be noted that this treatment deliberately omits any consideration of the properties of the high current arcs that characterise the post-breakdown regime, since this topic is adequately dealt with in the literature on plasma physics. An appendix has however been included that outlines the essential details of the associated breakdown phenomenon that can result from a "flashover" across the internal vacuum surface of the glass or ceramic insulators that invariably support high voltage electrodes.

Whilst most of the cited references have been taken from well known scientific periodicals, a considerable number have also been drawn from the Proceedings of the International Symposium on "Discharges and Electrical Insulation in Vacuum" - subsequently abbreviated as Proc. DEIV. These were initiated in 1964 at the Massachusetts Institute of Technology (Proc. DEIV-I) with subsequent two-yearly symposia being held at various other international centres in North America, Europe and the U.S.S.R. Since these proceedings have provided a regular up-dating of the major developments in the field, they could be a valuable source of detailed information for the reader who wishes to pursue the subject beyond the introductory level provided by this text.

Contents

Preface	v
Acknowledgements	viii
Author's Notes	ix
Symbols and Abbreviations	x
1. Introduction	1
2. The Operational Characteristics of a High Voltage Vacuum Gap	13
3. Breakdown Initiating Mechanisms I - Electron Emission Based	51
4. Breakdown Initiating Mechanisms II - Microparticle Based	83
5. Simulation Studies I - The Point-to-Plane Field Emitting Diode	117
6. Simulation Studies II - Microsphere Impact Phenomena	141
7. Diagnostic Studies of Electrode and Gap Phenomena	171
8. Recent Advances in the Understanding of Prebreakdown Electron Emission	211
Appendix - Flashover across Solid Insulators in a Vacuum Environment	229
Subject Index	241

Acknowledgements

I would like to extend my thanks firstly to those colleagues who kindly undertook the refereeing of this book, and in so doing, offered many valuable and constructive suggestions for its improvement. Principle among these are G.P.Beukema and B.Jüttner who shared the majority of this task; in addition, I am indebted to R.A. Anderson, J.P. Brainard, B.M. Cox, R.E. Hurley, O. Lloyd and H.C. Miller for their specialist opinion on specific chapters. I am also grateful to several of the above for providing original material for inclusion in the book, and to many other authors and publishers for their agreement to reproduce figures. In all instances, I have endeavoured to make full acknowledgement and apologise for any accidental omissions.

My thanks are also due to Sylvia Wallace for her patience and co-operation in the typing of both the draft and final copy of the manuscript.

Finally, I affectionately acknowledge the constant support and encouragement given by my wife, Jean, to whom I dedicate this book.

Author's Notes

1. Although SI units have been used consistantly throughout this book, it will be noted that "pressure" has been expressed in terms of the millibar, where 1 mbar $\equiv 10^2$ Pa. This choice is based on the current policy of vacuum equipment manufacturers who calibrate their pressure monitoring systems in the mbar since this unit is similar in magnitude to the more familiar *"torr"* (i.e. 1 torr = 133 Pa $\sim$ 1 mbar).

2. As already stated in the Preface, reference has frequently been made to papers appearing in the two-yearly Proceedings of the International Symposium on Discharges and Electrical Insulation in Vacuum. For simplicity, this source has been abbreviated to Proc. I, II ... IX-DEIV where I (1964) and II (1966) were held in the U.S.A. at M.I.T., III (1968) in Paris, IV (1970) at Waterloo, Canada, V (1972) in Poznam, Poland, VI (1974) in Swansea, UK, VII (1976) in Novosibirsk, USSR, VIII (1978) in Albuquerque, USA, and the most recent IX (1980) in Eindhoven, The Netherlands.

Similarly, in the Appendix, reference is frequently made to papers taken from the Annual Reports on Conferences on Electrical Insulation and Dielectric Phenomena held at the National Academy of Science, Washington, D.C., USA; these have been abbreviated Ann. Rpt. CEIDP.

Symbols and Abbreviations

SYMBOLS

A_e	effective emitting area of a micropoint electron source
α_v	pulse over-voltage coefficient
β	geometric enhancement factor of the electric field at a micropoint electron source
C	specific heat
C_c	Cranberg constant
γ	electron penetration depth
D	microcrater diameter
d	electrode separation (i.e. electrode gap)
δ_e	secondary electron yield coefficient
E	macroscopic electric field in an electrode gap
E_b	macroscopic d-c breakdown field
E'_b	macroscopic pulse breakdown field
E_c	critical microscopic field defining whether a breakdown event is cathode or anode initiated
E_g	microscopic electric field in the gap between a microparticle and an electrode
E_ℓ	microscopic field defining the onset of space-charge limited emission
E_m	microscopic field at the surface of a microemitter
E_o	operational macroscopic gap field
e	electronic charge
ε	dielectric constant
F_d	microparticle detachment force
F_{vw}	Van der Waals adhesive force

h	height of a microprotrusion
I	the prebreakdown current flowing across a high voltage gap
I_o	modified Bessel function
i_{EE}	"explosive" electron emission current
i_F	generalised field electron emission current from a single emitter
i_{OF}	low-temperature field electron emission current from a single emitter
i_{TF}	high-temperature field electron emission current from a single emitter
i_p	photomultiplier current
j_F	generalised field electron emission current density
j_{OF}	low-temperature field electron emission current density
j_{TF}	high-temperature field electron emission current density
K	Thermal conductivity
k	Boltzmann's constant
M_p	microparticle mass
μ_o	Fermi energy at $T = 0$
$\mu(T)$	chemical potential
ρ	density
ρ_t	tunnelling resistivity
Q_p	microparticle charge
Q_T	total charge transferred between a microparticle and an electrode
q_i	impact ionisation charge
R_a	radius of anode "hot-spot"
R_g	"Gaussian" radius of electron beam cross-section
R_p	microparticle radius
r	tip radius of microprotrusion
s	thickness of ambient oxide film on an electrode surface
σ	surface charge density
σ_y	yield strength of electrode material
T	temperature
T_b	temperature at the base of a microprotrusion

T_e	electron temperature
T_i	Nottingham inversion temperature
T_p	phonon temperature
T_r	temperature at the tip of a microprotrusion
$T(r,x)$	temperature distribution in an anode "hot-spot"
T_{oo}	temperature at the centre of an anode "hot-spot"
t	time
t_b	total breakdown time
t_c	contact time of a bouncing microparticle
t_d	breakdown delay time
t_p	pulse length
t_t	transit time of a microparticle across an electrode gap
τ	charge relaxation time
τ_A	thermal response time of an anode "hot-spot"
τ_c	thermal response time of a cathode microprotrusion
τ_γ	heat spread parameter in an anode "hot-spot"
τ_s	characteristic tip-sharpening time
τ_t	time constant of charge exchange process occurring during the bouncing impact of a charged microparticle
U_k	kinetic energy of a microparticle
V	externally applied d-c gap voltage
V_{ac}	externally applied a-c gap voltage
V_b	d-c breakdown voltage of a gap
V_b'	pulse breakdown voltage of a gap
V_{ip}	externally applied impulse gap voltage
V_o	operational voltage of a gap
V_p	potential of a charged microparticle relative to an electrode
v	microparticle velocity
v_c	critical microparticle impact velocity for plastic deformation of electrode
v_f	cathode flare velocity
v_i	impact velocity of a microparticle
W	total power in an electron beam
w	power density of an electron beam

$\Omega(T)$	electrical resistivity
Z	atomic number

ABBREVIATIONS

EEE	Explosive electron emission
EHT	Extra high tension
FEE	Field electron emission
FL	Fermi level
F-N	Fowler-Nordheim
HV	High Voltage
I-V	Current-voltage characteristic
M-FEE	Metallic field electron emission
SEM	Scanning electron microscopy
T-F	Thermally assisted field emission
UHV	Ultra high vacuum

1 Introduction

1.1 The Breakdown Phenomenon
1.2 Historical
1.3 Practical Considerations
1.4 Reviews and Bibliographics
1.5 References

1.1. The Breakdown Phenomenon

Although vacuum is used extensively for the insulation of high voltages in such devices as X-ray tubes, electron microscopes, power vacuum switches, particle accelerators and separators etc., the reliability of its performance is limited by the operational risk of an unpredictable "sparking" or "arcing" between the high voltage electrodes, when the insulating capability of the vacuum gap is suddenly lost and "electrical breakdown" is said to have occurred. For some devices, such as sealed-off high voltage vacuum diodes with oxide cathodes, a breakdown event is likely to be an irreversible process and catastrophic from both the operational and financial points of view since, not only will the cathode probably be damaged, but the high voltage gap is subsequently likely to break down at a very much lower voltage: at all events, the future performance of the device will almost certainly be permanently impaired. In other applications however, such as vacuum switches and particle separators, occasional breakdown events, although undesirable, can generally be tolerated without disasterous consequences, provided special precautions are taken; for example, by controlling the energy that is available in the external circuitry for dissipation in a gap during a breakdown event. Not surprisingly, this practical limitation of the insulating capability of vacuum has had a profound influence on the design of high voltage vacuum equipment: in the short term, the problem is conventionally tackled by such empirical and often expensive procedures as maximising the dimensions of vacuum gaps, using special electrode materials and surface polishing techniques, or incorporating sophisticated electronic protection circuitry. For the long term, there has been a considerable research investment directed towards obtaining an understanding of the fundamental physical processes that give rise to breakdown, so that by taking informed precautions the insulating capability of high voltage vacuum gaps can be improved. It is with the details of this research programme and the technological implications of its findings that this book is principally concerned.

The most serious hazard in the early applications of vacuum insulation was the presence of excessive residual gas, which manifested itself either directly as a relatively high ambient pressure in the gap, probably little better than $\sim 10^{-6}$-10^{-5} mbar, or indirectly as transient pressure bursts caused by the thermal desorption of gas from the electrodes and vacuum chamber walls by localised electron or ion bombardment processes. Thus, if the local pressure p in the gap approaches a value where the mean free path of electrons becomes less than the dimension of the electrode gap d, the necessary conditions will be created for avalanche ionisation and the spontaneous establishment of an arc between the electrodes. This situation has been quantified as the well known Paschen Law [1], which defines the sparking or breakdown potential V_b in terms of a function of the product pd whose detailed form can be found, for example, in the writings of Von Engel [2], Morgan [3] and Llewellyn-Jones [4] on the electrical properties of low pressure ionised gases. However, as a result of the many advances that have taken place in high vacuum technology, where it is now standard practice to use baked-out vacuum systems in which ambient pressures of $< 10^{-7}$ mbar can be guaranteed, this mechanism of electrical breakdown is no longer regarded as a threat and, accordingly, will receive no further treatment in this text.

Thus, whilst the use of relatively gas-free ultra high vacuum (UHV) conditions greatly improves the high-voltage insulating capability of a vacuum gap, its electrical breakdown is still ultimately initiated by some form of discharge process arising from the creation of an ionisable medium in the gap. Since this can now only be derived from an increase in the local metal vapour pressure, it follows that any physical explanation of this form of breakdown must be based upon electrode surface processes that lead to the vaporisation of electrode material.

1.2. Historical

The breakdown phenomenon was first investigated scientifically by Wood [5] in 1897 and somewhat later by Earhart [6], Hobbs [7] and Millikan and Sawyer [8]. From these early studies it was established that, even prior to breakdown, a vacuum gap has a small but finite conductivity as evidenced by the flow of "prebreakdown" currents whose magnitude increased rapidly with increasing gap voltage until breakdown occurred. For mm gap separations, it was found that the corresponding breakdown field was typically $\sim 10^8$ Vm^{-1}, although it depended somewhat on the electrode material. A further observation of considerable practical significance was that the breakdown voltage was independent of pressure in the range 10^{-8} - 10^{-5} mbar. Millikan and Sawyer [8] also discovered that the voltage hold-off capability of a given gap can be significantly improved if it is subjected to an initial "conditioning" procedure (see Section 2.3) whereby the voltage is increased in small steps such that all major prebreakdown current instabilities are allowed to decay before the next voltage increment is applied. In 1920, Millikan and his subsequent co-workers [9-11] embarked on a decade of study into the source of the noisy but reversible component of the prebreakdown currents that flow between a pair of broad-area high voltage electrodes. They established that they were electronic and originated from a cold emission process (now known as field electron emission FEE) at isolated points on the surface of the cathode which gave rise to complementary fluorescent spots on the anode. At this time, these emission sites were assumed to be localised regions of the electrode surfaces where there was either an "effective" reduction in the work function through the Schottky effect [12] at field-enhancing microfeatures associated with the intrinsic microscopic roughness of electrode surfaces, or to a "real" reduction in the work function due to the presence of isolated chemical impurities. The noisy nature of the currents was attributed to the back-sputtering of ions produced by electron collision processes in the gap. Millikan and Lauritsen [11] also established that this prebreakdown current I had a well-defined empirical dependence on the gap field E such that a graph of log I versus 1/E gave a reversible straight line, i.e.

$$I = A \exp\left(-\frac{B}{E}\right)$$

where A and B are constants. It was found however that the slope B and intercept A of such plots were very sensitive to the electrode surface conditions. Other early workers of note whose principal concern was with the origin and role of these highly localised cold emission processes included Hull and Burger [13], Snoddy [14], Beams [15] and Ahearn [16]. The initial conclusion to emerge from their studies was that breakdown was due to the intense localised heating and consequent vaporisation of the anode by the bombardment of electrons emitted from these point sources. However, Ahearn [16] extended the understanding of the phenomenon by considering the possibility of breakdown being cathode initiated following the field-induced rupture of current emitting projections.

One of the first really comprehensive investigations into how the operational breakdown voltage of a gap depends on such practical parameters as the electrode material, surface preparation and gap spacing etc. was undertaken by Anderson [17] in 1935. Although the general practical conclusions to emerge from this and many subsequent studies of its kind will be reviewed in chapter 2, special mention should be made in this historical context of Anderson's identification of the 'total voltage effect'.

This is associated with large cm-gap regimes supporting hundreds as opposed to tens of kilovolts, where it is found that breakdown tends to be voltage rather than field-dependent and not apparently related to the prebreakdown electron emission currents which are frequently absent or negligible in such regimes, i.e. where the macroscopic gap fields are significantly lower than those existing in the earlier mm-gap studies of cold emission processes. To illustrate this distinction, it can be pointed out that, whereas it is possible for a 0.5 mm vacuum gap to support ∿20kV without breaking down, a 10 cm gap will support less than 1MV. Another important observation associated with this type of large-gap breakdown event was that electrode material is transported across the gap, apparently arbitarily from either the cathode or anode. In these early experiments, this phenomenon was investigated by using dissimilar electrodes, say copper and aluminium, so that optical spectroscopy techniques could be used to identify the presence of traces of a "foreign" element on a given electrode. Although it was concluded from these findings that there was evidently some additional electrode surface process which was common to both cathode and anode, no satisfactory physical explanation for it emerged until 1952 when Cranberg [18] proposed his "clump" hypothesis. This breakdown model introduced for the first time the concept that loosely adhering microscopic particles ("clumps", or nowadays more frequently referred to as "microparticles") may be torn from an electrode surface by the applied field and, because of their charge, accelerated across the gap to impact on the opposite electrode as high velocity microparticles, causing localised fusion and vaporisation of electrode material that is sufficient to trigger the breakdown of the gap. The immediate appeal of this simple mechanism was that it provided an explanation of why breakdown events are unheralded, independent of the prebreakdown current and can result in material transfer between electrodes. There have subsequently been many refinements and developments of the original model: for example, there is the "trigger discharge" model of Olendzkaya [19], whereby a charged microparticle can give rise to a local breakdown initiating discharge between itself and an electrode at very close distances of approach. As a result, the concept of microparticle initiated breakdown is now firmly established and will be discussed at length in chapter 4. Apart from these theoretical considerations, there have also been extensive laboratory simulation studies using artificially generated microparticles to verify many of the theoretical predictions: in fact, chapter 6 is devoted to a full review of these investigations.

At about the same time that Cranberg proposed his microparticle initiated breakdown mechanism, Dyke and his co-workers in America [20-22] made the next major contribution to the subject with their publication of the first quantitative results from a controlled laboratory study on the electron emission induced breakdown mechanism identified by earlier workers. The approach followed by this group, which will be fully described in chapter 5, was to simulate the field emitting micro-protrusions thought to be present on broad-area electrodes by laboratory-etched micropoint emitters similar to those used in the field emission microscope pioneered by Müller [23]. With the much improved vacuum conditions available at that time, they were able to use such emitters to study the breakdown characteristics of a well defined point-plane diode and establish that there is a critical emission current density of about $1 \times 10^{10} Am^{-2}$ at which the emitting surface becomes thermally unstable, cathode material is vaporised and breakdown is consequently initiated. The relevance of these studies to the understanding of the breakdown mechanisms operating in a broad-area gap situation was further emphasized by the electron optical profile imaging of the surfaces of miniature electrodes by Bogdanovskii [24] in 1959, and later for broad-area electrodes by Little and Smith [25] and other workers, that positively confirmed the existence of micro-protrusions having a sufficiently "sharp" geometry to produce the required geometrical field enhancement for FEE to occur. Based on information of this kind, Tomaschke and Alpert [26] were then able to show that the measured macroscopic breakdown field of a thoroughly out-gassed broad-area tungsten gap corresponded to a microscopic breakdown field of $\sim 6\text{-}7 \times 10^{9}\ Vm^{-1}$ at the tip of a tungsten microprotrusion; i.e. in agreement with the value quoted earlier that was measured directly using control micropoint emitters.

By the mid 1960's it had been recognised that a given field emitting microprotrusion would also give rise to an associated anode "hot-spot" where the electrode surface becomes locally heated by the bombardment of the fine pencil of electrons emitted by the cathode protrusion. Thus, if the local power density of the beam reaches some critical value, it is possible for anode material to be vaporised and hence the initiation of an arc between the electrodes. Such a mechanism is conventionally termed "anode-initiated" breakdown, as opposed to "cathode-initiated" breakdown when the microprotrusion itself becomes thermally unstable. In order to be able to predict which of these initiating mechanisms is most likely to precipitate the breakdown of a gap, unified theories were developed firstly by Chatterton [27] and Slivkov [28] in 1966 and in a somewhat more complete form by Carbonnier et al [29] in 1967, which established the critical initiating criteria for the two mechanisms in terms of the gap field, the electron emitting properties of the microprotrusion, the cathode and anode thermal diffusion characteristics and finally, the material constants of the electrode material. The general qualitative conclusion to emerge from these theories is that a sharp thin microprotrusion will give rise to "cathode-initiated" breakdown whilst a more blunted geometry will favour the "anode-initiated" mechanism: for a quantitative evaluation of the criteria, the reader is referred to chapter 3. It must however be pointed out at this early stage that, in their original idealised form, these breakdown initiation models take no account of a number of other physical processes that must be assumed to occur in practical high voltage gap regimes. Thus, more recent analyses of gap behaviour have attempted to incorporate, for example, the effects of ion desorption, ion bombardment (sputtering), surface diffusion of contaminants, and the more dramatic changes in the microtopography of an electrode surface that can result from localised fusion processes.

To complement the development of these models for electron emission and microparticle based breakdown, there has also been a considerable effort to obtain experimental evidence supporting their validity. For example, electron optical imaging techniques have been developed for both identifying the position of cathode emitting sites and measuring the dimensions of their associated anode hot-spots; optical and X-ray techniques have been used to measure the temperature of "anode spots"; mass spectrometry has been employed to monitor both the desorption of gas and metal vaporisation due to thermal processes at both the cathode and anode; elemental analysis by optical spectroscopy and neutron activation techniques have confirmed that material is transferred between electrodes, presumably by microparticle processes; finally, scanning electron microscopy has played a major role in identifying significant features associated with the microtopography of electrodes. The main findings of these and other techniques will be reviewed in chapter 7 when the reader has become fully acquainted with the detailed theories of electrical breakdown.

1.3. Practical Considerations

In parallel with these fundamental studies of breakdown initiating mechanisms, there has been an on-going development programme in the technological practice of high voltage vacuum insulation, whose basic aim has been to improve the voltage hold-off capability of gaps. Accordingly, the experimental philosophy has generally been to follow the more "destructive" technique of measuring the breakdown voltage V_b of a given gap regime, rather than its prebreakdown behaviour, with particular emphasis being given to evaluating the reproducibility of such breakdown data. The considerations that have featured most prominantly in this programme have been the choice of electrode material, the detailed design of electrode profiles and the final preparation of their surfaces prior to assembly: once under vacuum, it then becomes equally important to consider the external circuit parameters and the available in situ preparatory procedures for gas desorption and electrode "conditioning". For some applications, it is also possible to consider the influence of the operating pressure of the gap and the residual gas species. The inescapable conclusion to emerge from most of these investigations is that it is very difficult to achieve a high level of performance reproducibility among a set of apparently identical experimental regimes. In practical terms, this has therefore meant that large "safety factors" have to be included in the design of commercial devices, such as adopting the often expensive procedure of increasing the separation and hence dimensions of electrodes. Whilst recognising this limitation, it is nevertheless possible to identify reproducible trends in behaviour among obviously different electrode regimes, and it is these that have converged to form the basis of modern high voltage engineering practice.

Although the details of such trends will be reviewed in the following chapter, some indication of their more important practical implications may be given at this stage. Thus, it is now common practice for commercial high voltage electrodes to be machined from stainless steel or titanium alloys with rounded edge profiles that are carefully chosen to avoid field-enhancing "edge effects". Their high-field surfaces are also mechanically polished to a sub-micron "mirror" finish followed by a final ultrasonic cleaning procedure immediately prior to assembly. The electrode separation d is set by the voltage hold-off requirements. For *short gaps* of $d \lesssim 2$ mm, where instabilities predominantly stem from electron emission processes, breakdown is *field-dependent*, with the minimum d-spacing being determined by a critical breakdown field that is typically $\sim 3\text{-}5 \times 10^7\ Vm^{-1}$; in practical terms, this therefore corresponds to 20 kV being safely supported across a 1 mm gap. On the other hand, for *large gaps* of $d \gtrsim 5$ mm, where microparticle processes are thought to take over the dominant role, breakdown becomes *voltage-dependent* so that the minimum d-spacing has to be determined from a power relation of the form $V_b \propto d^m$, where m typically takes a value in the range 0.4 to 0.7 [30]; thus, whereas on the short-gap field-dependent behaviour pattern, a 5 mm gap might be expected to support $\sim$ 150 kV, in practice it will only have a voltage hold-off capability of perhaps $\sim$ 100 kV. The choice of in situ electrode conditioning treatment depends very much upon the function of the high voltage device: for the more common "passive" type of application, where the principal aim is to avoid arcing between electrodes, a prebreakdown "current" conditioning procedure is generally followed, whereas for "active" applications such as the contacts of power frequency vacuum circuit breakers, where intermittent arcing has to be tolerated, "spark" conditioning is more appropriate. In all applications, however, it is essential to minimise any capacitive energy stored in the external circuit that can be dumped across the gap during a breakdown; wherever possible, it is also desirable to have large current-limiting resistors ($\sim$MΩ's) in series with high-voltage electrodes.

Apart from being the ultimate manifestation of electrical breakdown, the vacuum arc, as intimated above, is also of vital technological significance as a transient condition that severely limits the operational performance of high voltage vacuum switches [31-33]. It is not surprising therefore that the phenomenon has been the subject of an intense independent research effort to establish the underlying physical mechanisms that control it; in particular, how the regenerative processes operating at the complementary anode and cathode "spots" sustain its burning, and what parameters ultimately determine how rapidly it can be extinguished. Since, however, a detailed discussion of the properties of a vacuum arc would be beyond the scope of this book, the topic will be dealt with only briefly in chapter 5. For the interested reader, there are comprehensive review articles[34-36] or more extended texts [37,38], that would provide an ideal introduction to the subject, whilst an insight into the most recent developments of this subject can be found, for example, in the studies of Jüttner [39] and Hantzsche [40].

Before concluding these introductory remarks on practical considerations, attention must be drawn to a secondary technological problem associated with the use of high voltage vacuum gaps; viz. the possibility of breakdown across the solid insulating support (eg. glass or ceramic) that carries the high voltage electrode. In most "passive" application this presents little difficulty provided precautions are taken to ensure an adequate design length and that its surface is maintained free from contamination. However, in "active" applications where surfaces can become "sprayed" with molten electrode material, or where the surface may become permanently damaged by high energy particles, such as in accelerator tubes, serious difficulties can be encountered. In a practical situation where such a flash-over occurs, it is very probable that a favourable conducting "track" is formed along the surface of the insulator, so that its subsequent insulating capability is permanently impaired; under such circumstances, the most expedient solution to the problem may well be to replace the insulator. Since however this is liable to be a costly remedy in most applications, efforts are currently being made to develop insulators that can in fact survive a modest number of operational high voltage breakdowns without their performance being significantly impaired. The physical mechanisms responsible for this type of breakdown event are not fully understood and will only be dealt with briefly as an appendix since the phenomenon is not directly related to the processes occurring in the vacuum gap.

1.4. Reviews and Bibliographies

For the reader who requires a more concise initial introduction to this subject than offered by the present text, there have been a number of specialist review articles dealing with the mechanisms of vacuum breakdown. The most notable of these are by Alpert, Lee, Lyman and Tomaschke [41], Slivkov, Mikhaylov, Sidorov and Nastyukha [42], Rakhovskii [43], Davies [44]and Latham [45]; more recently, there are the reviews of Chatterton and Farrall that appear respectively in references [37]and [38] which are edited collections of writings on the broader topic of electrical breakdown of gases.

The first detailed bibliography devoted to the phenomena associated with the initiation of breakdown was compiled by Hawley and Maitland [46] in 1967. Whilst this was valued by research workers at that time, it has been successively superceded by the bibliographics of Bacon, Grissom, Mangan, McClure and Newton [47] in 1972, by Farrall [48-50] in 1972, 1974 and 1976, and most recently by that of Miller [51] in 1978 and its up-date [52] in 1980. Of these, the up-dated Farrall bibliography is undoubtedly the most comprehensive, since it covers not only prebreakdown and arc phenomena, but is also cross-referenced under a large number of "categories of interest". However the more up to date bibliography of Miller would be a particularly valuable adjunct for the research worker who requires the most recent collation of information on the topics covered in this book.

1.5. References

1. Paschen, F., *Weid. Ann.* **37**, 69-75, (1889).
2. Von Engel, A., "Ionised Gases". Oxford University Press, (1955).
3. Morgan, C.G., Fundamentals of Electrical Discharges in Gases. *In* "Handbook of Vacuum Physics (Vol.2 - Physical Electronics" Electronics"). Pergamon, New York, (1965).
4. Llewellyn-Jones, F., "Ionisation and Breakdown in Gases", Methuen, (1966).
5. Wood, R.W., *Phys. Rev. Ser. I*, **5**, 1-10, (1897).
6. Earhart, R.F., *Phil. Mag.* **1**, 147-59, (1901).
7. Hobbs, G.M., *Phil. Mag.* **10**, 617-31, (1905).
8. Millikan, R.A. and Sawyer, R.A., *Phys. Rev.* **12**, 167-70, (1918).
9. Millikan, R.A. and Shackelford, B.E., *Phys. Rev.* **15**, 239-240, (1920).
10. Millikan, R.A. and Eyring, C.F., *Phys. Rev.* **27**, 51-67, (1926).
11. Millikan, R.A. and Lauritsen, C.C., *Proc. Nat. Acad. Sci. (US)*, **14**, 45-49, (1928).
12. Schottky, W., *Z. Physik*, **14**, 63-106, (1923).
13. Hull, A.W. and Burger, E.E., *Phys. Rev.* **31**, 1121-8, (1928).
14. Snoddy, B., *Phys. Rev.*, **37**, 1678-85, (1931).
15. Beams, J.W., *Phys. Rev.*, **44**, 803-7, (1933).
16. Ahearn, A.J., *Phys. Rev.*, **50**, 283-53, (1936).
17. Anderson, H.W., *Elec. Eng.*, **54**, 1315-20, (1935).
18. Cranberg, L., *J. Appl. Phys.*, **23**, 518-22, (1952).
19. Olendzkaya, N.S., *Rad. Eng. Electron Phys.*, **8**, 423-9, (1963).
20. Dyke, W.P. and Trolan, J.K., *Phys. Rev.* **89**, 799-808, (1953).
21. Dyke, W.P., Trolan, J.K., Dolan, W.W. and Barnes, G., *J. Appl. Phys.*, **24**, 570-6, (1953).
22. Dyke, W.P., Trolan, J.K., Martin, E.E. and Barbour, J.P., *Phys. Rev.*, **91**, 1043-54, (1953).

23. Müller, E.W., *Z. Physik,* **106**, 541-50, (1937).
24. Bogdanovskii, G.A., *Sov. Phys.- Solid State,* 1, 1171-6, (1959).
25. Little, R.P. and Smith, S.T., *J.Appl. Phys.* **36**, 1502-4, (1965).
26. Tomasche, H.E. and Alpert, D., *J.Vac. Sci. Technol.* **4**, 192-8, (1967).
27. Chatterton, P.A., *Proc. Phys. Soc. (London)* **88**, 231-45, (1966).
28. Slivkov, I.N., *Sov. Phys. Tech. Phys.* 11, 249-53, (1966).
29. Charbonnier, F.M., Bennette, C.J. and Swanson, L.W., *J.Appl. Phys.* **38**, 627-33, (1967).
30. Maitland, A., *J. Appl. Phys.* **32**, 2399-2407, (1961).
31. Selzer, A., *IEEE Trans. Ind. Appl.* **1A-8**, 707-22, (1972).
32. Althoff, F.D., *Elektrotech, Z.A.* **92**, 538-43, (1971).
33. Farrall, G.A.,*IEEE Trans., Parts, Hybrids and Packaging,* **PHP-11**, 134-8, (1975).
34. Farrall, G.A., *Proc. IEEE,* **61**, 1113-36, (1973).
35. Rakhovskii, V.I., *IEEE Trans. Plasma Science,* **PS-4**, 81-102, (1976).
36. Miller, H.C., *IEEE Trans. Plasma Science,* **PS-5**, 181-96, (1977).
37. J.M. Meek and J.D. Craggs (eds), "Electrical Breakdown of Gases", John Wiley, New York and Chichester, (1978).
38. J.M. Lafferty (ed.), "Vacuum Arcs", John Wiley, New York and Chichester, (1980).
39. Jüttner, B., *Beiträge Plasmaphysik,* **19**, 25-48, (1979).
40. Hantzsche, E., *ZIE-Preprint* **79-10**, (1979).

Review Articles

41. Alpert, D., Lee, D.A., Lyman, E.M. and Tomaschke, H.E., *J. Vac. Sci. Technol.* 1, 35-50, (1964).
42. Slivkov, I.N., Mikhaglov, V.I., Sidorov, N.I. and Nastyukha, A.I., *Atomizdat,* Moscow: translation FTD-MT-24-123-71, NTIS Report AD745471, (1972).
43. Rakhovskii, V.I., *Nauka,* Moscow 1970: translation FTD-MT-24-718-73, NTIS Report AD773868 (1973).
44. Davies, D.K., *J. Vac. Sci. Tech.,* **10**, 115-21, (1973).
45. Latham, R.V., *Phys. Technol.* **9**, 20-25, (1978).

Bibliographies

46. Hawley, R. and Maitland, A., "Vacuum as an Insulator". Chapman and Hall, London (1967).
47. Bacon, F.M., Grisson, J.T., Mangan, D.L., McClure, G.W. and Newton, J.C., "A Bibliography on Arc Discharges", Sandia Labs. Report SC-B-72 3233, (1972).
48. Farrall, G.A., "A Cross-Referenced File on Vacuum Arc and Vacuum Breakdown Phenomena". General Electric CRD Report 72CRD169, (1972).

49. Farrall, G.A., First up-date of [47] above; General Electric CRD Report 74CRD178, (1974).
50. Farrall, G.A., Second up-date of[47] above; General Electric CRD Report 76CRD052, (1976).
51. Miller, H.C., "A Bibliography and Author Index for Electrical Discharges in Vacuum" (1897-1976), NTIS Report No. GEPP-366, (1978).
52. Miller, H.C., First up-date of [50] above (1897-1978), NTIS Report No. GEPP-366a, (1980).

2 The Operational Characteristics of a High Voltage Vacuum Gap

2.1 General considerations
2.2 The plane-parallel d-c gap
(i) Experimental regime
(ii) Current-voltage characteristic
(iii) Fowler-Nordheim representation of the current-voltage characteristic
(iv) Electrode separation
(v) Electrode polarity
(vi) Electrode temperature
2.3 Electrode conditioning
(i) "Current" conditioning
(ii) "Glow-discharge" conditioning
(iii) "Gas" conditioning
(iv) "Spark" conditioning
2.4 Residual gas pressure
(i) Dry air
(ii) "Foreign" gas species
(iii) The "ignition" phenomenon
2.5 Design criteria for "practical" high voltage gaps
(i) General considerations
(ii) Electrode geometry
(iii) Electrode separation
(iv) Electrode material
(v) Electrode surface preparation
(vi) External circuitry
2.6 Applied voltage waveform
(i) Sinusoidal voltages
(ii) Impulse voltages
(iii) Pulse voltages
2.7 References

2.1 General considerations

From the Introduction to this text, the reader will already have begun to appreciate the physical complexity of a high voltage vacuum gap. Not only does its behaviour depend on a large number of disposable macroscopic parameters, e.g. the electrode material, their geometry and separation, the residual gas pressure etc., but also upon the ill-defined microscopic properties of electrode surfaces as determined for example by their preparation procedures and the operational "history" of the gap. Equally, there is a wide range of physical phenomena, such as electron emission, microparticle, ionic, electrode heating and thermal diffusion processes, that can operate within such a complex regime and significantly influence the performance of a gap. Thus, although there is an extensive literature describing detailed investigations into the behaviour of both "experimental" and "practical" gap regimes, it is not surprising that unspecifiable microscopic differences frequently result in a large "scatter" between the findings reported from apparently identical systems. Nevertheless, it is possible to identify certain underlying and reproducible dependencies of the gap behaviour on its macroscopic parameters that may be used as design criteria by high voltage engineers. The aim of the present chapter is therefore to provide a survey of these general trends, with particular reference to the uniform-field, plane-parallel vacuum gap since this has been the most widely studied electrode geometry. We shall concentrate initially on the d-c insulating properties of gaps, leaving a discussion of the less well understood a-c regime until the end of the chapter.

2.2 The plane-parallel d-c gap

2.2(i) Experimental regime

The basic mechanical and electrical systems required for studying the behaviour of a high voltage vacuum gap under controlled laboratory conditions are illustrated schematically in Fig. 2.1. In the case of a plane-parallel geometry, the electrodes consist of two identical circular discs mounted on electrically insulated feed-throughs to a UHV chamber which nowadays is likely to be a demountable and bakeable stainless steel system capable of reaching a pressure $\lesssim 10^{-9}$ mbar: all components, particularly the electrical insulators, must therefore be unaffected by temperature cycling up to $\sim 250^{\circ}$C. Such a practical system is shown in the photograph of Fig. 2.2. One of the electrodes is generally designated the "high voltage" electrode HV (either positive or negative polarity) and accordingly has a specially designed mounting insulator capable of holding-off the maximum voltage that is to be applied across the gap. The mounting for the other "low voltage" or "earthy" electrode LV incorporates some form of bellows-linked translational manipulator for controlling the electrode separation d: it is sometimes desirable for this assembly to include an additional "tilt" manipulating facility for ensuring the accurate parallelicity of the electrodes. For further practical details of this type of electrode assembly, the reader is referred to a selection of published investigations [1-5]; fur-

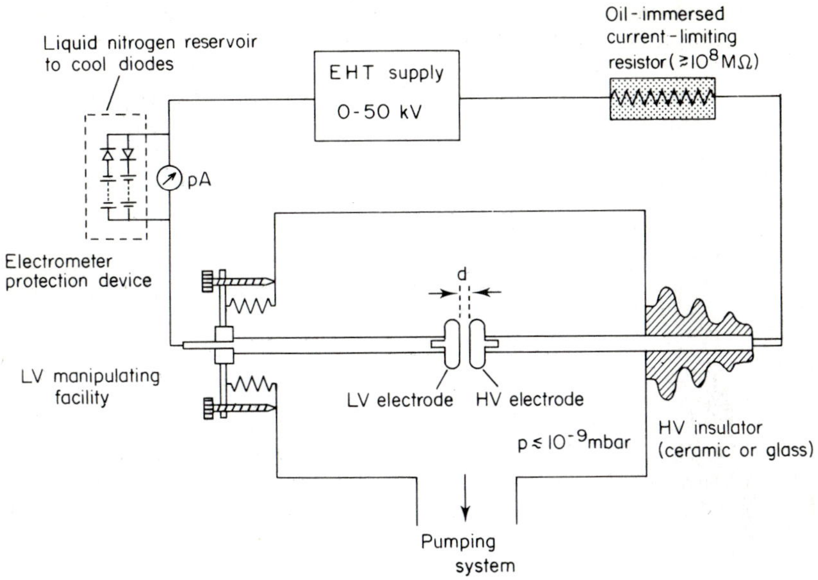

Fig. 2.1 A schematic representation of the experimental facility required for studying the current-voltage characteristi high voltage vacuum gap.

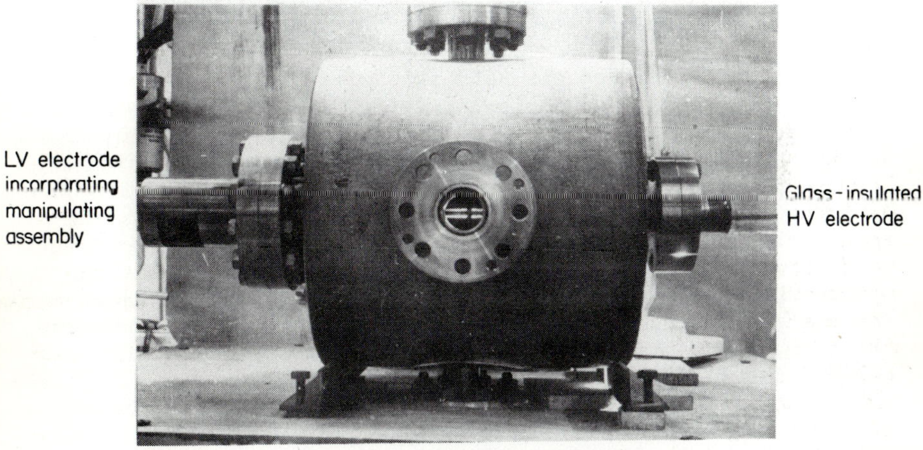

Fig. 2.2 An example of the type of UHV stainless steel experimental chamber shown in Fig. 2.1: one port has been removed in order to show the "test" electrode gap.

ther examples may be found in the bibliographies of Farrall and Miller cited in the Introduction.

To avoid the possibility of undesirable "edge effects", such as would arise from the local enhancement of the uniform gap field at a highly radiussed sharp edge of an electrode [6], it is essential to machine the outer edges of plane-parallel electrodes so that they have a rounded profile as shown in Figs. 2.1 and 2.2. The effect is illustrated in more detail in Fig. 2.3 which contrasts the distribution of electric field lines associated with pairs of unprofiled and profiled electrodes. In its ideal

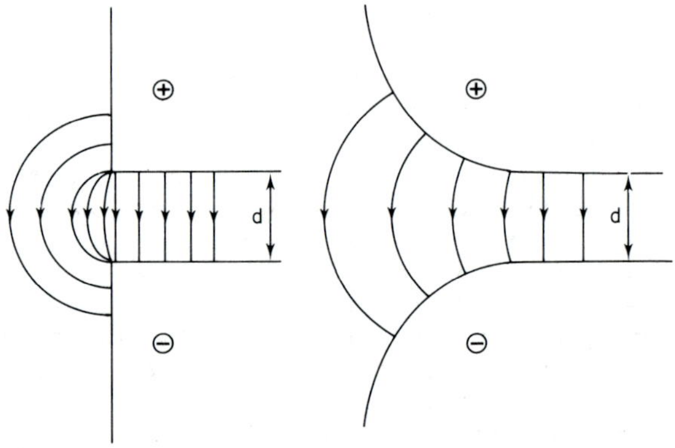

Fig. 2.3 The electric field lines associated with a planar electrode gap formed from (i) *unprofiled electrodes*, where the sharp edges result in a local enhancement of the gap field, and (ii) *profiled electrodes*, that give a uniform surface field.

form, this profile must ensure that the electrode surface field never exceeds its uniform mid-gap value. This generalised requirement has been quantified by detailed field computations as the Rogowski [7], Bruce [8], or Harrison [9] profiles which are defined in terms of the electrode separation d, such that short gaps require a more highly radiussed profile than large. As a result of the proven operational advantages to be gained from this precaution, electrode profiling has now been adopted as standard practice in high voltage engineering. It should also be noted at this stage that the elctrode surface preparation is of great importance in determining the performance of a gap; however, a detailed consideration of this topic will be delayed until section 2.5(v).

Since, as will be discussed in subsequent sections, the performance of a high voltage gap is extremely sensitive to the presence of residual gas and other contaminants, such as vacuum pump oil, it is essential to choose a suitable evacuating system. Thus, ion-getter or turbomolecular pumping systems are in common use since they employ no intermediate pumping medium that could potentially contaminate the experimental environment: ion-getter pumps do however have the disadvantage of having low pumping speeds, whilst turbo molecular pumps are currently very expensive. On the other hand, oil diffusion pumped systems are relatively cheap, fast, and if adequately trapped, can achieve the required performance: a carefully designed system employing a liquid nitrogen trapped, polyphenol-ether oil filled diffusion pump, a supplementary titanium sublimation pumping facility and a trapped rotary roughing pump can reliably achieve operating pressures of $\lesssim 5 \times 10^{-10}$mbar.

The associated external electrical circuitry required for d-c measurements is also shown in Fig. 2.1 and is seen to consist of a simple series combination of a conventional low-current ($\lesssim$ 1mA) EHT module having a continuously variable and internally monitored output voltage, an oil-immersed current-limiting resistor typically $\sim 10^8\ \Omega$) and a picoammeter for measuring the circuit current. The specifications of the EHT unit will depend upon the d-spacing of the electrodes; a 0-50 kV unit would be adequate for d $\lesssim$ 2 mm, but the maximum voltage requirement would rise steeply to $\sim$ 250 kV for a d $\sim$ 5 mm and to $\sim$ 0.5 MV for d $\sim$ 1 cm [2]. A particularly desirable feature of such units is a "fine" control of the output voltage through a continuously variable "helipot" arrangement. To protect the picoammeter against a flashover of the gap, it is desirable to shunt it by some form of protection device such as a pair of biased-off zener diodes connected back-to-back as shown in Fig. 2.1. If these components are also cooled to liquid nitrogen temperature it is possible to increase the residual resistance appearing across the combination to $\gtrsim 10^{12}\ \Omega$ when it will be greater than the input resistance of the picoammeter, so that only a negligible fraction of the total gap current will be shunted past the meter: this procedure also has the advantage of reducing the electronic noise generated in these components. For similar reasons, it is important to ensure that the resistance to earth of the low-voltage electrode should also exceed $10^{12}\ \Omega$.

2.2(ii) *Current-voltage characteristic*

It will be assumed in the following discussion that the vacuum chamber pressure is < 10^{-8} mbar which implies that the system has been baked to $\sim$ 250°C and that the "test" electrodes have therefore been partially out-gassed. To observe the general form of the current-voltage response, the applied voltage V derived from the EHT supply shown in Fig. 2.1 is slowly increased until the picoammeter records a small but continuous current of $\lesssim 10^{-10}$ A; i.e. as opposed to the transient displacement current ($\propto$ dV/dt) associated with the electrode capacitance. On further increasing V, Fig. 2.4 illustrates how this "prebreakdown" current I will rise rapidly and become progressively unstable (see insert) until, without warning, the gap will break down; i.e. an arc is struck between the electrodes so that the gap resistance falls to zero and the circuit current is only limited by the external resistance. The value of V at which this occurs is termed the breakdown voltage V_b of the gap. Although this general behaviour is

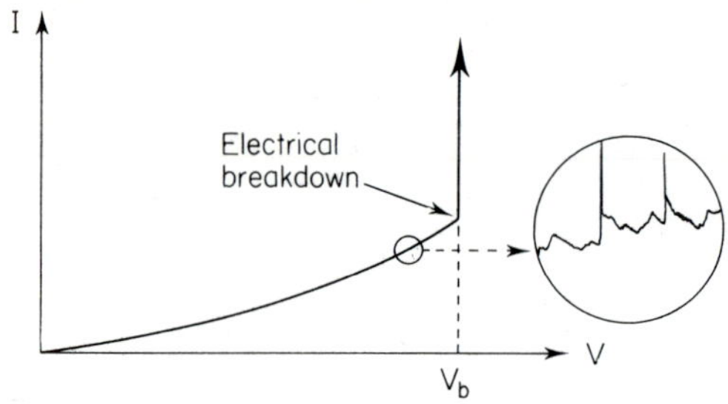

Fig. 2.4 The typical form of the non-ohmic current-voltage characteristic of a high voltage vacuum gap.

broadly common to all high voltage vacuum gaps, the detailed nature of the response, particularly the level of the prebreakdown currents and value of V_b, is very sensitive to the macroscopic parameters of the gap, the electrode surface preparation procedure and its operational "history".

With a pair of freshly prepared "virgin" electrodes, the I-V response is characterised firstly by large and very instable prebreakdown currents, and secondly, as shown in the insert to Fig. 2.3, by the superposition of frequent current spikes known as "micro-discharges" whose duration can vary from 50-1000μs, and whose magnitude can exceed the mean prebreakdown current by perhaps two orders; this latter phenomenon being most pronounced at higher voltages as $V \rightarrow V_b$. The physical origin of these microdischarge pulses has been considered by Arnal [10] and a number of other early authors [1,11-13], with several mechanisms offering a plausible explanation for their occurance. Firstly, they could be manifestations of sub-critical instances of the "explosive" electron emission or microparticle based breakdown mechanisms to be discussed respectively in Chapters 3 and 4. Secondly, they could stem from regenerative ionisation processes resulting from the local desorption of "pockets" of gas remaining in the electrode surface after the initial bake-out. Thirdly, there is the type of ion-exchange mechanism analysed by Gerasimenko [14] in which positive and negative ions are ejected from contaminant films on electrode surfaces. This latter mechanism is assumed to be initiated by say a random positive ion created in the gap that is then accelerated by the field to generate further negative ions on impact with the cathode, which subsequently generate more positive ions on impact with the anode etc. Thus, if the ion multiplication factor at the two electrodes is greater than unity, the process will develop in an avalanche fashion to give the observed microdischarge. The question of whether a microdischarge can lead to a spark (i.e. a breakdown) has been investigated by Berland et al. [15], who conclude that whilst there is a definite correlation between the two processes at low gap voltages, the same is not true at higher voltages. More recently, McKibben [16] has considered the practical significance of microdischarges in the context of the design and performance of accelerator tubes where electrodes tend to have large gaps (> 1 cm) which is the type of regime principally associated with the occurrence of microdischarges. He notes that the phenomenon can be partially eliminated by using electrodes made of titanium or its alloys, since these materials rank as having a "low ion exchange loading", especially in clean vacuum conditions where organic contamination is minimised. The operation of tubes containing an inert gas such as helium at a pressure of $\sim 10^{-5}$mbar is also beneficial (see Section 2.4)

Even with these advantageous design features, it is still important to take further precautions to control the remaining microdischarge events that will inevitably occur during the initial voltage application; otherwise, a virgin gap will almost certainly break down at a voltage that is significantly lower than that to be anticipated from its macroscopic specifications, and will thereafter be unlikely to ever achieve its maximum insulating capability. To avoid such an irreversible and operationally disastrous occurrence in practical applications, it is customary to subject virgin electrodes to one of the carefully controlled in situ "conditioning" treatments described in Section 2.3. These result in a gap that has not only a stable and reversible current-voltage characteristic as shown by the smooth curve in Fig. 2.4, but, more important, has the maximum possible voltage hold-off capability. However, as will be discussed in Section 2.3, the effectiveness of "conditioning" in stabilising prebreakdown currents and raising V_b varies considerably among electrode materials. For the most favourable regimes, it can reasonably be anticipated to achieve breakdown fields of $\gtrsim 50\text{MVm}^{-1}$ although this is still over two orders of magnitude below the theoretical value of $\sim 6.5 \times 10^9\text{Vm}^{-1}$ for a "perfect" vacuum gap [2].

2.2(iii) *Fowler-Nordheim representation of the current-voltage characteristic*

With the recognition that stable prebreakdown currents originate from "cold" electron emission processes at perhaps one or two points on an electrode surface, it was a natural progression to look for an interpretation of them in terms of the well established Fowler-Nordheim theory of field emission from metal surfaces. As explained in the Introduction, it was this line of reasoning that led to the concept of there being isolated microprotrusions on an electrode surface where the uniform gap field E is geometrically enhanced by a factor β to a microscopic value βE (see Fig. 3.2) that is above the threshold of $\sim 3 \times 10^9\text{Vm}^{-1}$ necessary for "metallic" field electron emission to occur. Although the theoretical development of this model will be delayed until Chapter 3, it is possible to anticipate the general form of the current-voltage characteristic. Thus, from the

Fowler Nordheim theory, the dependence of the low-temperature emission current density j_{OF} on the local surface field E given by equation 3.2 can be acceptably simplified by letting the functions t(y) and v(y) → 1, so that

$$j_{OF} = (B_1E^2/\phi)\ \exp\ (-B_2\phi^{\frac{3}{2}}/E) \tag{2.1}$$

where ϕ is the work function of the electrode material and B_1 and B_2 are known fundamental physical constants (see Section 3.1). With $E = \beta E = \beta(V/d)$ in the present case of a plane-parallel electrode geometry, and assuming there to be just one dominant site having an emitting area A_e, the total emission current or prebreakdown current I will be given by

$$I = A_e j_{OF} = (A_e B_1/\phi)(\beta V/d)^2\ \exp\ (-dB_2\phi^{\frac{3}{2}}/\beta V)$$

or taking logs

$$\ln(I/V^2) = -(dB_2\phi^{\frac{3}{2}}/\beta)(1/V) + \ln(A_e B_1\beta^2/d\phi) \tag{2.2}$$

It follows therefore that a plot of log I/V^2 against 1/V, known as a Fowler-Nordheim or F-N plot, should give a straight line if this type of field emission mechanism is responsible for the prebreakdown currents. As illustrated in Fig. 2.5, this is indeed confirmed experimentally for a wide range of applied fields, and has accordingly led to the general acceptance of the above explanation of the non-ohmic conductivity of a HV gap. It should however be added that F-N plots do sometimes depart from linearity at very high fields (as shown dotted in Fig. 2.5), but this behaviour can generally be attributed to subsidiary physical processes, such as the onset of space charge effects [see Section 5.1(ii)] rather than indicating false assumptions in the basic emission model.

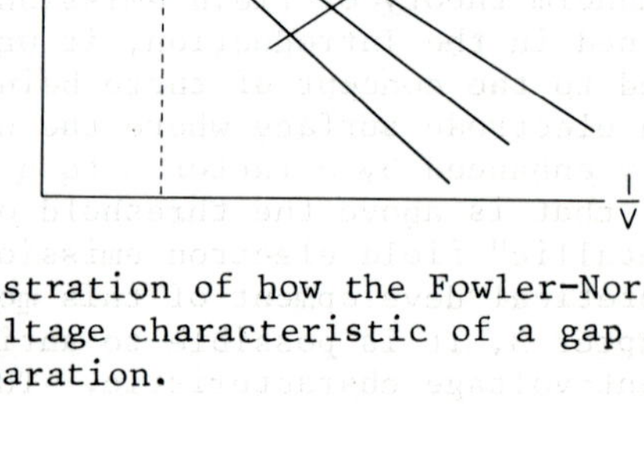

Fig. 2.5 An illustration of how the Fowler-Nordheim (F-N) plots of the current-voltage characteristic of a gap are influenced by the electrode separation.

The linearity of the F-N plot has the further advantage of providing information about both the local field enhancement β at an emission site and its apparent emitting area A_e. Thus, it will be seen from equation 2.2 that with B_1 and B_2 being known, and assuming an appropriate value for ϕ (which can be taken as an effective constant of ~ 4.5 eV for most electrode materials), β can be found from the slope of the F-N plot, and then used to find A_e from the intercept. It also follows that since β is inversely proportional to the slope, low-β "blunt" emitters (i.e. those that are likely to be stable in a practical situation) will be identified by their giving a steep-sloped F-N characteristic. Estimates of β and A_e taken from the extensive published literature on the behaviour of vacuum gaps, reveal that they can assume widely varying and apparently arbitary values within the typical ranges of $10 \lesssim \beta \lesssim 1000$ and $10^{-16} \lesssim A_e \lesssim 10^{-12} m^2$. It should be added however that there have also been occasional reports of much higher predicted values of A_e, even approaching the unlikely dimension of $10 m^2$ [17]. Whilst the lower values of these parameters, say $\beta \lesssim 150$ and $A_e \lesssim 10^{-15} m^2$, can readily be interpreted in terms of the above model, it becomes increasingly difficult to reconcile the higher β and A_e values with field emitting microprotrusions having realistic physical dimensions. In fact, this apparent anomaly will be considered further in the concluding chapter of this book in the light of recent experimental investigations that have provided further insight into the electron emission mechanisms operating on broad-area electrodes.

2.2(iv) Electrode separation

With the type of laboratory regime illustrated in Fig. 2.1, it can readily be demonstrated how the d-spacing of the electrodes has a strong controlling influence over the prebreakdown I-V characteristic of the gap. Experimentally, this is observed as a rapid fall in I with increasing d at constant V, whilst in terms of the associated F-N plot, the effect results in a systematic shift of the characteristic as illustrated in Fig. 2.5. This behaviour can be readily understood from equation 2.2, which shows how the slope of an F-N plot is directly proportional to d, whilst the intercept varies inversely with d. In practice, however, it is found that the measured variation in the F-N plots with d cannot be entirely accounted for in the above terms: it also appears that the field enhancement factor β appearing in equation 2.2. depends on d [1,2,18,19]. This effect is highlighted more dramatically by the experimental observation that the macroscopic gap field required to maintain a given prebreakdown current *decreases* with increasing d. Initially, this behaviour was attributed to the geometrical influence of the electrode edge profile [2]; however, using an anode probe hole technique to study individual sites in the centre of electrodes, Jüttner [18,20] was subsequently able to show that the phenomenon was in fact related to the voltage across the electrode gap and accordingly termed it the Total Voltage effect. He interpreted the effect in terms of the equilibrium that exists on an emitting surface between the sputtering of adsorbed oxygen by positive ions and the recovery of the surface by the migration of oxygen atoms. On this picture therefore, higher voltages would correspond to higher sputtering rates, and hence emission currents, since an oxygen-free surface has a lower work function. However, following a more recent model of Beukema [21], to be discussed in a different context in the following section, it is also possible that a voltage-dependent increase in emission could stem from the enhanced field-growth by surface migration of field emitting microprotrusions; i.e. such as could result from a rise in the cathode surface temperature following its bombardment by increasingly energetic positive ions. It should finally be noted that the published data [1,19,22] suggests that this effect is most marked with those electrode materials that give unstable gaps, e.g. copper and aluminium.

The important practical consideration of how the breakdown voltage V_b (see Fig. 2.4) depends on the electrode separation d will be dealt with formally in Section 2.5(iii). However, it can be said in summary here that at *small gaps* ($d \lesssim 0.5$mm), where breakdown is assumed to be initiated by an electron emission based mechanism, V_b is proportional to d, whereas at *large gaps* ($d \gtrsim 2$mm), where breakdown is assumed to be microparticle initiated, V_b shows a less steep dependence on d.

2.2(v) Electrode polarity

On the basis of the field emitting microprotrusion explanation of the reversible prebreakdown current-voltage characteristic, the behaviour of a given gap will be determined almost entirely by the microscopic detail of the electrode surface chosen to be the cathode. It follows therefore that since it is virtually impossible to prepare microscopically identical electrode surfaces, any gap will have two independent and frequently very different I-V characteristics, according to the alternative polarity arrangement of the electrode [23,24]. The operational stability of these two modes may be evaluated in terms of the respective emitting properties of the two surfaces as given by the β-values obtained from the associated pair of F-N plots: thus, the arrangement having the steeper sloped (low-β) plot can reasonably be assumed to have the higher voltage hold-off capability.

Beukema [21] has reported on another polarity effect that can occur with the present type of plane-parallel experimental gap regime, where one electrode is designed to carry the high voltage with the other being effectively earthed through some form of low-impedance current recording device (see Fig. 2.1). An analysis of the I-V characteristics of such systems reveals that, at any given operating pressure, there are consistantly higher emission current levels, and consequently lower hold-off voltages, where the "high voltage" electrode is made the cathode. This

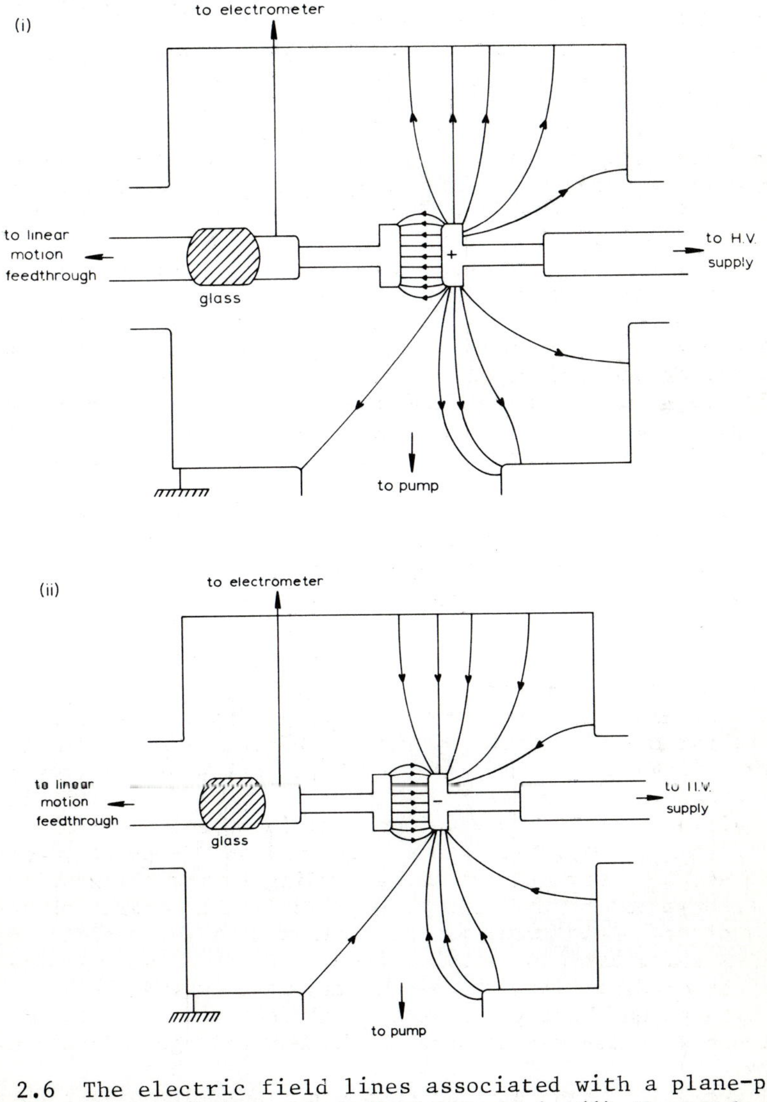

Fig. 2.6 The electric field lines associated with a plane-parallel gap when the "high voltage" electrode is (i) the anode (normal operating polarity) and (ii) the cathode. In case (ii), the chamber is effectively part of the anode and can therefore provide an additional source of positive ions through electron desorption process.
(From Beukema [21], with permission).

effect was attributed by Beukema [21] to a mechanism involving the electron desorption and ionisation of gas from the anode, the subsequent increase in the local temperature of the cathode by impinging ions, followed by the field-activated surface diffusion process described by Shrednik et al. [25,26] and Cavaille and Drechsler [27] which can lead to the build-up of field-enhancing facets that then act as new high-β electron emission centres. To understand how the influence of this mechanism can be sensitive to the electrode polarity, it is necessary to compare the field distribution for the two cases. Thus referring to Fig. 2.6, it is apparent that with arrangement (ii) i.e. the cathode at HV, the walls of the experimental chamber will also act as an anode, so that compared with arrangement (i), there will be a vastly increased surface area from which gas can be desorbed by electrons emitted from sites on the edges of the cathode. Although the practical significance of this effect has not been quantified, the evidence points to it being a potentially important consideration in the design of high voltage devices.

2.2(vi) Electrode temperature

Since this parameter can rarely be treated as a variable quantity in practical high voltage devices, there have only been a limited number of investigations into the temperature-dependence of the prebreakdown I-V characteristic of broad-area gaps, with the majority of these concentrating on low temperature superconducting regimes [24,28-34] for which there are associated device applications such as microwave cavities. On the assumption that gap currents stem predominantly from field electron emission processes at isolated metallic microprotrusions, i.e. as outlined above in Section 2.2(iii), it could be anticipated on theoretical grounds (see Chapter 3) that in the low temperature range $0 < T < 300K$, the I-V characteristic should be virtually independent of temperature. Such a behaviour has indeed been confirmed, for example, by Septier and his co-workers [30,31] for tantalum electrodes, where it was found that the F-N plots of the I-V characteristic at 4.2K, 11.7K and 77.3K were indistinguishable from one another. Similar findings have been reported by Cobourne and Williams [33,34] for niobium, vanadium, tantalum and aluminium electrodes, although these authors also reported that the F-N characteristic of virgin electrodes exhibits a reproducible discontinuity involving an abrupt increase in the slope in going from low to high fields; i.e. corresponding to either an increase in the work function ϕ or a decrease in the field enhancement factor β. Since however the discontinuity was found to disappear after $\sim$ 15-30 breakdown events, it was difficult to attribute the phenomenon directly to the superconducting state; rather, it appeared to stem from some form of conditioning process, such as discussed in the following section.

2.3 Electrode "conditioning"

As indicated in the previous section, this type of in situ treatment is an essential prerequisite if a HV gap is to achieve its full insulating capability. The basic concept behind any "conditioning" process is to safely quench as many as possible of the sources of prebreakdown current and "primary" microparticle events, so that the total number of potential hazards to the stability of the gap is significantly reduced. Since this objective is clearly of immense practical significance, there has been a considerable research effort directed towards developing techniques that can be relied upon to improve the voltage hold-off performance of gaps. As a result, four alternative procedures have been evolved.

2.3(i) "Current" conditioning

This is both the simplest and probably the most widely used technique, and is particularly suitable for the initial treatment of "virgin" electrodes that are to be used in "passive" applications. The procedure involves using the same basic circuitry illustrated in Fig. 2.1, whereby the applied voltage is increased in small discrete steps such that the prebreakdown current is allowed to stabilise at each stage before progressing. This sequence is illustrated schematically in Fig. 2.7, and highlights how there is a general fall in both the noise level of the continuous prebreakdown current and the frequency of random current "spikes" or "microdischarges": the time constant of this stabilisation process is typically $\sim$ 30 min. Another common feature of "current" conditioning is the sudden and irreversible

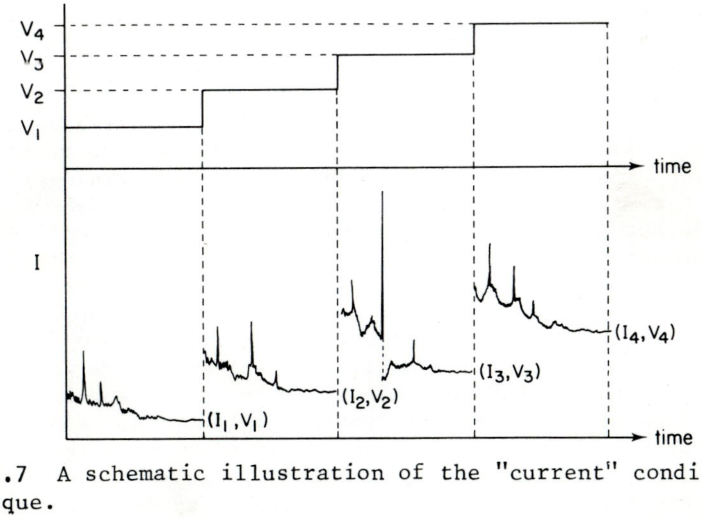

Fig. 2.7 A schematic illustration of the "current" conditioning technique.

fall in the mean level of the prebreakdown current such as follows a microdischarge in the V_3 conditioning stage. In this technique, the current-limiting series resistor plays the important role of a negative feedback element, in that if there is a random surge in the prebreakdown current, the voltage across the resistor will correspondingly increase and result in a lowering of the gap voltage, thus controlling the mechanism responsible for the surge. If the conditioning process is arrested at say the voltage V_4, where the stable prebreakdown current is i_4, the gap will have a stable and reversible current-voltage characteristic up to the limiting coordinates (i_4, V_4); i.e. similar to that shown by the smooth curve of Fig. 2.4. In practical applications, this conditioning procedure is of course continued until the intended operating voltage is reached, or more frequently exceeded by an acceptable safety margin of $\sim$ 25%. There is clearly a limit to the effectiveness of this treatment since the current drawn from the residual "stable" emitting sites will eventually reach the critical level for the onset of thermal instability and the consequent breakdown of the gap. However, with an optimum electrode design, coupled with the correct choice of electrode material and surface preparation (see the following section), it can be reasonably anticipated for example, that hold-off voltages of 10kV, 100kV and 1MV can be reliably achieved for gaps with d-values of 0.5, 5 and 50mm respectively. It should also be added that if the polarity of the gap is changed (or if it is intended for a-c operation), the above conditioning procedure has to be repeated for the other polarity connection.

There has been considerable speculation as to the physical processes that give rise to the stabilising effects of "current" conditioning [35]. Traditionally, this discussion has been mainly in terms of the influence of high fields on electrode microprotrusions, loosely adhering microparticles and microreservoirs of occluded gas, since these were thought to be the most important agencies responsible for the various components of the prebreakdown current. Thus, the sharpest field-emitting microprotrusions are assumed to be either thermally blunted following excessive electron emission or, if mechanically unstable, are removed altogether from the electrode surface by the strong electromagnetic forces associated with the applied field: such an event is clearly suggested by the type of sudden fall in the prebreakdown current that can occur during a conditioning "stage" (see Fig. 2.7). In the case of loosely adhering microparticles, it has been demonstrated experimentally [36] that, with a slowly increasing conditioning voltage, these will be detached at the lowest possible field and hence acquire only a minimum charge; as a result, their single-transit kinetic energies will be too low for a breakdown-initiating explosive impact. Instead, they will either be harmlessly removed from the gap by repeatedly bouncing between the electrodes as described in Section 4.8(i), or become permanently welded to an electrode surface by the modified trigger discharge mechanism of Beukema [36] discussed in Section 4.5(ii). The disappearance of random charge transients or "microdischarges" (see Fig. 2.7) from the prebreakdown current during its stabilisation in a conditioning stage is frequently cited as evidence in support of the suppression of microparticle activity in a gap. Similarly, the field-desorption of residual gas trapped in grain boundaries etc. will be more controlled under a slowly increasing field, so that the risk of a large gas burst sufficient to initiate a breakdown is minimised. The existance of such a gradual desorption process is directly confirmed by mass spectrometer measurements described in Section 7.1(iv), or indirectly as the general reduction in the "noise" on the prebreakdown current as conditioning proceeds. The involvement of gas in the conditioning process is further supported by the observation that the time constant associated with the decay of the prebreakdown current at a given voltage illustrated in Fig. 2.7 is pressure-dependent, even down to $\sim 10^{-10}$mbar. A detailed discussion of the effects related to the presence of residual gas will be given in Section 2.4.

2.3(ii) "Glow-discharge" conditioning

In this approach, the primary aim is to use the sputtering action of low-energy gas ions to remove contaminants from electrode surfaces and thereby, as discussed in Section 2.2(ii), minimise the incidence of microdischarges and possible breakdown events: a secondary improvement could also result from an increase of emitter work function following its coverage by inert gas atoms. The experimental procedure involves raising the pressure in the vacuum chamber to $\sim 10^{-3}$-10^{-2}mbar via a suitable gas-handling system so that a low-voltage a-c glow discharge can be struck between the electrodes. This low-current discharge can be conveniently derived from a 50 Hz source and, for optimum results, is typically run at $\sim$ 30 mA for up to $\sim$ 1 hr: longer periods of ion sputtering can often lead to a rapid degradation of the performance of a pair of electrodes. At the conclusion of this treatment, the electrode chamber is of course re-evacuated to $\lesssim 10^{-8}$mbar before making any high voltage measurements. Investigations into the effectiveness of this technique have shown it to be markedly dependent upon the residual gas species used to promote the glow discharge. Thus, from among the gases studied (H_2, D_2, He, Ar, N_2, SF_6 and "dry" air), helium, followed by nitrogen, consistently give the best results; i.e. as measured by the improvement in the hold-off voltage of the gap and the increase in the slope of the F-N plot of the current-voltage characteristic [37-39]. Considerable advantages are often claimed for this treatment over "current" conditioning, and so it is not surprising that it is common practice to subject such high voltage devices as particle-beam separators to an initial "glow-conditioning" treatment with helium at a pressure of $\sim 10^{-3}$mbar [38].

2.3(iii) "Gas" conditioning

In contrast to "glow-discharge" conditioning, which relies for its effect on the superficial "blanket" sputtering action of low-energy ions over the whole electrode surface, the "gas" conditioning technique aims at a more drastic sputtering action that is selectively localised to emitting sites on the cathode electrode. The experimental procedure, as originally reported by Lyman, Alpert and co-workers [40-42], and later used by Beukema [36,43], involves introducing an inert gas such as argon into the system at a pressure of $\sim 10^{-3}$mbar and then running a low prebreakdown current ($\sim$ 50μA) at a high voltage ($\gtrsim$ 20kV). Under such conditions, positive ions will be formed by electron impact in the high field region in the immediate vicinity of a field emitting microprotrusion such as shown in Fig. 3.4, and these will then be accelerated back to the emitter to blunt its tip by their sputtering action. A running check on the effectiveness of this treatment can be had by noting the fall-off in current at constant voltage: alternatively, its over-all effect can be quantified by comparing the β-values of the gap obtained from the "before" and "after" F-N plots of its current-voltage characteristics.

There have been contradictory reports as to the influence of this conditioning procedure on the breakdown voltage V_b of a gap. Thus, whilst Ettinger and Lyman [42], for example, found a 3 to 5 times improvement in V_b with tungsten and copper electrodes, which they assumed to be limited by the condition that the rate of blunting of existing protrusions was balanced by the rate of formation of new ones, Beukema [36] observed no significant improvement with stainless steel and titanium electrodes. Such inconclusive findings are not however surprising when it is appreciated that this, and indeed the "glow-discharge" conditioning procedure, cannot be expected to have a significant influence on the incidence of microparticle initiated breakdown events [36].

2.3(iv) "Spark" conditioning

In a situation where a previously "conditioned" high voltage gap has become "deconditioned" following an inadvertant breakdown, it is usually possible to retrieve a large measure of its original performance by subsequently subjecting it to repeated sparkings: equally, this same procedure can be applied to condition virgin polished electrodes up to their optimum insulating capability. This technique is also known as "spot-knocking", after the concept that its dominant aim is to remove localised high-β cathode emission sites or "spots" by arc erosion [44]; however, it is also efficient in eliminating microdischarges and diminishes the incidence of microparticle processes. For these reasons, it is widely used commercially as a method of maintaining the rating of high voltage vacuum devices. The electrical circuitry required for over-stressing the gap need be no more complicated than that shown in Fig. 2.1, although it might be necessary to reduce the series resistor to $\sim$ 100 KΩ in order to increase the rate of dissipation of energy in the spark. Alternatively, the effect can be achieved by an over-voltage pulse technique such as described by Miller and Farrall [44]. It is found that the number of sparkings required to achieve the maximum regeneration of a gap is unpredictable but usually varies between five and ten for common electrode materials such as copper [43,45], stainless steel [43] and molybdenum [46,47]; however, this number can be much larger for severely arced electrodes. With copper, for example, Cox [45] showed that the breakdown field increased with the number (up to 5) of low-current (< 1 A) conditioning arcs, and interpreted his findings in terms of a local hardening of the surface in the vicinity of emitting regions. In order to apply this conditioning technique effectively, it is important to note that the external capacitance associated with the gap should be minimised so that only a limited amount of energy ($\lesssim$ 10J) is dissipated in the gap during sparking [48]. From studies of the effectiveness of this type of conditioning in the important practical regime of the high voltage vacuum switch, Farrall [49] has shown that if a spark discharge is struck between the contacts during their closing sequence, they should in turn be opened with low-current arcing if the maximum voltage hold-off capability is to be subsequently achieved: with a "cold" opening (i.e. in which no arc current is drawn), the spark discharge is likely to have a deconditioning effect.

Using a more sophisticated form of spark conditioning, Jüttner [50] has recently shown that it is possible to achieve an electrode "polishing" effect using nanosecond discharges under UHV conditions, and that this procedure can lead to a dramatic improvement in the voltage hold-off capability of a gap. The change in the microtopography of an electrode surface brought about by this "polishing" procedure is vividly illustrated by the "before" and "after" scanning electron micrographs of Fig. 2.8. It was also shown that a similar "polishing" effect can be achieved with pulses as long as 500ns provided the current rise-rate is kept below a critical value of 0.5-1A ns^{-1}. From such observations it would appear that this approach to conditioning has considerable potentiality and therefore warrants further investigation.

Before concluding this discussion on electrode conditioning procedures, it should be pointed out that the above traditional interpretations of the associated physical processes occurring on the electrode surfaces may well be incomplete. Recent experimental observations to be discussed in Chapter 8 indicate that many emitting sites can have a more complicated physical structure than previously thought and that the effects of conditioning should more correctly be interpreted on an "atomic" as opposed to "microscopic" basis.

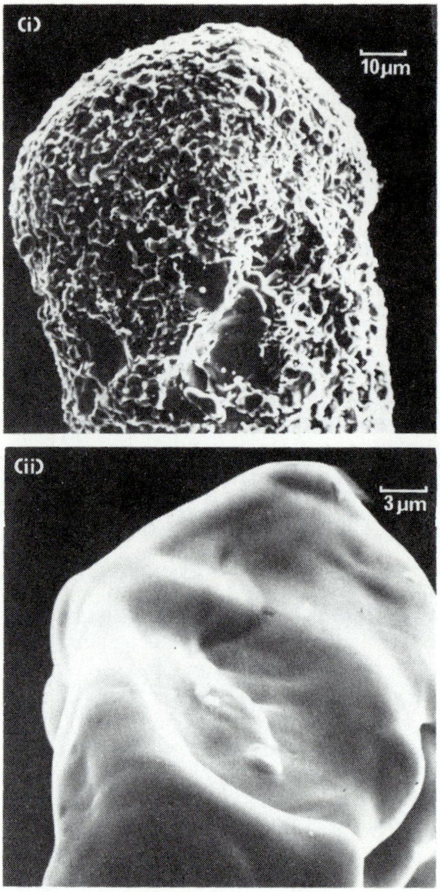

Fig. 2.8 Illustrating the electrode "polishing" effect of nanosecond discharges: (i) on an initially eroded copper cathode, and (ii) the same cathode after "polishing" with 2ns discharges. (From Jüttner [50], with permission).

2.4 Residual gas pressure

2.4(i) Dry air

It has long been known from practical experience, particularly with accelerator tubes [16], that there is a "pressure effect" associated with the insulating properties of a high voltage gap [51-59] that is particularly marked at large d-spacings [55-59]. This manifests itself most obviously by the existence of a characteristic pressure p* at which the breakdown voltage V_b of a gap reaches a maximum value V_b* that can be as much as 50% higher than its mean hold-off voltage at normal operating pressures. The value of p* will vary according to the electrode material, their geometry, the gap separation and the residual gas species, although it will typically be in the range (1-150) x 10^{-4}mbar: among the inert gases however, for which the effect is generally the most marked, it has been reported that there is no great dependency on the particular species [54]. Thus, in technological applications where such "semi-vacuum" conditions can be tolerated, the effect can be used to considerable advantage; in particular, there have been many reports of its application in particle accelerators and separators [16,38,56,57]. One of the earliest detailed studies of the "pressure effect" was due to Murray [54]; more recently, Hackam and his co-workers [59-62] have systematically investigated the behaviour of V_b with pressure and gap separation over a wide range of electrode materials. This later work has identified a number of general trends which are illustrated in Fig. 2.9.for the case of "commercially" polished plane-parallel copper electrodes having air as the residual gas medium. From this set of breakdown data, it will be seen that all of the plots are characterised by having a low-pressure plateau region ($V_b = \bar{V}_b$), a peak in the voltage hold-off capabil-

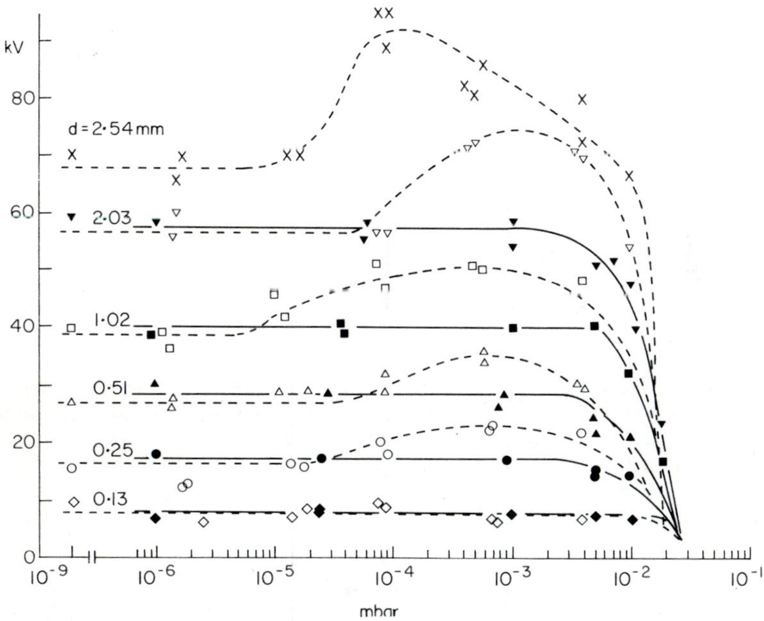

Fig. 2.9 The "pressure effect", illustrated by a family of plots showing how the d-c (dotted lines and open symbols) and a-c (solid lines and closed symbols) breakdown voltages of a pair of plane-parallel Cu-electrodes depend on the pressure and gap separation. (From Hackham and Altcheh [61], with permission).

ity ($V_b = V_b$*) and a final high-pressure region where the onset of collision ionisation processes result in a rapid fall in V_b. It is also apparent that whilst there is a general increase of V_b with gap separation, the optimum operating pressure p* corresponding to V_b* remains nearly constant for all but the largest gap separation plots. There are however bound to be significant variations of p* among electrode materials as is shown in Table 2.1 which collates the results obtained from this type of measurement.

TABLE 2.1

Material	p* (mbar)	V_b*	$(V_b^* - V_b)/V_b$ %
Aluminium	1.5×10^{-4}	48	11
OFHC Copper	1.0×10^{-3}	75	32
Nickel	2.0×10^{-6}	97	7
Niobium	5.0×10^{-4}	90	25

From this sample of data, it will be seen that both the value of V_b* for a given gap separation (2mm for the examples given),and its percentage enhancement through the "pressure-effect" over the constant low-pressure value V_b,show a significant dependence on the electrode material. Among this group of electrode materials, it is evident that copper and niobium are most susceptible to this effect, which suggest that they have surfaces that are particularly "active" to the gas species present in air, i.e. principally oxygen and nitrogen. Conversely, there have also been reports of electrode materials such as sterling-silver that do not exhibit a pressure effect [62]; in such cases, the electrode surfaces must be physically and chemically inert to the ambient gas species.

Another significant manifestation of the "pressure effect" is a general lowering of the prebreakdown current levels at any given gap field, and it is this observation that has been focussed upon as providing some insight into the fundamental phenomena that are responsible for the effect. However, because of the physical complexity of the electrode surface processes that are likely to occur in the pressure range 10^{-4}-10^{-3}mbar, it has to be recognised at the outset of this discussion that a complete interpretation of the observed behaviour must inevitably be very difficult and probably inconclusive. One explanation that has received wide support is due to Alpert et al. [41], and has been referred to already in Section 2.3(iii). This is based on the concept that in the pressure range being considered, it is possible for there to be a reduction in the local field enhancement at emitters, and hence a lowering of their β-factors (see equation 2.2), through the sputtering action of low-energy ions formed by electron collision processes in the vicinity of the tips of field emitting microprotrusions. Apart from obtaining verification of the essential features of this mechanism from simulation studies on single micropoint emitters, these same authors showed that the mechanism could also be used very effectively as the basis of the in situ "gas" conditioning technique previously described in Section 2.3(iii). There is however one feature of the pressure effect that cannot be explained solely in terms of this model, viz. its reversibility as the pressure is cycled, since this requires there to be either a re-sharpening of previously blunted emitters or the creation of new ones. Two further physical processes that have respectively been considered in this context are the surface diffusion mechanisms discussed by Shrednik et al. [25,26], Cavaille and Drechsler [27] and Litvinov et al. [63], and the welding impact of cathode-bound microparticles proposed by Beukema [36]; both of which will be referred to again in greater detail in the following two chapters. In an alternative approach, Trump [64] and Hackam [59] have attributed the "pressure effect" to an increase in the work function of an emitter following the physi-sorption of gas at the higher pressure. This interpretation is particularly attractive since it also provides an apparently plausible explanation for the reversibility of the phenomenon; viz. that gas previously adsorbed at high pressures will be field-desorbed at low pressures and thereby return the emission currents to their previous higher levels. However, this model must remain speculative at this stage since very little information exists on precisely how gas is adsorbed in the complex regime of a broad-area electrode surface: it is only for the very much simpler regime of small area emitters where, for example, Jüttner et al. [64] have been able to quantify how the emission mechanism is influenced by the adsorption of gas (see Section 7.1).

From the above discussion, it is evident that the "pressure-effect" should more specifically be associated with the properties of the cathode surface since this is the source of electron emission and hence determines the level of the prebreakdown current at any given field. It follows therefore that the breakdown characteristics of a gap having dissimilar electrode materials will show a pronounced polarity dependence: for example, Table 2.1 indicates that an aluminium-nickel combination would be markedly more stable with the aluminium electrode as the anode. Equally, for non-planar electrode geometries, where there is a large disparity between the electric fields acting on the two electrode surfaces, there will be a similar polarity effect. Thus, in experiments using a point-plane geometry [39], the breakdown strength of the gap is generally over 30% higher when operating with a positive-point polarity, i.e. where the planar cathode surfaces are subjected to a much reduced field. However, it is important to note that with this latter geometry the effect is observed at much smaller d-spacings than with planar electrodes.

2.4(ii) "Foreign" gas species

Investigations into the pressure-dependence of V_b have also been extended to other controlled gas environments [39,48], including hydrogen, helium, argon, nitrogen, oxygen, carbon monoxide and sulphur hexafluoride. These studies have shown that, with the possible exception of hydrogen, a "pressure effect" similar to that illustrated in Fig. 2.9 for dry-air is observed for the remaining gas species when used in conjunction with a wide range of electrode materials. There is however, a considerable variation in the magnitude of the effect, although the evidence tends to suggest that most of these isolated gas species provide a more favourable insulating medium than dry air, with the relatively inert gases of N_2, He and SF_6 generally giving the highest voltage hold-off characteristics. As discussed in the previous section for the case of dry air, the physical interpretation of these pressure effects is likely to be very complex, probably involving several physical processes. However, by referring to selected studies of how the residual gas species influences the insulating properties of high voltage gaps, it is possible to give a reasonably consistent explanation of the exper experimental data on the basis that an improved insulating capability stems predominantly from an increase in the emitter work-function [39]. Thus for systems in which chemisorption processes are likely to occur, such as those involving O_2 and CO on copper, nickel, molybdenum, tungsten and stainless steel, it has been shown that ϕ can typically increase in the range $0.3 \lesssim \Delta\phi \lesssim 1.8$ eV. Similarly, from the literature on ion bombardment phenomena [65,66], it is clear that physi-sorption processes can give rise to comparable increases in ϕ. He ions, for example, are known to be adsorbed more efficiently than Ar ions [65,66], and it has been suggested [39] that this could offer an explanation of why He gas gives a higher breakdown voltage than argon. It must however be emphasized that the actual changes in the work function associated with any given combination of electrode material and gas species can show a large scatter depending critically on the initial electrode preparation procedure and any subsequent in-situ treatments: for this reason, it is frequently very difficult to reproduce published data.

2.4(iii) The "ignition" phenomenon

This effect is associated with the pressure range 10^{-5}-10^{-4} mbar and is observed experimentally at some arbitrary voltage V_i as a sudden increase in the prebreakdown current by several orders of magnitude to a new "ignited" mode where the gap current becomes very much less dependent on the applied voltage. The phenomenon is illustrated schematically in Fig. 2.10, from which

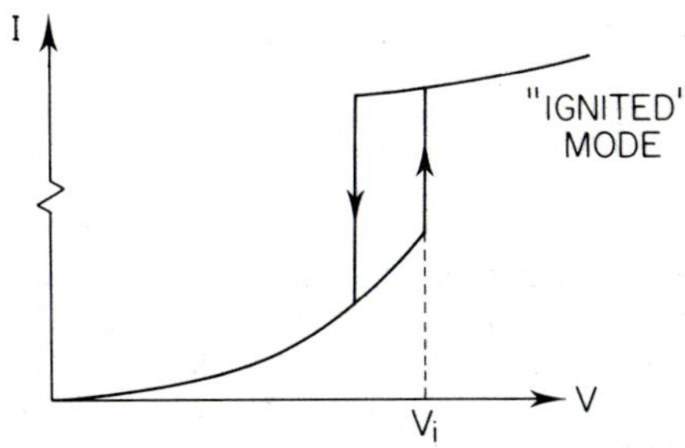

Fig. 2.10 A schematic illustration of how the "Ignition" phenomenon manifests itself on the current-voltage characteristic of a high voltage gap.

it is also seen that, when the gap voltage is cycled, there is an associated "hysteresis" of the I-V characteristic similar to that found with a low-pressure glow discharge where there are distinct "striking" and "extinction" voltages. Although most reports of the effect have been related to systems having a residual air medium [67-69] there is also evidence to suggest that it may be common to most gas species. Physical explanations of the phenomenon tend to be somewhat vague but are either based upon some form of localised regenerative ionisation process that stems from the selective desorption of gas at an anode "hot-spot", or in terms of the onset at a critical field of an enhanced electron emission resulting from resonance tunnelling via virtual energy states associated with adsorbed contaminant atoms.

In the context of this discussion on step-like discontinuities in the I V characteristic of a high voltage gap, mention should also be made of a recent observation by Cox [43] that it is also possible to observe a type of irreversible hysteresis effect under UHV conditions, where regenerative ionisation processes are unlikely to occur. Instead their origin has been associated with a "switching" phenomenon that is a characteristic feature of a more complex type of emission process to be discussed in Chapter 8.

2.5 Design criteria for high voltage electrode assemblies

2.5(i) General considerations

In practical applications of high voltage vacuum insulation, the design engineer is generally faced with the problem of evolving a compromise between two independent sets of design criteria. On the one hand he has to ensure that the operational principles of the device are satisfied, (e.g. the electric field requirements) and on the other, he has to have regard for the constraints imposed by the insulating capability of the vacuum gap. The former consideration will normally dictate the general form of the electrode geometry, e.g. apertured discs for the electrostatic lens systems of particle accelerators, whilst the latter will set a lower limit on the electrode separations which, for the example given, will determine the diameter of the lens apertures. Beyond this, there remains the choice of the electrode material, and surface preparation procedure, together with the optimisation of the edge profile and effective area of the electrodes. The relative importance of these factors have been investigated under controlled laboratory conditions in numerous "development" studies that have broadly followed one of two approaches. In the first, which includes the majority of such studies, the electrode geometry is reduced to its simplest symmetrical configuration, viz. the plane-parallel, uniform-field gap, so that the influence of the electrode material, surface preparation procedure, conditioning treatment and residual gas pressure on the I-V characteristic of the gap can more readily be assessed. The aim of the second approach is to more closely simulate the type of electrode geometries found in practical devices, so that it is possible to study the effects associated with non-uniform gap fields, such as would exist, for example, with sphere-sphere, sphere-plane, point-plane and concentric cylinder electrode combinations.

2.5(ii) Electrode geometry

Whilst the general form of a gap geometry is automatically decided by the function of the device involved, the final detailed design of the electrode profiles is determined by the physical operating requirements of the gap; e.g. a specific operational field E_o for the case of a particle separating module or a particular voltage hold-off capability V_o with say a HV vacuum switch. In practice, the design usually involves optimising the d-spacing of the electrodes (discussed in the following section) in conjunction with their effective area A_E, since both of these parameters have a strong but opposing influence on V_o (and hence E_o): thus, an increase in d at constant A_E will lower the gap field at a given applied voltage and hence result in a higher V_o, whereas an increase in A_E at constant d will generally lead to a lower V_o since more potential hazards in the form of emitting sites and microparticles will become exposed to the constant gap field [71]. This area-effect has also been shown to account for discrepancies in the published breakdown behaviour of plane-parallel electrode gaps of a given material, such as for example with stainless steel [72]. It must however also be appreciated that, because of the electrode edge-profiling requirements discussed in Section 2.2(i), an increase in d will correspondingly require an increase in the radius of the edge profile, so that, unless the overall dimensions of the electrodes are proportionally increased, there could be a sufficient fall off in the uniformity of the gap field to impair the operation of the device. This observation therefore explains why there has to be a general scaling-up of electrode dimensions in applications requiring say, a megavolt hold-off capability. It is also possible, that the violation of this requirement in experiments where the d-spacing of fixed geometry electrodes is varied, could give rise to a spurious d-dependence of the field enhancement factor β.

In the rare situation that the electrode geometry is not constrained by some specific operational requirement, and that the sole aim is to achieve the maximum hold-off voltage for a given gap spacing, laboratory experiments have shown that an impressive improvement can be derived from using a positive point-plane geometry [21,73,74]. In fact, from comparative measurements with stainless steel electrodes, Hackam [39] has shown that a three to four fold gain in the voltage hold-off capability can be achieved by this approach. Pivovar et al. [74] have also shown that there is still a small but significant gain when the above geometry "expands" to a sphere-plane configuration. One very plausible explanation for the favourable voltage hold-off characteristics of this type of regime is that, for any given applied voltage, the field on the planar cathode surface will be significantly lower than with a pair of similarly spaced plane-parallel electrodes. For example, a simple calculation using equations 2.3 to 2.5 below shows that for a geometry having a tip of radius $\sim$ 0.01mm and a d-spacing of 0.1mm, this difference will be nearly 20% [39]. Accordingly, there will be lower levels of electron emission from any potential sites and hence a much reduced risk of breakdown occurring. Beukema [21], on the other hand, has discussed an alternative explanation for the phenomenon in terms of how gas desorbed from the anode can augment field emission processes on the cathode surface: with such a model, small anode surface areas (as in the present case of a "point" anode) would therefore give rise to only a minimal effect. Also, with the combination of a low cathode field and the very small anode area associated with a "point" electrode, there will be less chance of microparticle processes occurring. It must however be emphasized that the above behaviour only applies to short gap regimes. At large gaps, microparticle processes become dominant, and there are plausible arguments given in Section 4.7(ii) which suggest that any polarity effect with non-uniform gap geometries will be reversed; i.e. it becomes more favourable to make the high field electrode the cathode.

In the course of designing gaps with non-uniform electrode geometries, it will normally be necessary to calculate the macroscopic field at the surface of an electrode to ensure that it does not exceed the critical breakdown value $\sim$ 6-8 x $10^7 Vm^{-1}$ given in Section 2.5(iii). Although such calculations are frequently very complicated, involving specialised mathematical techniques [75-79], some geometries can be treated analytically. Thus, in the case of a hemisphere-plane configuration, for example, the axial field is given to a good approximation [75] by

$$E_{oy} = 2dV[d^2(f + 1)+ y^2(f - 1)]\Big/[d^2(f + 1)-y^2(f - 1)]^2 \qquad (2.3)$$

where y is the axial coordinate, d the gap length, V the applied voltage and the function f is given by

$$f = \frac{1}{4}\left\{(2P - 1) + \left[(2P - 1)^2 + 8\right]^{\frac{1}{2}}\right\} \qquad (2.4)$$

where

$$p = 1 + d/R \qquad (2.5)$$

with R being the radius of the hemispherical electrode.

2.5(iii) Electrode separation

Although the electrode separation d is a crucial gap parameter, it is also very difficult to fix since its influence cannot be specified in absolute terms. This is because the voltage hold-off capability V_b of any given electrode geometry is not a simple function of d, but rather depends upon a number of parameters, some of which cannot be physically quantified. Under these circumstances, it is only possible to have a meaningful discussion of the dependence of V_b on d among gap regimes of a given electrode material and that have been prepared according to some standard procedure involving "optimum" surface polishing and in situ conditioning treatments (see respectively Sections 2.5(vi) and 2.3). However, even with a strict adherence to such recommended guidelines, there will still be a significant "scatter" in the insulating performance of identically prepared gaps. For this reason, it is important to incorporate "safety factors" of at least 25% when fixing the d-spacing of gaps in commercial devices.

As a consequence of this ill-defined behaviour of vacuum gaps, the design procedure for any specific application must almost inevitably involve a series of trial-and-error experiments with laboratory mock-ups to establish the correct gap spacing. Some initial guidance can however often be derived from published performance data or related experimental regimes, and to this end, the reader is referred to the extensive bibliographies cited in the Introduction to this text, which contain reports on numerous and diverse electrode combinations. The main unifying condition to emerge from such studies is that for *small gaps* ($d \lesssim 0.5$mm), breakdown tends to be field-dependent, whereas at *large gaps* ($d \gtrsim 2$mm) it becomes voltage-dependent. In physical terms, the "small-gap" behaviour corresponds to breakdown being initiated by one of the electron emission based mechanisms discussed in Chapter 3, whilst the "large-gap" behaviour becomes dominated by the microparticle processes discussed in Chapter 4. For the special case of plane-parallel gaps that have been prepared according to optimum specifications, the typical dependence of V_b on d will take the form illustrated in Fig. 2.11, where for $d \lesssim 0.5$mm the linear relation

$$V_b \propto d = E_b\, d \qquad (2.6)$$

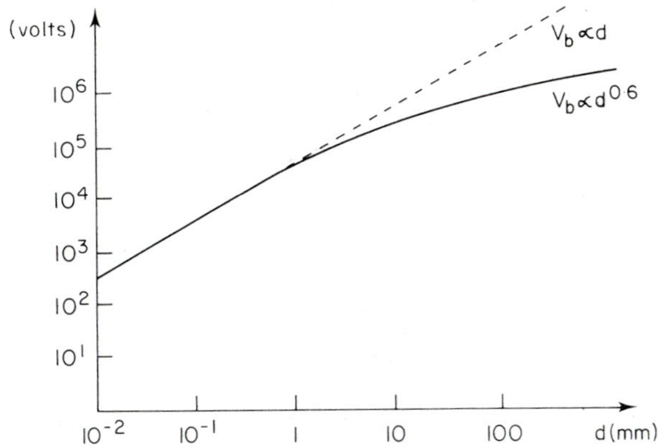

Fig. 2.11 Illustrating how the breakdown voltage V_b of a plane-parallel high voltage gap typically depends on the electrode separation d.

holds, and for $d \gtrsim 2.0$mm, i.e. beyond the transition region $0.5 \lesssim d \lesssim 2.0$mm, the power relation

$$V_b \propto d^\alpha = Kd^\alpha \qquad (2.7)$$

takes over [1,22,48,72,80-88]. Under favourable conditions the low-gap macroscopic breakdown field E_b will be in the range $6\text{-}8 \times 10^7 Vm^{-1}$ [1], whilst in the high field case, the constant of proportionality K and power α can vary respectively between $\sim$ 40-45 kV $m^{-\alpha}$ and 0.4-0.6, depending on the experimental conditions of the cited investigations.

2.5(iv) Electrode material

It has long been recognised that the correct choice of this parameter is of vital importance if a high insulating capability is to be achieved for a given gap design. Nowadays, this is facilitated by drawing on the past experience of numerous laboratory and practical studies that have led to the establishment of an approximate hierachy in the suitability of materials for use as high voltage electrodes. Thus, although there are many instances of "overlap" in the published data on the relative merits of materials, it is generally agreed that at one extreme there are materials such as copper and nickel, whose electrodes are particularly subject to instabilities, whilst at the other, there are stainless steel and titanium that consistantly give stable electrodes and hence have come to be the "accepted" materials of high voltage engineering: molybdenum should perhaps also be included in this latter group since it too is becoming more accepted for use in practical devices. A widely used type of stainless steel is AISI Spec. 304 (18/8 chrome/nickel alloy), whilst in the case of titanium there is the IMI alloy Ti - 318 ($\sim$ 89% titanium, 5-7% aluminium, 3-4.5% vanadium and 0.3% iron).

In attempting to identify the physical characteristics that single out these materials as being particularly suitable for high voltage applications, it can first be noted that they are all "physically hard" with numbers > 300 on the Vickers Scale. This property alone is not however a sufficient requirement, since there are other refractory materials such as tungsten that have never been found to give consistantly stable electrodes. A further significant property that is shared particularly by stainless steel and titanium is their resistance to corrosion effects such as oxidation, which, in part, is thought to be attributable to the fact that the surfaces of these materials are both characterised by having a strong insulating ambient oxide film $\sim$ 5nm thick [89]; i.e. as opposed to the semiconducting ambient oxide films that are commonly found on metals such as copper [90]. This type of surface property is thought to be a particularly important prerequisite for high voltage electrodes and will be considered in greater detail in Section 4.8(ii) when discussing the behaviour of microparticles in HV gaps. Another important property of these "accepted" high voltage materials is that they are equally the "accepted" materials of UHV technology; i.e. they have the property of being non-gassy. Finally it should be noted that the most recent findings discussed in Chapter 8 could well indicate that there are other material properties, such as the distribution and composition of surface impurities, that might eventually prove to be of crucial importance in determining the behaviour of high voltage electrodes.

2.5(v) Electrode surface preparation

According to the established models for breakdown initiation, the "ideal" electrode surface would be one that is free of both microprotrusions and superficially adhering microparticles. This therefore indicates the need for an electrode "finishing" treatment in which the operational surface is first subjected to some sort of microscopic polishing procedure and then to a final cleaning treatment for removing all traces of superficial debris. Attempts have therefore been made to evaluate the relative effectiveness of standard metallurgical polishing techniques viz. those based on mechanical, chemical and electrochemical processes. It was found in fact by Williams and Williams [91] that whilst the latter two techniques could occasionally produce very stable high voltage electrodes, the mechanical polishing approach was generally the most reliable and has consequently been adopted as standard practice in high voltage engineering. Electrodes whose preparation is based on this technique are said to be "commercially" polished.

The first stage of this polishing procedure is to take the freshly machined electrodes and further smooth their operational surfaces by grinding them with progressively finer carborundum grits. After a thorough washing, they are then polished to a ¼ μm "mirror" finish using a succession of alumina-based diamond pastes. The final and very vital stage in their preparation is to immerse them for long periods in an ultrasonic bath successively filled with trichloroethylene, acetone, methanol and distilled water to ensure that all traces of grease and polishing material are removed from their surface. Great care also has to be taken to avoid any re-contamination during the handling procedures involved in their final assembly: it is therefore particularly important that these latter operations are conducted in a "clean room" environment so that, for example, the risk of dust particles collecting on their surface is minimised. Despite these precautions, an electrode surface prepared in this way will still have a very complex microscopic structure, as illustrated by the scanning electron micrograph of Fig. 2.12 which shows a

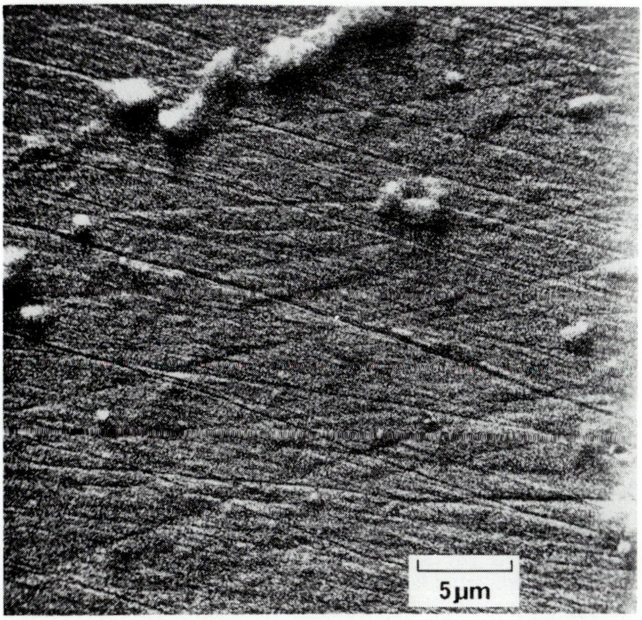

Fig. 2.12 A scanning electron micrograph showing the typical microtopography of a ¼-micron "commercially" polished planar copper electrode.

typical $(25\mu m)^2$ area of a virgin, mechanically polished copper electrode. Apart from its evident non-planar microtopography, it is also likely to have non-uniform micro-mechanical properties due to varying degrees of work-hardening within the highly disturbed upper surface layer. Similarly, there will be wide variations in the local levels of oxidation and contamination (e.g. decomposed hydrocarbons), and this will result in the surface also having non-uniform micro-electric properties. In addition, there will be many isolated non-metallic micro-inclusions, derived for example from the polishing treatment, that represent potential electron emission sites (see Chapter 8), and hence a hazard to the stability of a gap.

An alternative approach to the problem of producing an "ideal" electrode surface is to use surface coating techniques, since these would apparently offer the immediate advantages of "smoothing-out" the microtopography and "burying" loosely adhering particles. Accordingly, there have been investigations into the effectiveness of not only evaporated metal films [92] but also dielectric films [84,93-95], since these would have the further advantage of lowering the electric field over an electrode surface. However, the general conclusion of these studies is that whilst there may be initial advantages in the form of lower and more stable prebreakdown currents, the ultimate voltage hold-off capability of such gaps is not significantly increased, and, more important, that after a breakdown it is virtually impossible to apply standard conditioning procedures to recover the insulating performance of the gap. This type of irreversible change is attributed to a rupturing of the film by the strong electro-mechanical forces associated with the gap-field, where they locally overcome the non-uniform adhesive forces between the film and electrode. Such an event would not only give rise to a highly unstable microtopography, but it would also inject "foreign" debris into the gap that could either act as breakdown initiating microparticles or become attached to an electrode surface to form field emission centres: as will be discussed in Chapter 8, this latter possibility is particularly likely in the case of dielectric material. It is possible however that with more sophisticated metal film deposition techniques where, for example, greater care is taken to achieve a uniform expitaxial growth of the deposited film over the substrate electrode, this approach may ultimately prove to be very profitable.

2.5(vi) External circuitry

The breakdown of a gap is always accompanied by the rapid dissipation of capacitive energy stored in both the gap itself and the associated external circuitry [96], where normally this latter contribution is much the larger since gap capacitances rarely exceed a few pF, particularly at large d-spacings. In fact, it is this energy that plays a vital role in "feeding" the growth of the initiating arc and hence determining the extent of the surface damage ultimately sustained by electrodes during a breakdown event. To avoid this process leading to an irretrievable loss in the voltage hold-off capability of a gap, it is imperative to take precautionary measures, firstly to limit the available energy, and secondly, to control its rate of dissipation [48]. In practical terms, this means on the one hand ensuring that all stray capacitance associated with the electrode mountings and connecting leads is reduced to a minimum, and on the other, inserting a current-limiting resistor in the HV line (such as shown in Fig. 2.1) to protect the gap against the dissipation of the reservoir of capcitive energy associated with the EHT generator. Experimental investigations into optimum spark conditioning procedures discussed in Section 2.3(iii) have indicated in fact that provided the value of this series resistor exceeds some limiting value, which is typically in the range 1-3 kΩ, its influence on the d-c breakdown voltage of the gap falls off very significantly [39,83,97]. Physically, this requirement appears to correspond to the situation where the time constant of the external circuit, which controls the rate of dissipation of the capacitive energy, should be greater than ∿ 10ns which is the characteristic time constant associated with the current growth during the initiation of a vacuum arc (see Section 5.3). For most d-c and low-frequency a-c applications, this condition presents no problem; in fact, to limit any discharge current and hence the resulting electrode damage, it is conventional to increase the external resistance to ∿ MΩ's. It is only in the case of high frequency a-c ($\gtrsim$ 100 MHz) or nanosecond pulse applications that the external circuit becomes critical.

2.6 Applied voltage waveform

There are many practical devices, such as magnetrons, klystrons, vacuum switches and high voltage electronic rectifiers [98-102], where it is necessary to use the insulating capability of vacuum for holding off time-dependent voltages. Probably the simplest example of such a waveform would be the 50 Hz sinusoidal voltage derived from a mains-driven high voltage transformer; others would be RF signals, square wave pulse trains and impulse voltages. Although it is clearly of immense technological importance to know in detail how vacuum gaps respond to these types of voltage waveform, there is only a limited selection of analytical data available. Accordingly, the following survey will be inevitably limited in scope and, in many instances, inconclusive.

2.6(i) Sinusoidal voltages

From comparative measurements of the low-frequency ($\lesssim$ 250 Hz) a-c and d-c breakdown characteristics of plane-parallel "conditioned" gaps of a given electrode material and gap spacing [48,61, 83,103,104], it can generally be concluded that the peak a-c breakdown voltage tends to be somewhat higher than the corresponding d-c value. However, the effect is not very marked and frequently only involves a difference of ∿ 10% in the two breakdown voltages; the magnitude of the discrepancy also appears to be independent of frequency up to ∿ 250 Hz. These observations should be further qualified by noting that a more lengthy preparatory procedure is required for gaps that are to be used for a-c experiments, since in this case both electrodes have to be conditioned; e.g. a larger number of sparkings will be required to achieve a comparable level of conditioning [48]. In common with the d-c behaviour of gaps, these studies show that the a-c response is similarly sensitive to the choice of electrode material, and that from the limited sample of data, there appears to be a common hierachy of electrode materials and a common optimum design specification for both d-c and a-c applications.

The dependence of the peak a-c breakdown voltage $(V_b)_{ac}$ on the d-spacing of plane-parallel gaps has been investigated by Hackam and Altcheh [48,61] for a range of materials, including aluminium, copper, nickel, niobium and sterling silver. It was found that, as with the d-c experiments, there is a clear transition between the small-gap and large-gap behaviour, being particularly marked with sterling silver, for example, which followed the empirical dependence

$$(V_b)_{ac} = 45d^{0.85} \qquad \text{for } 0.05 \lesssim d \lesssim 1.5\text{mm} \tag{2.8}$$

and

$$(V_b)_{ac} = 57d^{0.3} \qquad \text{for } 1.5 \lesssim d \lesssim 2.8\text{mm} \tag{2.9}$$

with $(V_b)_{ac}$ being given in kV; i.e. differing significantly from the d-c behaviour defined by equations 2.6 and 2.7. Since however the other members of this small sample of materials had a nearly linear small-gap dependence coupled with a large-gap power dependence that more closely approximated to the d-c behaviour, it has to be concluded that there is insufficient evidence to establish the existence of a distinct a-c breakdown characteristic.

The same authors also investigated whether there is an a-c "pressure effect" [61] comparable to that illustrated in Fig. 2.9 for d-c gaps. Their findings indicate that whilst a similar phenomenon does occur, it is less general among electrode materials, where, from a sample set of measurements with aluminium, copper, nickel and niobium electrodes, a "pressure effect" was only observed with the latter two materials. There also appears to be no correlation between the optimum pressure values associated with the d-c and a-c operation for a given electrode material, so that in the case of nickel, the "optimum" d-c pressure is $\sim 3 \times 10^{-6}$mbar, whilst for the a-c case it is $\sim 2 \times 10^{-3}$mbar: in fact, the available data indicates that any "pressure effects" with a-c regimes only occur above $\sim 10^{-5}$mbar.

There is very little published information about the a-c breakdown behaviour of gaps at high frequencies. Experiments at RF frequencies [103,104] have shown that gap performances are indistinguishable from their low-frequency characteristics. However, at MHz frequencies [105], it has been found that the gap-dependence of the breakdown voltage (in kV) takes the form $V_b = 31d^{0.7}$ over the range $1 \lesssim d \lesssim 3.5$mm, which begins to show some departure from the low-frequency behaviour defined by equations 2.8 and 2.9. This trend is further reinforced by the findings of Halpern et al. [106] who showed that the breakdown voltage of a 5mm gap at a frequency of $\sim$ 2800 MHz was significantly higher than its equivalent d-c value.

2.6(ii) Impulse voltages

Farrall [107] has considered the breakdown behaviour associated with this type of ramp waveform from both a theoretical and experimental point of view. His analysis, which applies to large gap situations ($d \gtrsim$ 1mm), where breakdown is assumed to be initiated by the Cranberg [80] microparticle based mechanism, distinguishes between experimental regimes using constant *rise rate* and constant *rise time* pulses, and shows that the gap-dependence of $(V_b)_{ip}$ for these respective regimes should take the form

$$(V_b)_{ip} \propto d^{5/6} \tag{2.10}$$

and

$$(V_b)_{ip} \propto d^{5/2} \tag{2.11}$$

From a review of the available data from pulsed over-voltage experiments [83,108], he was able to tentatively confirm that these types of breakdown event followed the above relations and were therefore very probably the result of microparticle processes.

More recently Lloyd and co-workers [109,110] have made a detailed study of the behaviour of vacuum switches under impulse voltage testing. They concluded that fully conditioned switch contacts generally exhibit a distinct "small" and "large" gap behaviour, where for $d \lesssim 1.5$mm

$$(V_b)_{ip} \propto d \simeq 40d \tag{2.12}$$

and for $d \gtrsim 2$

$$(V_b)_{ip} \propto d^{\frac{1}{2}} \simeq 64d^{\frac{1}{2}} \tag{2.13}$$

with $(V_b)_{ip}$ given in kilovolts. Whilst recognising that such a transition has traditionally been attributed to a change in the breakdown mechanism from field emission initiated at "small" gaps ($d \lesssim$ 1mm) to microparticle initiated at "large" gaps ($d \gtrsim$ 1mm), they make the important point that the time scale of large-gap breakdown events is too short to involve any mechanism requiring the particle to make a complete transit of the gap. Accordingly, they suggest that large-gap events could result from the trigger discharge mechanism described in Section 4.8(ii), which is associated with the *launching* of a microparticle. However, in the light of more recent findings to be discussed in Chapter 8, it is possible that such events could also have resulted from a thermal instability following the rapid "switching-on" (i.e. within tens of nanoseconds), of a more complex type of non-metallic electron emission mechanism associated with insulating microinclusions.

2.6(iii) Pulse voltages

The response of a high voltage gap to a fast-rise "square" voltage pulse has been extensively studied. In particular, microsecond and nanosecond pulse techniques have been used to investigate the fundamental physical processes responsible for initiating a high voltage vacuum arc. However, in view of the importance of this topic, a full discussion of these experiments will be delayed until Chapters 3 and 5 for the respective cases of the plane-parallel and point-plane electrode geometries.

2.7 References

1. Pivover, L.J. and Gordienko, V.I., *Sov. Phys-Tech. Phys.I.* 908-12, (1963).
2. Alpert, D., Lee, D.A., Lyman, E.M. and Tomaschke, J., *J. Vac. Sci. Technol.*, 1, 35-50, (1964).
3. Bennette, C.J., Swanson, L.W. and Charbonnier, F.H., *J. Appl. Phys.*, **38**, 634-40, (1967).
4. Roherbach, F., *Report CERN*, 71-38 (NTIS), (1971).
5. Hackam, R. and Salman, S.K., *Vacuum*, **23**, 9-20, (1973).
6. Donaldson, E.E. and Rabinowitz, M., *J. Appl. Phys.* **34**, 319-22, (1963).
7. Rogowski, W., *Archiv. für Elektrotechnik*, **12**, 1-15, (1923).
8. Bruce, F.M., *J.I.E.E.*, **94**, 138-49, (1947).
9. Harrison, J.A., *Brit. J. Appl. Phys.*, **18**, 1617-22, (1967).
10. Arnal, R., *Ann. Phys. (France)*, **10**, 830-73, (1955).
11. Mansfield, W.K., *Brit. J. Appl. Phys.*, **11**, 454-61, (1960).
12. Boersch, H., Hamisch, H. and Wiesner, S., *Z. Agnew. Phys.*, **13**, 450-6, (1961).
13. Powell, H.P.S. and Chatterton, P.A., *Vacuum*, **20**, 419-29, (1970).
14. Gerasimenko, V.I., *Sov. Phys-Tech. Phys.*, **13**, 107-12, (1968).
15. Berland, R., Bert, M., Favrel, J. and Arnal, R., *Proc. IV-DEIV*, **56-60**, (1970).
16. McKibben, J.L., *Los Alamos Report. LA-5376MS*, (1973).
17. Hurley, R.E., *J. Phys. D: Appl. Phys.*, **13**, 1121-8, (1980).
18. Jüttner, B. and Wolff, H., *Proc. 7th Int. Conf. Phenom. Ionised Gases (Beograd 1965)*, 1, 226-9, (1966).

19. Davies, D.K. and Biondi, M.A., *J. Appl. Phys.* **37**, 2968-77, (1966).
20. Jüttner, B., Wolff, H. and Pech, P., *Proc. 8th Int. Conf. Phenom. Ionised Gases*, **70**, (1967).
21. Beukema, G.P., *J. Phys. D: Appl. Phys.* **6**, 1455-66, (1973).
22. Hackam, R. and Salman, S.K., *Proc. I.E.E.*, **119**, 377-84 and 1747-50, (1972).
23. Williams, D.W. and Williams, W.T., *J. Phys. D: Appl. Phys.* **7**, 1173-83, (1974).
24. Allan, R.N. and Salim, A.J., *J. Phys. D: Appl. Phys.* **7**, 1159-69, (1974).
25. Shrednik, V.N., Pavlov, V.G., Rabinovich, A.A. and Shaikhin, B.N., *Phys. Stat. Sol. (a)*, **23**, 373-81, (1974).
26. Pavlov, V.G. and Shrednik, V.N., *Proc. VII-DEIV*, 209-216, (1976).
27. Cavaille, J.V. and Drechsler, M., *Proc. VII-DEIV*, 217-221, (1976).
28. Looms, J.S.T. Meats, R.J. and Swift, D.A., *J. Phys. D: Appl. Phys.*, **1**, 377-9, (1968).
29. Williams, W.T., *Nature: Phys. Sci.*, **231**, 42-4, (1971).
30. Septier, A. and Bergeret, H., *Rev. Gen. Electricite*, **80**, 565-7, (1971).
31. Bergeret, H., Nguyen Tuong Viet and Septier, A., *Proc. VI-DEIV*, 112-7, (1974).
32. Gomer, R. and Hulm, J.K., *J. Chem. Phys.* **20**, 1500-5, (1952).
33. Cobourne, M.H. and Williams, W.T., *Proc. VI-DEIV*, 279-84, (1974).
34. Cobourne, M.H. and Williams, W.T., *Proc. IX-DEIV, Physica*, **104c**, (1981), In press.
35. Maitland, A., *Brit. J. Appl. Phys.*, **13**, 122-5, (1962).
36. Beukema, G.P., *J. Phys. D: Appl. Phys.*, **7**, 1740-55, (1974).
37. Danloy, L. and Simon, P., *Proc. V-DEIV*, 367 72, (1972).
38. Steib, G.F. and Moll, E., *J. Phys. D: Appl. Phys.*, **6**, 243-55, (1973).
39. Hackham, R. and Govindra Raju, G.P., *J. Appl. Phys.*, **45**, 4784-94, (1974).
40. Lyman, E.M., Lee, D.A., Tomaschke, H.E. and Alpert, D., *Proc. II-DEIV*, 33-39, (1966).
41. Alpert, D., Lee, D.A., Lyman, E.M. and Tomaschke, H.E., *J. Appl. Phys.*, **38**, 880-1, (1967).
42. Ettinger, S.Y. and Lyman, E.M., *Proc. III-DEIV*, 128-33, (1968).
43. Beukema, G.P., *Physica C.*, **61**, 259-74, (1972).
44. Miller, H.C. and Farrall, G.A., *J. Appl. Phys.*, **36**, 1338-44 and 2966 , (1965).
45. Cox, B.M., *J. Phys. D:Appl. Phys.* **7**, 143-51, (1974).
46. Williams, D.W. and Williams, W.T., *J. Phys. D: Appl. Phys.* **5**, 1845-54, (1972).
47. Williams, D.W. and Williams, W.T., *J. Phys. D: Appl. Phys.* **6**, 734-43, (1973).

48. Hackam, R., *J. Appl. Phys.*, **46**, 3789-99, (1975).
49. Farrall, G.A., *IEEE Trans. Parts, Hybrids, Packag.* **PHP-11**, 134-8, (1975).
50. Jüttner, B., *Beitr. Plasmaphys.* **19**, 259-65, (1979).
51. Turner, C.M., *Phys. Rev.* **81**, 305, (1951).
52. McKibben, J.L and Boyer, K., *Phys. Rev.* **82**, 315-6, (1951).
53. Linder, E.G. and Christian, S.M., *J. Appl. Phys.* **23**, 1213-6, (1952).
54. Murray, J.J., *UCRL Report*, No. 9506, (1960).
55. Prichard, B.A., *J. Appl. Phys.* **44**, 4548-54, (1973).
56. Cooke, C.M., *Proc. II-DEIV*, 181-93, (1966).
57. Morgan, C.G., *Proc. IV-DEIV, Addenda*, (1970).
58. Germain, C. and Rohrbach, F., *Proc. 6th Int. Conf. Phenom. Ionised Gases*, 111-7, (1963).
59. Hackham, R., *Int. J. Electron Phys.* **28**, 79-87, (1970).
60. Govindra Raju, G.R. and Hackham, R., *Proc. IEEE*, **120**, 927-36, (1973).
61. Hackham, R. and Altcheh, L., *J. Appl. Phys.* **46**, 627-36, (1975).
62. Hackham, R. and Salman, S.K., *IEEE Trans. Electr. Insul.* **EI-10**, 9-13, (1975).
63. Litvinov, E.A., Mesyats, G.A., Proskurovsky, D.I. and Yankelevitch, E.B., *Prov. VII-DEIV*, 55-57, (1976).
64. Jüttner, B., Wolff, H. and Altrichter, B., *Phys. Stat. Sol.* **27a**, 403-12, (1975).
65. Carter, G. and Colligon, J.S., *In* "Ion Bombardment of Solids" (p.363), Heinemann, London, (1968).
66. Kaminsky, M., *In* "Atomic and Ionic Impact Phenomena on Metal Surfaces", (Chapter 1), Springer-Verlag, Berlin, (1965).
67. Chatterton, P.A., *Proc. II-DEIV*, 195-206, (1966).
68. Powell, H.P.S. and Chatterton, P.A., *Vacuum*, **20**, 419-29, (1971).
69. Hackam, R., *Proc. IEE*, **119**, 377-84, (1972).
70. Cox, B.M., *CEGB Res. Report*, R/M/N1021, (1979).
71. Rabinowitz, M. and Donaldson, E.E., *J. Appl. Phys.* **36**, 1314-19, (1965).
72. Hackam, R. and Salman, S.K., *J. Appl. Phys.* **45**, 4384-92, (1974).
73. Leader, D., Proc. IEE, **100 2A**, 138-40 and 181-6, (1953).
74. Pivover, L.I., Tubaev, V.H. and Gordienko, V.I., *Sov. Phys-Tech. Phys.*, **2**, 909-10, (1959).
75. Mason, J.H., *Proc. IEEC*, **102**, 254-62, (1955).
76. Thwaites, R.H., *Proc. IEEC*, **109**, 600-9, (1962).
77. Loeb, L.B., *In* "Electrical Corona, their Basic Physical Mechanism", University of California Press, Berkeley, (1965).
78. Abou-Seada, M.A. and Nasser, E., *Proc. IEEE*, **56**, 813-18, (1965).
79. Ryan, H. McL., *Proc. IEEE*, **117**, 283-9, (1970).
80. Cranberg, L., *J. Appl. Phys.*, **23**, 518-22, (1952).

81. Boyle, W.S., Kislink, P. and Germer, L.H., *J. Appl. Phys.* **26**, 720-5, (1955).
82. Slivkov, I.N., *Sov. Phys-Tech. Phys.*, **2**, 1928-34, (1957).
83. Denholm, A.S., *Can. J. Phys.* **36**, 476-93, (1955).
84. Hawley, R. and Zaky, A.A., *Prog. Dielectri.* **7**, 115-21, (1967).
85. Maitland, A., *J. Appl. Phys.* **32**, 2399-407, (1961).
86. Davies, D.K. and Biondi, M.A., *J. Appl. Phys.* **37**, 2969-77, (1966).
87. Kranjec, P. and Buby, L., *J. Vac. Sci. Technol.* **4**, 94-6, (1967).
88. Bloomer, R.N. and Cox, B.M., *Vacuum*, **18**, 379-82, (1968).
89. Fane, R.W., Neal, W.E.J. and Latham, R.V., *J. Appl. Phys.* **44**, 740-3, (1973).
90. Butcher, E.C., Dyer, A.J. and Gilbert, W.E., *J. Phys. D: Appl. Phys.* **1**, 1673-87, (1968).
91. Williams, D.W. and Williams, W.T., *J. Phys. D: Appl. Phys.* **5**, 1845-54, (1972).
92. Sudan, R.N. and Gonzalez-Perez, F., *J. Appl. Phys.* **35**, 2269-70, (1964).
93. Jedynak, L., *J. Appl. Phys.* **35**, 1727-33, (1964).
94. Rohrbach, F., *Proc. I-DEIV*, 393-401, (1964).
95. Bolin, P.C. and Trump, J.G., *Proc. III-DEIV*, 50-53, (1968).
96. Rabinowitz, M., *Vacuum*, **15**, 59-66, (1965).
97. Simon, D.J. and Michelier, R., *Proc. III-DEIV*, 263-6, (1968).
98. Armstrong, T.V. and Headley, P., *Electron Power*, **20**, 198-203, (1974).
99. Barken, P., Lafferty, J.M., Lee, T.H. and Talento, J.L., *IEEE Trans. Power Appar. Syst.* **PAS-90**, 350-9, (1971).
100. Slade, P.G., *IEEE Trans. Parts Hybrids and Packaging*, **PHP-10**, 43-50, (1974).
101. Borgers, S.J., *Proc. IEE*, **99 III**, 307-15, (1952).
102. Venable, D., *Rev. Sci. Instrum.* **33**, 456-62, (1962).
103. Wijker, W.J., *Appl. Sci. Res.* **B9**, 1-20, (1961).
104. Kustom, R.L., *J. Appl. Phys.* **41**, 3256-68, (1970).
105. Hill, C.E., *Proc. IV-DEIV*, 137-41, (1970).
106. Halpen, J., Everhart, E., Rapuano, R.A. and Slater, J.C., *Phys. Rev.*, **67**, 688-95, (1946).
107. Farrall, G.A., *J. Appl. Phys.* **33**, 96-99, (1962).
108. Rosanova, N.B. and Granovskii, V.L., *Sov. Phys-Tech. Phys.* **1**, 471-8, (1956).
109. Lloyd, O. and Hackam, R., *Proc. Inst. Electr. Eng.* **122**, 1275-8, (1975).
110. Lloyd, O. and Fairfield, J.H., *CEGB Res. Report*, R/M/N937, (1977).

3 Breakdown Initiating Mechanisms I – Electron Emission Based

3.1 "Metallic" Field Electron Emission (M-FEE)
(i) Low-temperature theory
(ii) Temperature-dependent theory
(iii) Space charge limitation
3.2 M-FEE from Broad-area High-voltage Electrodes
(i) Localised emission sites
(ii) Field enhancing properties of idealised microprotrusions
(iii) FEE properties of idealised microprotrusions
3.3 DC "Cathode" and "Anode" Initiated Breakdown Mechanisms
(i) Cathode stability
(ii) Anode stability
3.4 Stability Considerations Under Pulsed Field Operation
(i) Cathode processes
(ii) Anode processes
3.5 Practical Breakdown Criteria: "Cathode" versus "Anode" Initiation
3.6 References

The concept of "cold" electron emission occurring at isolated sites on broad-area cathodes where the macroscopic gap field is locally enhanced by the presence of metallic microprotrusions was first outlined in the Introduction to this book and subsequently used in the last chapter as a basis for interpreting the current-voltage characteristic of HV gaps. We now have to enquire more closely into the physical basis of this type of emission process and the mechanisms by which it can initiate electrical breakdown.

3.1. "Metallic" Field Electron Emission (M-FEE)

The theory of this emission mechanism was originally formulated by Fowler and Nordheim in 1928 [1] and described the quantum mechanical tunnelling of electrons through the modified potential barrier illustrated in Fig. 3.1 that results from the presence of a high external electric field E acting on an atomically-clean metal surface.

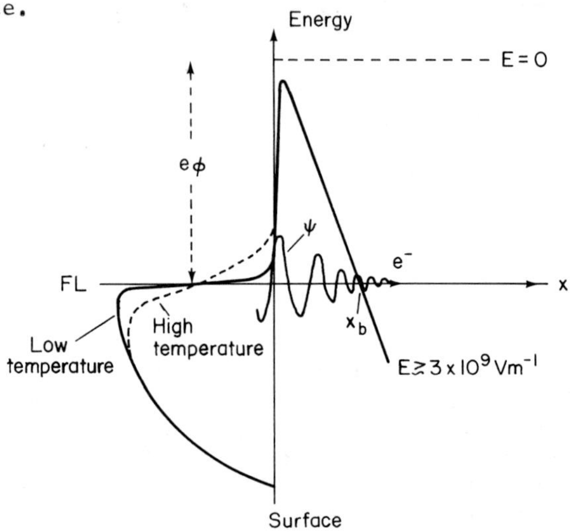

Fig. 3.1 A schematic representation of the quantum mechanical tunnelling mechanism by which a field emitted electron escapes from the surface of a metal. It shows the low and high-temperature electron energy distributions within the metal and the modified high-field potential barrier outside the surface.

For tunnelling to occur, the wave function ψ of an electron in the surface of the metal must still be finite beyond the barrier, despite its rapid attenuation. This concept may alternatively be formulated in terms of the Heisenberg Uncertainty Principle [2], $\Delta x . \Delta p \simeq h/2\pi$, where in the present context, Δx is the uncertainty in the position of the electron, viz. the barrier width, and p is the uncertainty in the electron momentum within the barrier, viz. $\sim (2m\phi)^{\frac{1}{2}}$. Both approaches lead to the requirement that an electron at the Fermi level FL shall "see" a barrier width $\Delta x \lesssim 1$ nm, which in practical terms requires an external field $E \gtrsim 3 \times 10^9$ Vm^{-1}. It should also be appreciated that in this emission mechanism the electrons leave the surface with the same initial energy as they had within the metal.

3.1(i) Low-temperature theory

The derivation of the Fowler-Nordheim (F-N) expression for the field-dependence of the emission current density j is based on "free electron" theory and involves three main stages of mathematical development. Firstly, the electron Supply Function $N(W_x)dW_x$ is obtained, which gives the flux of electrons incident on the barrier from within the metal that have normal energy components between W_x and W_x+dW_x. Next, the electron Transmission Coefficient $D(W_x)$ is derived, which gives the probability that an electron with an energy W_x will be transmitted by the barrier: the product of these functions $N(W_x)\ D(W_x)\ dW_x$ then gives the number of electrons with energies between W_x and $W_x + dW_x$ that will tunnel through the barrier. Finally, the total number of electrons that tunnel through the barrier is obtained by integrating the above expression over all energies, so that the actual field electron emission current density ($A.m^{-2}$) will be given by

$$j_F = e \int_{\substack{\text{all}\\ \text{energies}}} D(W_x)N(W_x)\,dW \tag{3.1}$$

where e is the electronic charge. Since the detailed evaluation of $W(W_x)$, $P(W_x)$ and this final integral is an extended and largely mathematical exercise that is not directly relevant to the development of the main theme of this text, it will be sufficient to quote the final result; for the interested reader, however, there are comprehensive modern treatments [3,4].

At *low temperatures* ($T \lesssim 300^oK$) where few electron states above the Fermi level are occupied, as shown by the low-temperature Fermi-Dirac electron energy distribution of Fig. 3.1, the basic Fowler-Nordheim equation is usually expressed in the form

$$j_{OF} = \frac{1.54 \times 10^{-6}E^2}{\phi t^2(y)} \exp.\left[\frac{-6.83 \times 10^9\phi^{1.5}v(y)}{E}\right] \tag{3.2}$$

where j_{OF} is the low-temperature FEE current density, E is the surface electric field (Vm^{-1}) and ϕ the work function of the emitting surface (eV); t(y) and v(y) are tabulated dimensionless elliptic functions [3-6] of the parameter y which is related to E and ϕ by

$$y = 3.79 \times 10^{-5}\ E^{\frac{1}{2}}/\phi \tag{3.3}$$

In practice, t(y) is a very slowly varying function of y and can reliably be taken as unity for the field range likely to be encountered at the tips of microprotrusions in high voltage gaps, i.e. $3 \times 10^9 \lesssim E \lesssim 10^{10}\ Vm^{-1}$; v(y), on the other hand, shows a significant field-dependence which can be closely approximated by the relation [7]

$$v(y) = 0.956 - 1.062y^2 \tag{3.4}$$

for the field range $2 \times 10^9 \lesssim E \lesssim 5 \times 10^9\ Vm^{-1}$ which is appropriate to stable field emission regimes. Now if the field E acts over an emitting area A_e, the emission current i_{OF} from this region will be given by $i_{OF} = j_{OF}A_e$ which, after substituting for j_{OF} from equation 3.2, and re-expressing in logarithmic form becomes

$$\log \frac{i_{OF}}{E^2} = \log \left[\frac{1.54 \times 10^{-6} A_e}{\phi t^2(y)} \right] - 2.97 \times 10^9 \phi^{1.5} v(y) . \frac{1}{E} \quad (3.5)$$

Substituting lastly for v(y) from equation 3.4 and letting $t(y) \simeq 1$ leads to the most useful form of the F-N equation,

$$\log \frac{i_{OF}}{E^2} = \log \left[1.54 \times 10^{-6} A_e . \frac{10^{4.52\phi^{-\frac{1}{2}}}}{\phi} \right] -2.84 \times 10^9 \phi^{1.5} . \frac{1}{E} \quad (3.6)$$

indicating that if the value of E is known, a graph of log i_{OF}/E^2 against 1/E would give a straight line with a slope

$$\frac{d(\log i_{OF}/E^2)}{d(1/E)} = -2.84 \times 10^9 \phi^{1.5} \quad (3.7)$$

and an intercept

$$\left[\log \frac{i_{OF}}{E^2} \right]_{E=\infty} = \log 1.54 \times 10^{-6} A_e . \frac{10^{4.52\phi^{-\frac{1}{2}}}}{\phi} \quad (3.8)$$

This observation will be returned to later in section 3.2(iii). From this discussion, it follows that the F-N equation 3.6 may be conveniently expressed in a simplified form similar to that used in Chapter 2, viz.

$$j_{OF} = C_1 E^2 \exp(-C_2/E) \quad (3.9)$$

where C_1 and C_2 are fundamental constants that have the values

$$C_1 = 1.54 \times 10^{-6} \times 10^{4.52\phi^{-\frac{1}{2}}}/\phi \quad (3.10(i))$$

$$C_2 = 6.53 \times 10^9 \phi^{1.5} \quad (3.10(ii))$$

It should be noted that many authors ignore the field-dependence of v(y) and, instead, use an approximate form of the F-N equation with t(y) = v(y) = 1 in equation 3.2. Thus, whilst this procedure only introduces errors of 5-10% in the slope of such a plot, the intercept can be affected by as much as two orders of magnitude through the factor $10^{4.52\phi^{-\frac{1}{2}}}$, so that only a limited physical significance can be attributed to measurements based on this parameter.

3.1(ii) Temperature-dependent theory

At higher temperatures ($T > 300^{o}K$), more electrons begin to occupy states above the Fermi level FL, as shown by the high-temperature electron energy distribution of Fig. 3.1. Clearly, these electrons will "see" a narrower barrier than those at the FL and will therefore have a higher tunnelling probability which, in practical terms, implies that the FEE current density would be expected to show a strong temperature dependence at high temperatures, which is not accounted for in the basic F-N theory. This effect has been considered by several authors in the course of developing unified theories of electron emission, notably Murphy and Good [8], Dyke and Dolan [9] and more recently Christov [10]. For $T \lesssim 1500^{o}K$, the temperature-assisted FEE current density j_{TF} can be accurately described by the analytic expression [9]

$$j_{TF} = j_{OF} \frac{\pi p}{\sin \pi p} \tag{3.11}$$

where p is a dimensionless temperature and field dependent parameter given by

$$p \simeq 9.3 \times 10^{5} \phi^{\frac{1}{2}} T/E \tag{3.12}$$

However, at higher temperatures where $p > 2/3$, the approximations leading to the above expression become invalid and the tabulated data of the more recent analyses of Christov [10] has to be used.

3.1(iii) Space charge limitation

The validity of the Fowler-Nordheim theory was first investigated experimentally by Haeffer [11], and later in more detail by Dyke and his colleagues [12] using a point-plane diode geometry resembling a simple field emission microscope, where the dimensions of the laboratory-fabricated micropoint emitter were accurately known so that the microscopic cathode field could be reliably defined. This type of measurement showed that there is a wide range of field for which there is a good agreement between theory and experiment, as evidenced by the linearity of the F-N plot of the diode current-voltage characteristic. However, at fields $\gtrsim 6 \times 10^{9} Vm^{-1}$, corresponding to $j_F \sim 6 \times 10^{11} A.m^{-2}$, the F-N plot begins to fall away from linearity, indicating the onset of some form of current-limiting mechanism. In a combined theoretical and experimental investigation, Dyke et al. [13] showed that the field-emitting diode characteristic closely followed a "three-halves" power law at these higher emission current densities, which could be satisfactorily interpreted in terms of a space-charge current limitation similar to the well known Child-Langmuir phenomenon that operates in planar and cylindrical diodes. The limiting field E_{ℓ} at which the low-temperature F-N theory breaks down because of the onset of space charge effects has been estimated by Chatterton [14] as

$$E_{\ell} \lesssim 8 \times 10^{8} \phi^{1.5} \tag{3.13}$$

which is in good agreement with the experimental findings of Dyke et al. [12,13]. Mention should also be made however of an alternative theoretical explanation of the phenomenon by Nagy and

Cutler[15]. Their basic assumption was that the classical image force barrier model cannot be used at small distances from the emitting surface. Accordingly, they re-formulated the F-N emission theory by applying quantum modifications to the electronic potential in the surface region of the metal, and were able to show that a plot of $\log(i_{OF}/E^2)$ against I/E can be expected to depart from linearity at fields $\gtrsim 5 \times 10^9 Vm^{-1}$.

3.2.M-FEE from Broad-area High Voltage Electrodes

For this electron emission mechanism to provide a satisfactory explanation of the pre-breakdown currents that flow between high voltage electrodes, it is first necessary to reconcile the apparent paradox that such currents are observed at gap fields that are frequently more than two orders of magnitude lower than the theoretical threshold field of $\sim 3 \times 10^9$ Vm^{-1} required for the mechanism to provide significant electron emission.

3.2(i) Localised emission sites

The clue to resolving this difficulty was provided by the experimental finding (see Chapter 7) that prebreakdown emission was confined to a few isolated microscopic sites on an extended cathode surface, where, evidently, either the field or surface conditions showed some favourable anomaly. It was then recognised that the microtopography of an electrode surface is far from planar and that, in consequence, there could be large variations in the microscopic surface field over the electrode: e.g. field lines would converge on protruding microstructures to give a geometrically enhanced local field. From these general considerations there emerged the widely accepted microprotrusion or metallic "whisker" model for explaining the origin of M-FEE prebreakdown currents. This model is based on the assumption that a a freshly polished electrode surface will almost certainly have one or more "whisker-like" features with geometries that would provide the necessary field enhancement. It can well be imagined for example how mechanical polishing could create filamentary structures lying initially in the plane of the electrode, but that could subsequently be erected normal to the surface by the strong electromechanical forces associated with the gap field and so provide the necessary field enhancing features: in fact, electron optical evidence for such a process will be described in Chapter 7.

3.2(ii) Field enhancing properties of idealised microprotrusions

In order to analyse the physical properties of this model, it is necessary to assume that the microprotrusion has an idealised symmetrical geometry and is orientated normal to a planar electrode, such as shown in Fig. 3.2 for the example of a semi-ellipsoidal microstructure. This figure also illustrates how, by the

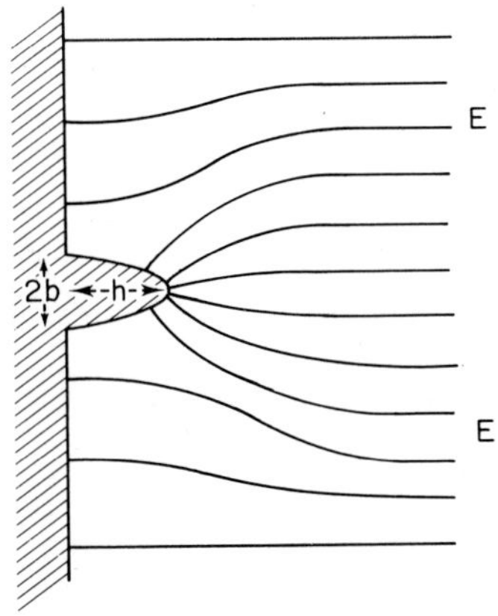

Fig. 3.2 An illustration of how a uniform *macroscopic* gap field E is geometrically enhanced to a higher *microscopic* value E_m at the tip of a microprotrusion projecting from a planar electrode surface.

convergence of the field lines, the uniform *macroscopic* gap field E is geometrically enhanced to a higher *microscopic* value E_m at the tip of the protrusion. The ratio of the microscopic to macroscopic fields is defined as the field-enhancement factor β, i.e.

$$E_m = \beta E \tag{3.14}$$

where the magnitude of β depends on the geometry and dimensions of a given protrusion. For the semi-ellipse of revolution illustrated in Fig. 3.2, the β-factor is given by the detailed expression [16]

$$\beta = \frac{(\lambda^2 - 1)^{1.5}}{\lambda \ln[\lambda + (\lambda^2 - 1)^{\frac{1}{2}}] - (\lambda^2 - 1)^{\frac{1}{2}}} \tag{3.15}$$

where $\lambda = (h/b)$; i.e. the ratio of the semi-major to semi-minor axes of the ellipse. For needle-like geometries, where $\lambda >> 10$, the above expression can be approximated by

$$\beta \simeq \frac{\lambda^2}{\ln\lambda - 0.3} \tag{3.16}$$

Alternatively, β may be expressed in the form [17]

$$\beta = \frac{2\ell^3}{(1-\ell^2)\ln\frac{1+\ell}{1-\ell} - 2\ell} \tag{3.17}$$

where $\ell = [1 - (b/h)^2\,]^{\frac{1}{2}}$ is the eccentricity of the ellipse. Several other idealised protrusion geometries have been analysed in equal detail, particularly those shown in Fig. 3.3 that are

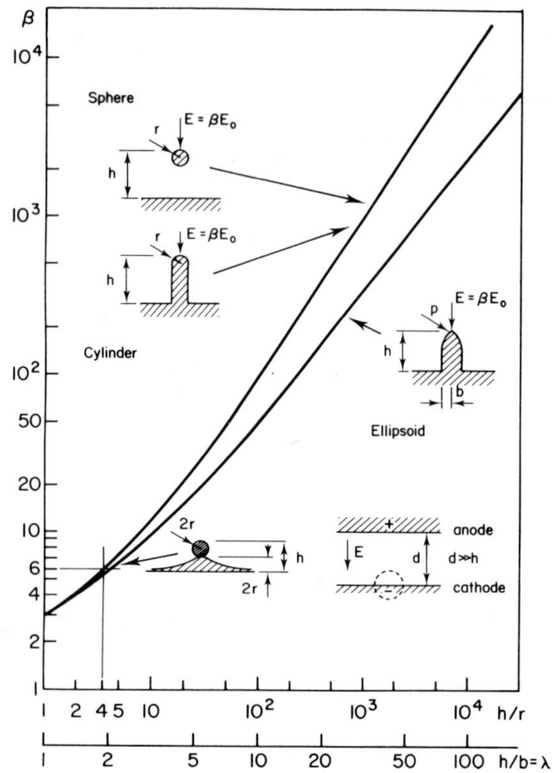

Fig. 3.3 A collated representation of the field enhancement factors β associated with various idealised microprotrusion geometries.
(From Rohrbach [16], with permission)

based on a spherical emitting surface [16]. Generally however, it has been shown that if the β-factors are computed as a function of h/r, the ratio of their height h to tip radius of curvature r, they can all be characterised to a good approximation by the unifying expression [18]

$$\beta \simeq 2 + \frac{h}{r} \qquad (3.18)$$

provided h/r $\gtrsim$ 5. It has to be added that Miller [19] has shown that β also depends on the electrode separation d through the relation

$$\beta = \beta_\infty \left(1 - \frac{h}{d}\right) \qquad (3.19)$$

where β_∞ is the value of β when d >>h; i.e. the conditions assumed in the above discussion.

3.2(iii) FEE properties of idealised microprotrusions

Consider now a typical practical situation in which the pre-breakdown current I flowing between broad-area electrodes is derived from a single microprotrusion at which the electric field is enhanced by a factor β over the macroscopic value E it would have had at a perfectly smooth cathode surface. From elementary electrostatic field theory, E will be generally defined by a relation of the form $E = V/fd$ where V is the voltage applied between the electrodes, d is their separation and f is a dimensionless function of the geometrical parameters of the electrodes: for a plane-parallel geometry $f = 1$, for concentric cylinders having cathode and anode radii R_c and R_a respectively, one has $f = R_c/(R_a - R_c)\ell n\, R_a/R_e$, whilst for concentric spheres $f = R_c/R_a$. Assuming, as in previous discussions, that this single micro-emitter is associated with a plane-parallel electrode geometry, it follows that the microscopic field E_m acting at its tip will be given by

$$E_m = \beta E = \beta\frac{V}{d} \tag{3.19}$$

If this equation is now used to substitute for E in equation 3.6, we obtain the logarithmic form of the F-N equation expressed in terms of the externally measurable parameters I and V,

$$\log\frac{I}{V^2} = \log\left[\frac{1.54\times10^{-6}\,A_e\beta^2 10^{4.52\phi^{-\frac{1}{2}}}}{\phi d^2}\right] - \frac{2.84\times10^9 d\phi^{1.5}}{\beta}\cdot\frac{1}{V} \tag{3.20}$$

It follows therefore that if the current-voltage data of such a single-emitter gap is presented in the form of an F-N plot, viz. $\log I/V^2$ versus $1/V$, it will give a straight line with a slope

$$\frac{d(\log I/V^2)}{d(1/V)} = -\frac{2.84\times10^9 d\phi^{1.5}}{\beta} \tag{3.21}$$

and an intercept

$$\left[\log(I/V^2)\right]_{V=\infty} = \log\left[\frac{1.54\times10^{-6}A_e\beta^2 10^{4.52\phi^{-\frac{1}{2}}}}{\phi d^2}\right] \tag{3.22}$$

Thus if d is known and the work function ϕ of the emitter is assumed to have the same value as the bulk electrode material, the slope of such an F-N plot provides an indirect measure of the β-factor of the emitter; it follows that this value may then be used to determine the emitting area A_e from the intercept of the plot.

For the more complicated situation where there are n emitters distributed over the cathode surface, each with its own enhancement factor β_i and emitting area $(A_e)_i$, the total prebreakdown current I will be given from equation 3.8 by

$$I = C_1(V/d)^2 \sum (A_e)_i \beta_i^2 \exp.(-C_2\beta_i d/V) \tag{3.23}$$

indicating that an F-N plot will no longer be expected to give a straight line. In practice, however, the reverse is found to be true, with a non-linear plot being the exception rather than the rule. An explanation for this apparent paradox was subsequently provided by multi-emitter computer simulation studies, first by Tomaschke and Alpert [20] and later by Farrall [21], which showed that the prebreakdown regime will always be dominated by one of a group of high-β emitters whose β and A_e characteristics will accordingly be reflected in the associated F-N plot [20,21].

3.3. M-FEE induced breakdown mechanisms

Having established the physical basis of the field emitting microprotrusion model, it is now necessary to extend the analysis to a consideration of the factors affecting the stability of the regime: in particular, to enquire whether any of the associated physical processes are likely to lead to the creation of a microplasma, since this is the essential "seed" of a breakdown event. The prerequisite of such a phenomenon is the formation of an ionisable medium and this, under good vacuum conditions, can only be derived from localised melting or vaporisation processes at the electrode surfaces. Accordingly, it is necessary to consider the energy dissipating mechanisms that can lead to thermally activated instabilities on either cathode or anode.

For the microprotrusion model illustrated in Fig. 3.4, there are two such "primary" mechanisms to be considered. *Cathode initiated breakdown* results from the spontaneous vaporisation of the tip of a microprotrusion following its excessive resistive (Joulian) heating by the current i_{0F} flowing towards the emitting surface. The onset of this instability will therefore be associated with a critical microscopic field E_c acting at the tip of the emitter. *Anode initiated breakdown* can occur if the local surface temperature of the electron bombarded region (i.e. the anode "hot spot") approaches the melting point of the electrode material, since under these conditions the metal vapour pressure can become high enough for the onset of regenerative ionisation processes. This type of instability will therefore be associated with a critical power loading W_c in the electron beam. (N.B. There is also a third indirect mechanism involving the in-flight vaporisation of a microparticle released from the anode "hot-spot" but this will be discussed in section 4.6(iii) of the following chapter as a microparticle initiating mechanism). We shall now consider a number of steady-state theoretical analyses of these mechanisms that have been based on the type of idealised micro-

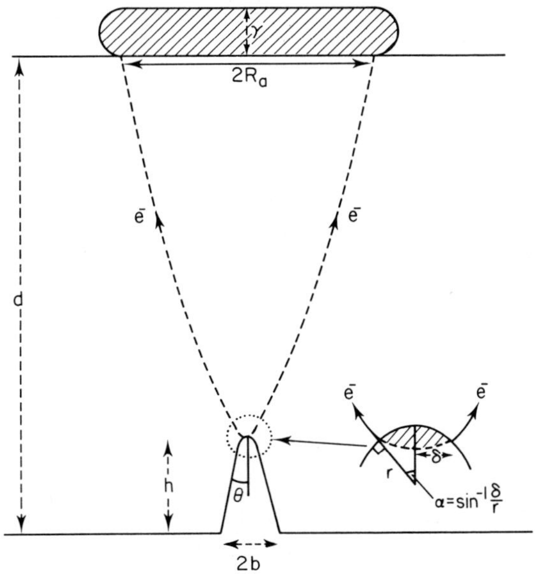

Fig. 3.4 The geometrical relationship between an idealised field-emitting microprotrusion and its associated anode "hot-spot" of radius R_a: δ is the radius of the spherical cap from which the electrons are emitted, and γ is the penetration of the electrons in the anode.

protrusion geometries shown in Fig. 3.3, and whose common objective has been to obtain expressions for E_c and W_c so that quantitative predictions can be made as to which of these instabilities is likely to occur in a given d-c practical situation.

3.3(i) "Cathode" initiated breakdown

For a complete analysis of the thermal stability of a cathode microprotrusion it would be necessary to consider four energy exchange mechanisms:

(a) internal resistive heating resulting from a high current density flowing into the tip of the emitter,

(b) thermal cooling by heat conduction down the shank of the protrusion into the "cold" reservoir provided by the bulk of the cathode electrode,

(c) thermal cooling by radiation losses from the surface of the emitter, and finally,

(d) the internal heating or cooling that can result from the Nottingham effect.

This latter process has a similar physical basis to the well-known cooling effect associated with thermionic emission, viz. that the energy of an emitted electron will be higher than that of its replacement conduction electron which is supplied at the

Fermi level. In the case of low-temperature FEE ($T \lesssim 300^oK$), electrons will be emitted from states below the Fermi level so that there will be a heating effect, where the energy dissipated in the lattice $(\Delta E)_N$ for each field emitted electron is given by Charbonnier et al. [22] as

$$(\Delta E)_N = 1.475 \times 10^{-29} E\phi^{-\frac{1}{2}} \tag{3.24}$$

Hence, if it is assumed that all electrons leave the surface with the same energy, as would correspond to the low-temperature approximation, the Nottingham power density dissipated in the surface of an emitter by an emission current density j_{OF} will be

$$W_{ON} = 9.2 \times 10^{-11} j_{OF}\ E\phi^{-\frac{1}{2}} \tag{3.25}$$

At high temperatures, electrons will tunnel from populated states above the Fermi level and so give rise to a cooling effect: the transition between heating and cooling is characterised by an inversion temperature T_i (defined later in this section by equation 3.30) which depends on the work function of the emitter and the applied field.

In the original analysis by Dolan et al. [23] of the thermal properties of the micro-emitter model, only two of the above energy exchange mechanisms were included in their computations, viz. resistive heating and conduction cooling; radiation cooling was also considered, but shown to play an insignificant role. For this restricted model, the temperature difference ΔT between the tip and base of the conical protrusion shown in Fig. 3.4 is given by [14]

$$\Delta T = \frac{j_F^2 \Omega(T) r^4}{4K(1-\cos\theta)^2}\left(\frac{h - r\cot\ \theta}{hr\cot\ \theta}\right) \tag{3.26}$$

where j_F is the emission current density, $\Omega(T)$ the electrical resistivity and K the thermal conductivity of the emitter. It soon became apparent however that this was an inadequate approach for obtaining reliable predictions; in particular, this model is inherently unstable at high emission current densities and therefore cannot explain the stable behaviour found in practice for clean emitters under strongly emitting conditions [9] where j_F can approach values of $\sim 10^{12} A.m^{-2}$. Accordingly it was superceded by more rigorous treatments that took account of the Nottingham contribution.

The earliest of these was due to Martin and his colleagues [24] in 1960 with important follow-up contributions from Levine [25], Charbonnier et al. [22], Vibrans [26], Brodie [29], Swanson et al. [28], Slivkov [29] and Chatterton [14]. All of these analyses were based on the assumption that any thermal instability will be initiated at the tip of the emitter where the temperature is a maximum; they therefore had as their common central aim the derivation of an expression for the temperature distribution in the vicinity of the apex of the microprotrusion. This hence involves setting up a differential energy exchange equation and solving it for the boundary conditions appropriate to the chosen protrusion geometry. In practice, this is generally a very complex procedure, particularly if a time-dependent solution is required. However, for slowly varying d-c gap voltages, where the sub-microsecond thermal time constant of the microemitter has no significance in controlling the temperature distribution, it is permissible to simplify the problem by using a steady-state solution. Thus, for the case of the truncated-cone type of emitter shown in Fig. 3.4, where radiation losses are assumed negligible compared with the heat dissipation by conduction, the solution of Martin et al. [24] for the steady-state temperature difference between the tip and base of the emitter takes the form

$$\Delta T = T_r - T_b = [\Omega(T)/2K](j_F r/b)^2 + (\pi k T_r r j_F/Kb)\cot\pi p \qquad (3.27)$$

where j_F, K and $\Omega(T)$ have the same significance as in equation 3.26, k is Boltzmann's Constant, and p is the same field and temperature dependent parameter defined by equation 3.11; T_r and T_b are respectively the tip and base temperatures of the emitter. Alternatively, this same temperature difference may be given in a more practical form as a function of the total emission current i_F [28], viz.

$$\Delta T = T_r - T_b = [\Omega(T)/2K\pi^2](i_F/\alpha r)^2 + (kT_r i_F/K\alpha r)\cot\pi p \qquad (3.28)$$

where α is the cone half-angle. It has to be appreciated however that the value of ΔT attained for a given emission current will be very sensitive to the microprotrusion geometry: for example, the thermal coupling of the conical emitter of Fig. 3.4 will clearly be more efficient than for a cylindrical emitter of similar h/r ratio, so that the latter will attain a higher tip temperature. The general conclusion from this observation is therefore that long thin microprotrusions will be less stable than those having a broad-base tapering geometry.

The first term in equation 3.28 accounts for the resistive heating and, being proportional to $\Omega(T)i_F^2$, increases rapidly with both emission current and temperature. The second term of this equation is due to the Nottingham effect and, because of its direct proportionality to i_F, is clearly less sensitive to increases in the emission current; more important however, it is sensitive to T, falling to zero at the invertion temperature T_i when $\cot\pi p = 0$ or $p = \frac{1}{2}$, thereafter going negative as the effect starts to provide a cooling contribution. The value of T_i, which is defined by the condition $p = \frac{1}{2}$, is based on a theoretical consideration of how the total energy distribution of field emitted electrons varies with temperature [22,25], and from equation 3.11 leads to

$$T_i = 5.4 \times 10^{-7} E\phi^{-\frac{1}{2}} \tag{3.29}$$

or more exactly

$$T_i = \frac{5.4 \times 10^{-7} E}{\phi^{\frac{1}{2}} \; t(y)} \tag{3.30}$$

where $t(y)$ is defined for equation 3.2. For most clean metallic emitters that are delivering a high emission current density, E and ϕ can be taken to be typically $\sim 6 \times 10^9 Vm^{-1}$ and ~ 4.5 eV respectively which gives a value for $T_i \sim 1500K$ that is almost independent of electrode material. Clearly, if any benefit is to be gained from Nottingham cooling, i.e. by it thermally stabilising the tip so that higher emission current densities can be drawn, T_i must be significantly lower than the melting temperature T_m of the emitter material, as is the case for refractory metals such as tungsten or molybdenum. For less refractory metals such as copper, whose melting point is $\sim$ 1360K, emission cooling can never come into operation which explains why emitters of this type of material are generally more susceptible to instabilities and hence breakdown events. The fall-off in the Nottingham heating contribution as $T \rightarrow T_i$ is due to an increasing number of electrons tunnelling from states above the Fermi level, so that the low-temperature approximation for the power dissipation W_{ON} given by equation 3.25 becomes increasingly invalid. Brodie [27] has considered this aspect of the mechanism analytically and gives tabulated data for the high-temperature Nottingham power dissipation W_{TN}. These computations show that for $T/T_i \lesssim 0.9$, the ratio of $W_{TN}/W_{ON} \gtrsim 0.5$ and that it is only when T is very close to T_i that W_{TN} begins to fall off rapidly. It should however be pointed out that this analysis by Brodie [27] is open to criticism [28] since he used the normal instead of the total energy distribution of the field emitted electrons.

The energy exchanges associated with the Nottingham effect have been studied experimentally under controlled laboratory conditions by two techniques. In the first, as pioneered by Dreschler [30] and later used by Charbonnier et al. [22], a clean tungsten emitter is welded to a low thermal capacity mounting, usually a thin wire, whose temperature variation can be accurately monitored as heat is either dissipated in or extracted from it. The second technique was developed by Swanson et al. [28,31] and was aimed at investigating the influence of emitter work function ϕ on the effect. To this end, they employed low-ϕ coatings (e.g. zirconium-oxygen on tungsten, giving $\phi \sim 2.7$ eV) to show that, as a result of emission cooling, larger current densities could be drawn from such emitters: they also used other low-ϕ coatings, whose desorption was temperature-dependent (e.g. barium on tungsten, giving $\phi \sim 2.1$ eV), to selectively identify the highly localised region of an emitter where the heating effects are greatest. Whilst both types of experiment confirmed that the predicted energy exchange processes do occur, including the existence of a Nottingham inversion temperature T_i, there was only limited agreement between theory and experiment. In particular, the values of T_i were found to be very much lower than anticipated from the theoretical relation of equation 3.29. Thus for a clean tungsten emitter with a field of $4.6 \times 10^9 Vm^{-1}$, T_i was found to be 550K compared to the theoretical value of 1165K: similarly, the experimental value of T_i for a zirconium-oxygen coated tungsten emitter with a field of $2.4 \times 10^9 Vm^{-1}$ was $\sim$ 475K as opposed to 775K predicted from theory. Although no detailed explanation is available for this discrepancy, there are strong indications that the free-electron based theoretical value used for the average energy of a field emitted electron relative to the Fermi level may be in error [31]. These same revised theoretical considerations also suggest that the values of ΔT predicted by equations 3.27 and 3.28 are likely to be too high. In practical terms, the existence of these lower inversion temperatures provides an explanation for the high stable FEE current densities ($\sim 5 \times 10^{11} A.m^{-2}$) that can be drawn from clean tungsten emitters under controlled conditions (see Chapter 5). Recognising therefore the evidently important role played by the Nottingham effect in determining the limiting conditions for stable electron emission, particularly in the case of the sites found on broad-area electrodes, it should be remarked that the subject warrants further theoretical and experimental investigation aimed at resolving the anomalies outlined above.

3.3(ii) Anode stability

The general topic of localised electron bombardment heating by focused beams of impact radius R_a and total beam power W was first treated analytically by Oosterkamp [32]; more recently, Vine and Einstein [33] have developed a more complete theory to cover the case of high energy beams where the effects of electron penetration in the target have to be taken into account. To apply this type of analysis to the specific regime of an anode "hot-spot" associated with a field-emitting microprotrusion in a high voltage gap, such as shown in Fig. 3.4, it is first necessary to have a knowledge of the electron spot diameter $2R_a$ at the anode. This will be determined firstly by the angular divergence of the electron emission as it leaves the cathode surface and secondly by the magnitudes of the initial transverse velocity components of the electrons i.e. those parallel to the emitting surface. The emission angle α will depend on the geometry of the emitter [14], but can be taken as $\sim 40^o$ for the representative truncated cone model of Fig. 3.4. If we follow the analysis of Chatterton [14] and assume as a first approximation that electrons are emitted normally to the cathode surface (i.e. neglecting their transverse velocity components) and that there are no space charge effects, the electrons will follow the field lines, in which case

$$R_a = \beta^{\frac{1}{2}}\delta \qquad (3.31)$$

or from equation 3.18 where h/r>> 2

$$R_a \simeq (h/r)^{\frac{1}{2}}\delta \qquad (3.32)$$

Here δ is the radius of the emitting area, as shown in the inset of Fig. 3.4. When account is taken of the initial transverse velocity components, which is essential in most practical situations, it can be shown that [14]

$$R_a = \beta^{\frac{1}{2}}\delta + 2d^{\frac{1}{2}}(\beta\delta\ \sin\alpha)^{\frac{1}{2}} \qquad (3.33)$$

In fact, R_a is normally dominated by the second term so that

$$R_a \simeq 2d^{\frac{1}{2}}(\beta\delta\sin\alpha)^{\frac{1}{2}} \qquad (3.34)$$

or finally, after substitution for $\sin\alpha = \delta/r$ (Fig. 3.4),

$$R_a \simeq 2\delta(d\beta/r)^{\frac{1}{2}} \qquad (3.35)$$

As an example, electron emission from a truncated-cone microprotrusion such as shown in Fig. 3.4, with dimensions h = 0.5μm, r = 5nm and hence $\beta \simeq 100$ (from equation 3.18), where it is assumed $\alpha = 40^o$ and $\delta \sim r/2 \sim 2.5$nm, the associated anode spot for a 2mm gap would have a diameter $2R_a \sim 30$μm.

The surface volume of the anode electrode in which the beam energy is dissipated (shown shaded in Fig. 3.4) will be determined by the electron penetration depth γ which is given by the Thomson-Whiddington Law [34] as

$$\gamma = \frac{V^2}{C} \qquad (3.36)$$

In this equation, V is the accelerating potential of the electron, which in this case corresponds to the gap voltage, and C is a constant defined by

$$C = \frac{g\rho Z}{A}$$

where Z, A and ρ are respectively the atomic number, atomic weight and density of the target material, with the fundamental constant $g = 7.8 \times 10^{10}$ (eV.m^2.Kg^{-1}). Thus, 10 and 50 kV electrons striking a copper anode would penetrate $\sim$ 0.3 and 8.0μm respectively, which illustrates the strong voltage-dependence of γ.

Two analytical approaches have been used to compute the steady-state temperature distribution in the anode hot-spot resulting from a constant electron bombardment power loading. The first, as followed by Oosterkamp [32] is really a low-energy approximation applicable to gap voltages $V \lesssim 25$ kV, where it is assumed that there is negligible electron penetration with $R_a >> \gamma$, so that the problem reduces to the classic thermal diffusion problem of a surface disc heat source of uniform power loading on a semi-infinite solid, as treated by Carslaw and Jaeger [35]. For the more realistic situation of an electron beam having a Gaussian current-density distribution, Vine and Einstein [33] gave the steady-state axial and surface temperature distributions, $T(0,x)$ and $T(R,0)$ respectively as

$$T(0,x) = T_{oo} \exp(x^2/1.44R_g^{\ 2}) \text{ erfc. } (x/1.2R_g) \tag{3.37}$$

$$T(R,0) = T_{oo} \exp(-r^2/2.88R_g^{\ 2}) I_o(r^2/2.88R_g^{\ 2}) \tag{3.38}$$

where T_{oo} is the temperature at the origin of coordinates, i.e. on the beam axis in the surface of the target. Clearly, T_{oo} will correspond to the highest temperature reached in the "hot-spot" and is therefore a central parameter in the present discussion of anode initiated breakdown. The value of T_{oo} will be given by

$$[T_{oo}]_1 = 0.414W/\pi^{\frac{1}{2}}KR_g \tag{3.39}$$

In equations 3.37 to 3.39, W is the total beam power in watts, K is the mean thermal conductivity of the anode material over the temperature range being considered ($W.m^{-1}\ K^{-1}$) and R_g is defined for a Gaussian beam as the radius at which the current density is half the maximum. To account for the power losses through radiation and backscattered electrons, it is necessary to replace W by the actual absorbed power W_a in equations 3.37 to 3.39, where W_a can be conveniently expressed in the form

$$W_a = aW \tag{3.40}$$

in which a is termed the power-retention factor and is a constant for a given material, ranging from 0.97 for the low atomic number element aluminium to 0.62 for the high atomic number tungsten [33]. Accordingly, the corrected steady-state temperature at the origin of coordinates $[T_{oo}]_2$ will be given by

$$[T_{oo}]_2 = 0.414aW/\pi^{\frac{1}{2}}KR_g \tag{3.41}$$

The second and more general treatment of the temperature distribution in an anode "hot-spot" is particularly relevant to high voltage electron beams ($V \gtrsim 25$ kV) where electron penetration becomes significant, i.e. $\gamma \to R_a$, so that it is no longer permissible to use the surface disc heating model. Thus, from a detailed analysis by Vine and Einstein [33], which considered a volume-distributed heat source, the corrected temperature at the origin of coordinates in the surface of the anode is given by

$$[T_{oo}]_3 = \xi[T_{oo}]_2$$
$$= (0.25aW/\pi K\gamma)\left[\log(1 + 1.4\gamma^2/R_g^{\,2}) \Big/ 1 - (0.8R_g/\gamma)\tan^{-1}(1.2\gamma/R_g)\right] \quad (3.42)$$

where $[T_{oo}]_2$ has been substituted from equation 3.41. The complicated geometric function ξ will always be <1, i.e. $[T_{oo}]_3 < [T_{oo}]_2$ and has been computed by Vine and Einstein for a wide range of $\gamma/2R_g$; however, Chatterton [14] has shown that it may be closely approximated by the simplified empirical functions:

$$\xi = 0.7(2R_g/\gamma)^{0.77} \qquad \text{for } \gamma/2R_g > 1$$
$$\xi = \exp(-0.3\gamma/R_g) \qquad \text{for } \gamma/2R_g < 2 \quad (3.43)$$

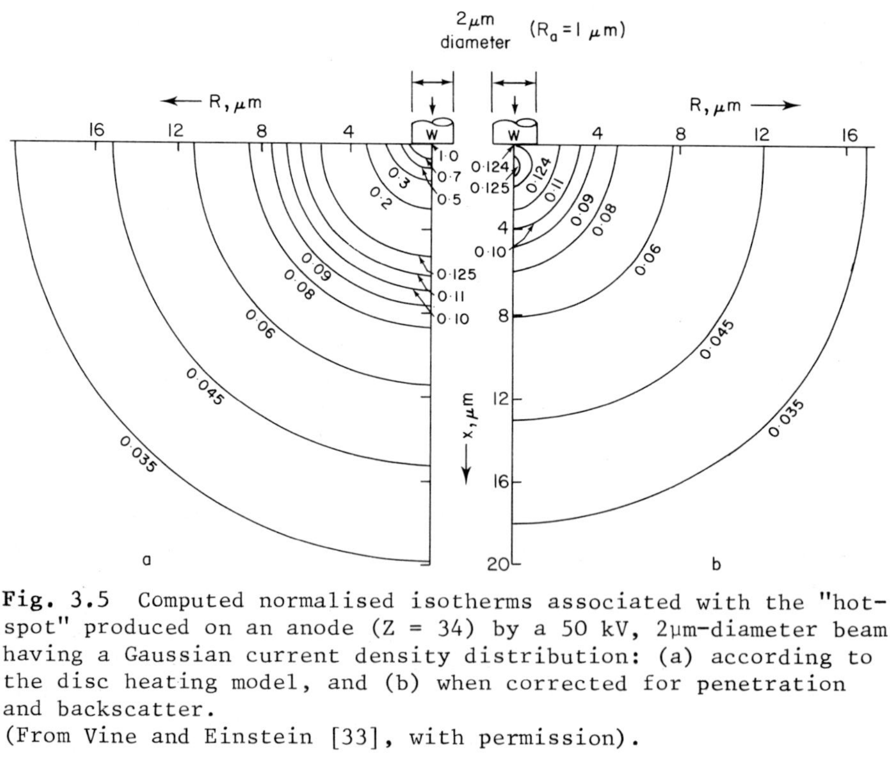

Fig. 3.5 Computed normalised isotherms associated with the "hot-spot" produced on an anode (Z = 34) by a 50 kV, 2μm-diameter beam having a Gaussian current density distribution: (a) according to the disc heating model, and (b) when corrected for penetration and backscatter.
(From Vine and Einstein [33], with permission).

As an illustration of the differing predictions of the "approximate" disc heating model and the more complete latter model, where account is taken of electron penetration and back-scatter losses, Fig. 3.5 compares their respective normalised isotherms, $[T/T_{oo}]_2$ and $[T/T_{oo}]_3$, for a 2μm-diameter, 50 kV beam impinging on a copper target for which the penetration depth $\gamma \sim 15.5$μm. From this figure, it is clear that the largest discrepancies occur within the penetration volume, where the disc model predicts much lower temperature gradients with, consequently, a higher temperature at any given point.

To conclude this discussion, it should be noted that a more complete treatment of this topic would have to take into account the influence of the various electron scattering processes that occur in the target, with particular attention being paid to how the dissipation of the incident electron beam energy varies with depth. An early review of these considerations, as they apply to "massive" targets, was given by Spenser [36]. Subsequently, Bishop [37] used an analytical approach based on Monte Carlo simulation techniques to investigate the energy dissipation in targets of finite thickness such as are encountered in electron microscopy. More recently, Vyatskin et al. [38] have developed experimental techniques for directly measuring the energy dissipation in massive targets. The important fact revealed by these studies is that, as a result of electron back-scattering processes, there is a characteristic depth for a given impact regime at which the rate of energy dissipation is a maximum; its value depending not only on the incident energy of the electrons, but also on the target material, since this determines the range of the electrons. As an example, we can compare the cases of 20 and 30 keV electrons impacting on a copper target, where the maximum rate of energy dissipation will occur respectively at depths of $\sim$ 300 and 600nm [38]. The practical implications of this sort of finding become progressively more important at higher energies, i.e. higher gap voltages, where an increasing fraction of the electron beam energy will be dissipated at a greater depth from the surface. For instance, under these circumstances there is the possibility of an explosive "bubble-like" anode process involving the ejection of showers of molten microdroplets from the anode hot-spot such as required for the breakdown initiating mechanism to be described in section 4.5(iii).

3.4 Stability Considerations under Pulsed Field Operation

In this section we shall be considering the transient response of the cathode microemitter and its associated anode "hot-spot" under non-equilibrium conditions; in particular, where a gap is subjected to a fast-rise pulsed voltage whose duration t_p is comparable or less than the thermal response times of both the cathode and anode microregimes. If this technique is extended to the use of variable-length, over-voltage pulses, i.e. whose amplitude is sufficient to initiate a breakdown, it is possible to study the temporal evolution of the processes occurring in the gap. The practical importance of such a pulsed-field operational regime is that it offers the possibility of applying higher gap voltages than under d-c conditions, and hence drawing higher emission current densities, without the cathode or anode temperatures having time to rise to their critical values for the initiation of thermal instabilities. As will be described later in Chapter 5, this effect has been impressively demonstrated under controlled laboratory conditions for the case of a point-plane electrode geometry. In practice, it is used to advantage, for example, in high power "flash" X-ray tubes.

3.4(i) Cathode response

This has been studied extensively by Mesyats and his co-workers [39-46,48-51] using both theoretical methods and the type of fast-rise, nanosecond over-voltage pulse technique referred to above. Their findings have led to a three-stage breakdown model involving, firstly, the heating of the cathode emitting site to the point of thermal instability and the onset of an "explosive" electron emission regime; secondly, the formation and expansion across the gap of the microplasma or "cathode flare" created from the vaporised cathode material; and thirdly, the subsequent formation of "anode flares" that cross the gap in the reverse direction and thus help to bridge it with an arc. A detailed account will be given in Chapter 5 of the experimental investigations into these fundamental processes as they occur under controlled laboratory conditions with a microscopically well defined point-plane electrode geometry. However, this brief description of the model is sufficient to indicate that the total breakdown time t_b, defined as the time taken for the gap voltage to collapse, can be expressed as

$$t_b = t_1 + t_2 \tag{3.44}$$

where t_1 corresponds to the emitter heating time, and t_2 to the time taken for the plasma to cross the gap and strike an arc. The parameter t_2 , which is often referred to as the "commutation time", is principally determined by the properties of the cathode-flare, with only a small correction included to take account of the contribution made by the secondary anode flares.

Experimental studies [39] have established that the delay time t_1 to the initiation of pulse breakdown obeys the empirical relation

$$j^2 t_1 = \text{constant} \tag{3.45}$$

where the value of the "constant" depends on the cathode material. It therefore follows that t_1 will be very strongly influenced by the explosive electron emission current density j, and hence the gap voltage: typically, t_1 varies in the range 0.1-100ns according to the level of over-voltaging. A close approximation to the commutation time t_2 may be obtained experimentally by using high-speed optical techniques [40,41] to measure the time taken for a cathode flare to cross the electrode gap d, where in terms of the cathode flare velocity v_f,

$$t_2 \sim d/v_f \tag{3.46}$$

Anode flares on the other hand have been shown by these techniques to develop at a time $\sim 0.5d/v_f (\simeq t_2/2)$ after the initiation of a cathode flare [40-43].

From such optical studies with both broad-area electrodes, and those to be described in Chapter 5 using a point-plane configuration, it has been shown that the magnitude of v_f is principally determined by the space charge density within the flare which, in turn, is closely related to the explosive emission current I(t) that is feeding the flare. Since however in practice v_f shows only a small variation over a wide range of experimental conditions, equation 3.46, indicates that t_2 will be very sensitive to the electrode gap d, typically varying between 20-500ns for d-values in the range 0.5-10mm; the corresponding flare velocity is $\sim 2 \times 10^4 ms^{-1}$. For most electrode regimes, I(t) will be space-charge limited and given by the expression [44]

$$I(t) = A\,V(t)^{1.5}\,v_f t\,(d - v_f t)^{-1} \tag{3.47}$$

where $A \sim 3 \times 10^{-5} AV^{-1.5}$ and V(t) is the gap voltage whose time-dependence will be governed by the external circuitry. By establishing an appropriate circuit equation and solving this in conjunction with equation 3.47, it is possible to obtain an analytical expression for t_2 [40,45]. For the cases considered, which are representative of most conventional experimental regimes, it emerges that

$$t_2 = (d/v_f) f(Z,V_p) \tag{3.48}$$

where $f(Z,V_p)$ is a slowly varying function of an appropriate input circuit parameter Z and the over-voltage pulse amplitude V_p. However, since $f(Z,V_p)$ is of the order unity, it follows that the approximation of equation 3.46 was justified. An exception to this rule is where a large gap (>3mm) is being fed from a discharging capacitor whose value is <30pf: in this case, the voltage collapse time is less than the commutation time, i.e. the capacitor is discharged before the gap is bridged by the plasma. It should also be added that equations 3.46 and 3.47 are also valid for d-c breakdowns when the gap length is $\lesssim$6mm and the applied voltage is $\lesssim$ 120 kV [46,47].

Returning to a further consideration of equation 3.44, it must be pointed out that it is liable to become invalid with low over-voltage pulses, where it is frequently found that t_b can exceed

$t_1 + t_2$ (as calculated respectively from equations 3.45 and 3.46) by several orders of magnitude. Under these circumstances, it is believed that the initial emission current density is too low to cause significant vaporisation of the tip, but is high enough to lower the self-diffusion activation energy of its surface atoms to the point where they can migrate under the influence of the applied field and give rise to a tip sharpening mechanism, and hence the critical conditions necessary for the formation of a microplasma. The characteristic time τ_s associated with such a sharpening process is given by [48]

$$\tau_s = 10 r_o \rho^{\frac{1}{2}}/E \tag{3.49}$$

where r_o is the initial radius of the emitter (cm), ρ the density of the cathode material ($g.cm^{-3}$) and E the macroscopic gap field ($V.cm^{-1}$). Thus, taking $r_o = 10^{-5}$cm, $\rho = 10$ $g.cm^{-3}$ and $E = 10^6$ $V.Cm^{-1}$ as being representative of typical gap conditions, equation 3.49 predicts $\tau_s \sim 10^{-7}$s, which is of the correct order to account for the high values found for t_b with low-overvoltage pulses.

The first complete theoretical analysis of the temperature response of a field emitting micropoint is due to Litvinov et al. [48,49] and was based on a model that assumed the important thermal processes and hence instabilities, occur in the surface layers of an emitter. Accordingly, their approach was first to establish a differential equation describing the thermal balance in a surface volume following the application of a step-function impulse field and then to solve this for a set of boundary conditions that closely approximated to those existing in typical experimental situations. To highlight the various physical processes involved, it is convenient to express the basic differential equation in the form

$$\rho C\,\frac{\partial T}{\partial t} = j_F^2\Omega(\tau) + \nabla\left\{(\lambda_e \nabla T_e) + \frac{3j}{5e}F.\mu_o\left[1 + \frac{5\pi^2}{12}\left(\frac{kT}{\mu_o}\right)^2\right]\right\} \tag{3.50}$$

$$\equiv \quad \text{I} \quad + \quad \text{II} \quad + \quad \text{III}$$

Here, the left hand side corresponds to the nett heat gained per unit volume as a result of electron-phonon interactions, and is expressed in terms of the total thermal capacity C which includes both the electronic and phonon contributions, C_e and C_p respectively: thus

$$\rho C(\partial T/\partial t) = C_e(\partial T_e/\partial t) + C_p(\partial T_p/\partial t) \tag{3.51}$$

where T_e and T_p are respectively the electron and phonon (or lattice) temperatures, with $T_e = T_p = T$ at $t = 0$ and as $t \to \infty$. The right hand side of equation 3.50 accounts for the energy dissipating mechanisms in which term I corresponds to the Joulian heating ($\Omega(T)$ being the temperature-dependent resistivity) and terms II + III represent the Nottingham heating effect discussed in section 3.3(i); i.e. where term II is the mean energy removed by electrons that are field emitted from the cathode surface (λ_e is an electron transport parameter), and term III is the mean energy of the replacement or "supply" electrons (μ_o is the Fermi energy defined at T = 0). The detailed form of term II has been given as [48]

$$\lambda_e \nabla T_e = (2kT_i j_F/e)\left[\pi^2 kT_e^2/4\mu(T)T_i + (\pi T_e/2T_i)\mathrm{ctg}(\pi T_e/2T_i)\right] \tag{3.52}$$

where T_i is the Nottingham inversion temperature defined by equation 3.30 and $\mu(T)$, the temperature-dependence of the chemical potential function, is given by

$$\mu(T) = \mu_o[1 - (\pi^2/12)(kT/\mu_o)^2] \tag{3.53}$$

in which μ_o is the Fermi energy at T = 0. Equations 3.44 to 3.47 have been solved for the type of idealised micro-emitting geometries discussed in section 3.2(ii) where the temperature is sufficiently low for j_F to be defined by equation 3.10 or its alternative form

$$j_{TF} = j_{OF}(\pi T_e/2T_i)/\sin(\pi T_e/2T_i) \tag{3.54}$$

At emission current densities $\lesssim 10^{13}\mathrm{Am}^{-2}$, it is found that both the electron and lattice temperatures, T_e and T_p, approach equilibrium values with comparable time constants $\tau_e \sim \tau_p \gtrsim 10^{-10}$s, i.e. indicating that under these conditions there is an efficient exchange of energy between the electrons and the lattice, so that it is therefore permissible to take $T_e = T_p = T$ and to treat the system as having a single thermal capacitance with $C_p = C$. However at emission current densities $\gtrsim 10^{13}\mathrm{Am}^{-2}$, where T_e can reach several tens of thousands of degrees, the above time constants assume values of $\tau_e \lesssim 10^{-12}$s and $\tau_p \sim 10^{-11}- 10^{-10}$s, thus indicating that there is a significant lag between the lattice and electron temperatures. However, when these times are compared with the values for the cathode response time t_1 measured experimentally, it is evident that lattice relaxation effects can be neglected in most practical situations. Applying this and a number of other simplifying assumptions, equation 3.50 may be solved [51] to yield the following analytical expression for t_1

$$j^2 t_1 = a\rho C/H_o \tag{3.55}$$

Here, $H_o = (\Omega(T)/T)$, and a is a material constant which depends weakly on the work function; in the case of tungsten, for example, a = 55. If the values of t_1 predicted by equation 3.55

are compared with those obtained from the empirical expression of equation 3.45 established from experimental data, agreement is generally very good. Thus, taking again the case of tungsten, experiments give $j^2 t_1 = 4 \times 10^{17} A^2 sm^{-4}$, whilst equation 3.55 gives $4.5 \times 10^{17} A^2 sm^{-4}$. It should also be noted that a similar value for the thermal response time of a microemitter was obtained from a computer simulation study by Mitterauer and Till [52] that used a simplified model in which the influence of the Nottingham effect was ignored.

3.4(ii) Anode response

The problem of extending the steady-state analysis of section 3.3(ii) to include the temporal response of the anode hot-spot temperature distribution under pulsed heating conditions has been considered by Charbonnier et al. [53], and in more detail by Dudek [54], who also conducted a complementary experimental investigation. However, to gain an insight into the essential features of the characteristic temperature response of this complex thermal regime, we shall refer here to the findings of the simplified approach of Charbonnier et al. [53] which is appropriate to conditions where the pulse length is less than or comparable to the thermal response time of the anode. In this treatment, the surface disc source diffusion model is solved for the special situation where times are short enough for the flow of heat to remain uni-directional, i.e. normal to the anode surface. The model was further simplified by considering an idealised circular cross-section beam having a uniform power loading w, where space charge effects and backscattered losses are ignored. For such a regime, two functions may be defined that give the temperature increase in the anode.

(i) For $0 \lesssim x \lesssim \gamma$ i.e. for points within the electron range γ of the target surface

$$T_1(x,t) = \frac{w}{2K\gamma}\left[(\gamma + x)^2 f(\alpha_1) + (\gamma - x)^2 f(\alpha_2)\right] \qquad (3.56)$$

where $f(\alpha_1)$ and $f(\alpha_2)$ are complicated functions defined by

$$f(\alpha) = \left[\exp.\left(\frac{-\alpha^2}{2}\right)\right]\left[\alpha(2\pi)^{\frac{1}{2}}\right]^{-1} + \alpha^{-2}\mathrm{erf}(\alpha) + \mathrm{erf}(\alpha) - 0.5 \qquad (3.57)$$

with

$$\alpha_1 = (\gamma + x)(2Kt/C\rho)^{-\frac{1}{2}}$$
$$\alpha_2 = (\gamma - x)(2Kt/C\rho)^{-\frac{1}{2}} \qquad (3.58)$$

In these equations, erf signifies the standard "error" function, whilst K, C and ρ are respectively the thermal conductivity, specific heat and density of the target.

(ii) For $x > \gamma$, i.e. for points inside the bulk of the target and outside the electron penetration range

$$T_2(x,t) = \frac{w}{2K\gamma}\left[(\gamma + x)^2 f(\alpha_1) - (x - \gamma)^2 f(\alpha_2)\right] \tag{3.59}$$

The highest anode surface temperature will occur at the centre of the hot-spot ($x = 0$) which, from equation 3.56, will be given by

$$\begin{aligned} T_1(0,t) &= \frac{w}{2K\gamma}\left[\gamma^2 f(\alpha_{01}) + \gamma^2 f(\alpha_{02})\right] \\ &= \frac{w\gamma}{K} f(\alpha_0) \end{aligned} \tag{3.60}$$

since $\alpha_{01} = \alpha_{02} = \alpha_0 = \gamma(2Kt/C\rho)^{-\frac{1}{2}}$ in this special case.

It will be seen from equations 3.56 and 3.59 that the time-dependence of T_1 and T_2 only appears through the quantities α_1 and α_2 in equation 3.57 for $f(\alpha)$, and that this is basically an exponential function in α^2. Accordingly the quantity $(\gamma \pm x)^2(2K/C\rho)^{-1}$ can be identified as the heat spread parameter which determines how rapidly the thermal diffusion process can dissipate heat energy; alternatively, it is possible to define a local thermal time constant for any point x which gives a measure of the time taken for the temperature at that point to approach its steady-state value. Thus, at $x = \gamma$, i.e. at the inner boundary of the disc heat source, we have from equation 3.58 that $\alpha_2 = 0$ and

$$\tau_\gamma - \frac{2\gamma^2 \rho C}{K} \tag{3.61}$$

Because of the dependence of τ_γ on γ, it follows from equation 3.36 that $\tau_\gamma \propto V_0^4$ and is consequently very sensitive to the energy of the bombarding electrons, where typically, $\tau_\gamma \sim$ nano-seconds for a 10 kV beam and $\sim$ milliseconds for a 1 MV beam. The changing temperature distribution in the surface of the anode as predicted by this pulsed heat source model can be conveniently illustrated in terms of the normalised variables (x/γ) and (t/τ_γ). Thus, Fig. 3.6 shows a family of normalised temperature distributions corresponding to increasing time intervals up to $t = 16\tau_\gamma$ following the application of a heat pulse [53].

Finally, the model can be used to provide approximate expressions that indicate how the temperature rise in the surface of the anode depends on the duration of the heat pulse t_p.

For very short pulses ($t_p \ll \tau_\gamma$), there will be an adiabatic situation with virtually no heat spread, so that at the end of the pulse there will be a uniform temperature rise throughout the disc given by

$$T(0,t_p) \simeq \frac{wt_p}{\gamma C\rho} \tag{3.62}$$

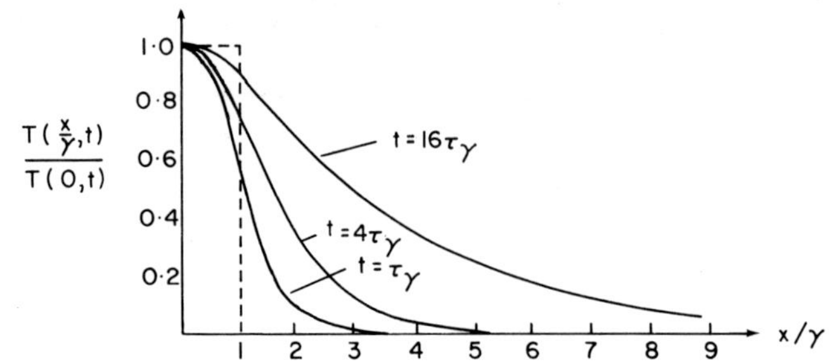

Fig. 3.6 Normalised axial temperature distributions associated with an anode "hot-spot" formed by a pulsed electron beam of varying duration t_p.
(From Charbonnier, Bennette and Swanson [53], with permission).

For intermediate pulses ($t_p \gtrsim \tau_\gamma$), there will be an appreciable diffusion of heat into the anode with the surface temperature being given by equation 3.60. However, for situations where t_p is significantly greater than τ_γ, so that $\alpha_1 << 1$, equation 3.60 can be approximated by [53]

$$T_1(0,t_p) \simeq 2wt_p^{\frac{1}{2}}/(\pi K C \rho)^{\frac{1}{2}} \tag{3.63}$$

For very long pulses ($t_p >> \tau_\gamma$); equilibrium conditions will be approached and the anode temperature rise will correspond to the steady-state limit calculated by Oosterkamp [32] viz.

$$T_1(0,t_p) \simeq wR_a / K \tag{3.64}$$

3.5 Practical breakdown criteria: "cathode" versus "anode" initiated

As stated in the introductory remarks to this chapter, the basic criterion for the breakdown of a vacuum gap is that the temperature of either a cathode microprotrusion or anode hot-spot should approach their respective melting points. Thus, in the preceeding sections these critical conditions have been independently quantified for the anode and cathode processes. For example, equations 3.27 and 3.28 may be solved to determine the critical (i.e. maximum) emission current density j_{FC} that may be drawn from a conical microprotrusion of known material and geometry before its tip temperature approaches to within $\sim$ 0.8-0.9 of its melting point when there is a high risk of breakdown being initiated through thermal or mechanical instabilities: the corresponding critical field E_c is then obtained from equations 3.10 to 3.18. Similarly, equations 3.41 or 3.42 may be used to define the critical power loading W_c that can be sustained at the anode hot-spot associated with this same conical microemitter; furthermore there will clearly be a critical emitter current, and hence cathode field, corresponding to W_c. The initiation of each of these breakdown mechanisms will therefore be associated with a critical gap field, say E_{c_1} and E_{c_2}, but the question however arises as to whether, for a given microemitter, breakdown will be initiated by the cathode or anode process, i.e. whether $E_{c1} \gtrless E_{c2}$ Qualitative reasoning suggests that long, thin and sharp protrusions will become thermally unstable before they can deliver sufficient emission current for the beam power loading at the anode to approach W_c, so that such a regime will give rise to cathode initiated breakdown: on the other hand, short, thick-shanked and rounded protrusions will have good thermal coupling to their base electrode and will therefore be capable of sustaining the necessary emission currents for the anode power loading to approach W_c and so precipitate anode initiated breakdown. This type of reasoning prompted Chatterton [14] and Charbonnier et al. [53], to recognise that there will be a critical protrusion geometry, defined by a critical field enhancement factor β_c, which will set the boundary between the initiation of the two mechanisms. Thus, for $\beta > \beta_c$, breakdown will be cathode-initiated, whilst for $\beta < \beta_c$, it will be anode-initiated. Following the analytical approach of Charbonnier et al. [53], which is based on a hemispherically-capped emitting protrusion, and uses the approximation of an anode disc heat source model referred to above, the steady-state anode power density is given by

$$w \simeq i_F V/\pi R_a^2$$

which, after making the substitutions $i_F \simeq \pi r^2 j_F$, $E = \beta(V/d)$ and $R_a = 2(\beta r d)^{\frac{1}{2}}$ becomes

$$w \simeq r j_F E/4\beta^2 \tag{3.65}$$

Introducing now the limitations imposed by the critical current density j_{FC} and field E_c (typically $6 \times 10^{11} Am^{-2}$ and $\gtrsim 5 \times 10^9 Vm^{-1}$ respectively) that can be sustained at a given cathode surface, together with the critical anode power loading w_c, equation 3.58 predicts that for *cathode initiated breakdown*,

$$\frac{r j_{FC} E_c}{4\beta^2} > w_c \tag{3.66}$$

and for anode-initiated breakdown

$$\frac{r j_{FC} E_c}{4\beta^2} < w_c \tag{3.67}$$

The boundary between the two processes will therefore be defined by $r j_{FC} E_c/4\beta^2 = w_c$, which allows a critical value of the field enhancement factor β_c to be defined for which both processes would be simultaneously initiated, viz.

$$\beta_c = \left(rj_{FC}\, E_c/4w_c\right)^{\frac{1}{2}} \tag{3.68}$$

Noting that $w_c \simeq KT_m/R_a$ from equation 3.64 and $R_a \simeq 2(\beta_o rd)^{\frac{1}{2}}$ from equation 3.35 with $\delta \simeq r, \beta_c$ may be alternatively expressed in the more practical form

$$\beta_c = r\ [j_{FC}E_c d^{\frac{1}{2}}/2KT_m]^{2/3} \tag{3.69}$$

A similar approach may be used to obtain equivalent expressions for β_c for pulse field operation [53], where it is generally found that these conditions favour cathode initiated breakdown. Reference should also be made to the experimental investigation of Utsumi [55] which broadly confirmed the conclusions of the above analysis, viz. that high-β emitters ($\beta \gtrsim 500$) invariably lead to cathode-initiated breakdown, whilst low-β emitters ($\beta \lesssim 30$) are found to precipitate anode-initiated breakdown.

When considering the practical implication of the above limiting conditions, it should be noted that calculations of the critical cathode current density and anode power density only vary by a factor of ~ 5 over a wide range of electrode materials from say alumina to tungsten [53]. Accordingly, there will only be a small spread in the values of β_c, and hence the macroscopic breakdown field E_b ($=E_c/\beta_c$), among commonly used electrode materials. These considerations alone would suggest however, that high conductivity metals such as copper, that can dissipate heat rapidly, would be more effective as anode materials, whilst refractory metals such as tungsten are to be favoured for cathodes on the grounds of their having lower inversion temperatures [31] with consequently more stable emitting characteristics.

Apart from the inherent approximations of this analysis of breakdown criteria, of which the neglect of space charge effects at high emission current densities is probably the most notable, the approach also suffers from the serious disadvantage of taking no account of protrusion shape; i.e. that there can be a wide range of geometries corresponding to a given β-value. This aspect was however considered by Chatterton [14] in a computational analysis that compared the critical behaviour of conical and cylindrical protrusions of similar tip radii r. The main conclusion to emerge from this investigation was that, whereas there is a large reduction in the value of β_c for the thinner cylindrical type of protrusion, with a consequent increase in the likelihood of cathode initiated breakdown, the critical anode condition is much less sensitive to protrusion geometry. This is not perhaps a surprising finding when it is remembered that a conical protrusion has a better thermal coupling with its base electrode and will therefore be inherently more stable. In assessing the importance of protrusion shape in practical situations it has to be noted that most direct electron optical evidence of protrusions (see Chapter 7) indicates that the conical geometry is very much more typical. For this reason, the analytical expression for β_c of equation 3.69 can still be regarded as a good approximation.

Note should finally be taken of an important observation by Jüttner [47] that although the traditional criterion for anode initiated breakdown used throughout this chapter is a fundamental requirement, it is not in itself a sufficient condition for there to be a 100% probability of a breakdown occurring. The reason for this is that, in order to explain the origin of the very high currents flowing during a breakdown (10-100A), it is necessary to assume the occurrence of a secondary process involving the formation of an explosive emission cathode spot through a breakdown between the advancing anode plasma and the cathode surface: an event that could be expected to be extremely rapid, since it is known that cathode spots have nanosecond formation times [56]. However, the probability of this secondary process occurring is less than unity, as can be demonstrated by using a triggering spark to artificially produce an anode plasma in an electrically stressed gap, and noting that this does not always result in the breakdown of the main gap: in contrast, if a similar experiment is performed using a cathode triggering spark, the probability of a breakdown is unity. This observation therefore implies that a breakdown event initiated by an anode microplasma involves a more complicated mechanism than previously assumed, and that statistically, it is less likely to occur than a cathode initiated event.

3.6 References

1. Fowler, R.H. and Nordheim, L., *Proc. Roy. Soc.* **A119**, 173-81, (1928).
2. Gomer, R., "Field Emission and Field Ionisation", Oxford University Press, Oxford, (1961).
3. Good, R.H. and Müller, E.W., *In* "Handbuck der Physik" Springer-Verlag, Berlin , **21**, 176-231, (1956).
4. Van Oostram, A.G.J., Philips Research Reports Supplements, No.1, (1966).
5. Miller, H.C., *J.Franklin Inst.*, **282**, 382-8, (1966).
6. Miller, H.C., *J.Franklin Inst.*, **289**, 347-51, (1969).
7. Beukema, G.P., *Physica*, **61**, 259-74, (1972).
8. Murphy, E.L. and Good, R.H., *Phys. Rev.*, **102**, 1464-73, (1956).
9. Dyke, W.P. and Dolan, W.W., *Adv. Electronics Electron Phys.*, **8**, 90-180, (1956).
10. Christov, S.G., *Phys. Stat. Sol.*, **17**, 11-26, (1966).
11. Haeffer, R., *Z. Physik*, **116**, 604-22, (1940).
12. Dyke, W.P., Trolan, J.K., Dolan, W.W. and Barnes, G., *J.Appl. Phys.*, **24**, 570-6, (1953).
13. Dyke, W.P., Trolan, J.K., Martin, E.E. and Barbour, J.P., *Phys. Rev.*, **91**, 1043-54, (1953).

14. Chatterton, P.A., *Proc. Phys. Soc.*, (London), **88**, 231-45, (1966).
15. Nagy, D. and Cutler, P.H., *Phys. Lett.*, **10**, 263-4, (1964).
16. Rohrbach, F., CERN Report, 71-5/TC-L, (1971).
17. Fursey, G.N. and Vorontsov-Vel'yaminov, P.N., *Sov. Phys: Tech. Phys.* **12**, 1370-6, (1968).
18. Vibrans, G.E., Tech. Report 353, Lincoln Lab., MIT (NTIS ESDTDR 64-327), (1964).
19. Miller, H.C., *J. Appl. Phys.*, **38**, 4501-4, (1967).
20. Tomaschke, H.E. and Alpert, D., *J. Appl. Phys.*, **38**, 881-3, (1967).
21. Farrall, G.A., *J. Appl. Phys.*, **41**, 563-71, (1970).
22. Charbonnier, F.M., Strayer, R.W., Swanson, L.W. and Martin, E.E., *Phys. Rev. Lett.*, **13**, 397-401, (1964).
23. Dolan, W.W., Dyke, W.P. and Trolan, J.K., *Phys. Rev.*, **91**, 1054-7, (1953).
24. Martin, E.E., Charbonnier, F.M. and others, WADD Techn.Rep. 59-20, Linfield Research Inst., (1960).
25. Levine, P.H., *J. Appl. Phys.*, **33**, 582-7, (1962).
26. Vibrans, G.E., *J. Appl. Phys.*, **35**, 2855-7, (1964).
27. Brodie, I., *Int. J. Electronics*, **18**, 223-33, (1965).
28. Swanson, L.W., Crouser, L.C. and Charbonnier, F.M., *Phys. Rev.*, **151**, 327-340, (1966).
29. Slivkov, I.N., *Sov. Phys: Tech. Phys.*, **11**, 249-53, (1966).
30. Drechsler, M., *Z. Naturforsch*, **18a**, 1376-80, (1963).
31. Swanson, L.W., Strayer, R.W. and Charbonnier, F.M., *Surface Sci.*, **2**, 177-82, (1964).
32. Oosterkamp, W.J., Philips Res. Rep. **3**, pp. 49, 160, 303, (1948).
33. Vine, J. and Einstein, P.A., *Proc. IEEE*, **111**, 921-30, (1964).
34. Whiddington, R., *Proc. Roy. Soc.*, **89**, 554-9, (1914).
35. Carslaw, H.S. and Jaeger, J.C., "Conduction of Heat in Solids", Oxford University Press, (2nd Edition), (1959).
36. Spenser, L.V., "Energy dissipation by fast electrons", National Bureau of Standards Monograph, No.1, (1959).
37. Bishop, H.E., *Brit.J. Appl. Phys.*, **18**, 703-15, (1967).
38. Vyatskin, A.Ya, Kabanov, A.N., Smirnov, B.P. and Khramov, V.Yu, *Rad. Eng. and Electron Phys. (USA)*, **22**, 80-4, (1977).
39. Kartsev, G.K., Mesyats, G.A., Proskurovsky, D.I., Rotshteyn, V.P. and Fursey, G.N., *Sov. Phys.- Dokl.*, **15**, 475-7, (1970).
40. Mesyats, G.A. and Proskurovsky, D.I., *Sov. Phys. J.*, **11**, 49-51, (1968).
41. Bugaev, S.P., Mesyats, G.A. and Proskurovsky, D.I., *Sov. Phys. - Dokl*, **14**, 605-6, (1969).
42. Bugaev, S.P., Koshelev, V.I. and Timoleev, M.N., *Sov. Phys. J.*, **17**, 193-196, (1974).
43. Baksht, R.B., Kokshenov, V.A. and Manylov, V.I., *Sov. Phys: Tech. Phys.*, **20**, 1069-71, (1975).

44. Bugaev, S.P., Litvinov, E.A., Lopatin, V.V. and Mesyats, G.A., "Nanosecond High Power Electron Pulses", Nauka, Novosibirsk, p.52, (1974).

45. Mesyats, G.A., *Zhurn, Tekhn. Fiz.*, **44**, 1521-4, (1974).

46. Proskurovsky, D.I. and Urike, Ya.Ya., *Proc. IV-DEIV*, 78-81, (1970).

47. Jüttner, B., Private Communication, (1980).

48. Litvinov, E.A., Mesyats, G.A., Shubin, A.F., Buskin, L.M., and Fursey, G.N., *Proc. VI-DEIV*, 107-111, (1974).

49. Litvinov, E.A., Mesyats, G.A., Proskurovsky, D.I. and Yankelevitch, E.G., *Proc. VII-DEIV*, 55-67, (1976).

50. Litvinov, E.A., Mesyats, G.A. and Shubin, A.F., *Sov. Phys. J*, **13**, 537-40, (1970).

51. Bugaev, S.P., Litvinov, E.A., Mesyats, G.A. and Proskurovsky, D.I., *Sov. Phys. Usp.*, **18**, 51-61, (1975).

52. Mitterauer, J. and Till, P., *Proc. VI-DEIV*, 95-100, (1974).

53. Charbonnier, F.M., Bennette, C.J. and Swanson, L.W., *J. Appl. Phys.*, **38**, 627-33, (1967).

54. Dudek, H.J., *Z. Angow. Phys.*, **31**, 243-50 and 331-7, (1971).

55. Utsumi, T., *J. Appl. Phys.*, **38**, 2989-97, (1967).

56. Jütner, B., *Beiträge Plasmaphysik*, **19**, 25-8, (1979).

4 Breakdown Initiating Mechanisms II – Microparticle Based

4.1 Origin of Microparticles
4.2 Early Theories
4.3 "Primary" and "Secondary Microparticles
4.4 Microparticle Charge Aquisition and Electromechanical Detachment Criteria
4.5 In-flight Phenomena
   (i) Particle charge modification by electron emission
   (ii) The "Trigger Discharge" breakdown mechanism
   (iii) The "Particle Vaporisation" breakdown mechanism
4.6 Single-transit Impact Phenomena
   (i) Low impact velocities
   (ii) Intermediate impact velocities
   (iii) High impact velocities
4.7 Multi-transit Impact Phenomena
   (i) Particle bouncing
   (ii) Particle kinetic energy enhancement
   (iii) Theoretical basis of charge exchange process
4.8 Microparticle Behaviour under Impulse Voltages
   (i) Impact-initiated breakdown
   (ii) The "detachment" trigger discharge
4.9 References

4.1 Origin of Microparticles

One of the inevitable consequences of the standard electrode preparation procedures described in chapter 2 is that a pre-operational electrode surface will be characterised by having a finite number of microscopic particles loosely adhering to it. These may originate from the various stages of mechanical polishing and be in the form of either partially embedded impurity particles of the polishing medium (e.g. alumina or diamond) or filamentary structures that have been torn from the surface:some idea of the complex microscopic structure of a typical "virgin" electrode is given by the scanning electron micrograph of Figure 2.11. Alternatively, they can be merely dust particles that become attached to an electrode surface by Van der Waals forces during the many handling manipulations of its final assembly. Another important source of microparticles that has to be added to this list are those originating from thermal instabilities at either the cathode or anode "hot spots" associated with isolated electron emission processes (see chapter 3). However, for "commercially" polished electrodes, it could reasonably be argued that embedded impurities and dust particles probably provide the most prolific source of microparticles: this is particularly true with large gaps where electron emission currents have generally become negligibly small.

It also has to be pointed out that the electrode geometry can have an important influence in determining the origin and multiplicity of microparticles. Thus for a symmetric plane-parallel gap formed by identically prepared electrodes having a separation d and supporting a voltage V there will be a uniform gap field E=V/d so that each electrode will, on average, donate a similar number of microparticles per unit area. Consider on the other hand the case of an asymmetric electrode pair that has a non-uniform gap field, say a sphere-to-plane geometry with an axial separation d and supporting a similar voltage V, it is clear that the higher field on the surface of the sphere will result in a selectivity for microparticles to originate from this electrode. It must be added however that this simple argument breaks down if dissimilar materials are used for the electrodes or their methods of surface preparation differ in any way.

4.2 Early Theories

The important role that can subsequently be played by such microparticles in initiating the electrical breakdown of a vacuum gap was first appreciated by Cranberg and quantified in his famous "clump" hypothesis [1], which was the name he coined to describe such microparticles. He recognised that in the presence of a high gap field there would be strong electro-mechanical forces tending to detach such protruding microfeatures from their highly charged parent electrode and that if this occurred they would enter the gap as charged particles to be accelerated to high velocities during their transit to the opposite electrode. At impact, these micro-projectiles would dissipate their kinetic energy U_k as either heat or mechanical shock energy and that if the impact energy density exceeds some critical value, dependent on the colliding materials, there would be sufficient vaporisation tion of the particle and target electrode to form a localised microplasma that could initiate the breakdown of the gap. Thus, for a particle of given charge Q_p and mass M_p crossing a gap d to which the applied voltage is V

$$U_k = \frac{1}{2} M_p v_i^2 = Q_p V \qquad (4.1)$$

where v_i is the terminal or impact velocity. It follows that if the cross-sectioned area of the particle is A, the impact energy density U_k/A will be given by

$$\frac{U_k}{A} = \frac{Q_p}{A} . V$$

where Q_p/A is the charge density on the particle. Now as will be discussed shortly, the charge density acquired by a particle will be proportional to the macroscopic field E, (i.e. $Q_p/A \propto E$), and since in general $E \propto V$, the above can be expressed as

$$\frac{U_k}{A} \propto EV = C'EV$$

where C' is a constant. In the particular case of a plane-parallel gap $E = V/d$ so that

$$\frac{U_k}{A} = C'\frac{E^2}{d} = C'V^2d$$

For a critical impact, where the impact energy density approaches some critical value $(U_k/A)_c$ with $E \to E_b$ and $V \to V_b$, E_b and V_b being respectively the breakdown field and potential, Cranberg's hypothesis will be expressed as

$$\left.\frac{U_k}{A}\right|_c \geqslant C'E_bV_b \geqslant C'dE_b^2 \geqslant C'V_b^2/d$$

or

$$E_b \geqslant C_c^{\frac{1}{2}}\, d^{-\frac{1}{2}} \qquad (4.2(i))$$

and $$V_b \geqslant (C_c d)^{\frac{1}{2}} \qquad (4.2(ii))$$

where $C_c = (1/C'(U_k/A)_c$ is the critical constant as originally defined by Cranberg. The value of C_c clearly involves several numerical constants, including a factor to account for any local field enhancement at the electrode surface where the particle became detached: it will also vary somewhat with the mechanical and thermal properties of the electrode surface. However, a typical value quoted by Cranberg as being appropriate to a wide range of experiments was $C_c \sim 10(\mathrm{MV})^2\mathrm{m}^{-1}$ for d measured in meters and V_b in megavolts.

In support of his theory, Cranberg [1] collated several sets of independent breakdown data and showed that V_b had the required mean $d^{\frac{1}{2}}$ dependence. He also cited some a-c breakdown measurements previously referred to in section 2.6, where a 2800 MHz, 2MV source was applied across 5 cm gaps and resulted in very much higher breakdown voltages than could be achieved with similar amplitude d-c voltage: a finding that can be readily explained when it is appreciated that in such an experimental regime, particles would have insufficient time to be accelerated across the gap during any half-cycle of the applied field so that particle-initiated breakdown would tend to be suppressed. Another important feature of this theory noted by Cranberg was that it satisfactorily accounted for the spontaneous breakdown events observed with large gaps where there was no measurable pre-breakdown currents and no possibility of electron emission-based breakdown mechanisms operating.

The basic Cranberg hypothesis just described was further refined by Slivkov [2] who introduced two physical constraints to make the model more physically realistic. Firstly, he assumed that the particle must have sufficient energy to be totally vaporised on impact: this implies that there will be a critical impact velocity and hence a maximum particle radius R_{max} for which this requirement will be satisfied. Secondly, he proposed that the impact must generate sufficient vapour to create the necessary conditions for initiating a localised discharge: this requirement therefore indicates a particle radius R_{min} for breakdown to be initiated. The precise numerical values of R_{max} and R_{min} will inevitably depend upon the particular experimental regime being considered; however their probable range for typical experimental conditions will be discussed in greater detail later in this chapter (Section 4.5). With the above two constraints incorporated in the basic particle impact model, the modified Slivkov breakdown criterion takes the form

$$V_b = C_s d^{0.625} \qquad (4.3)$$

where C_s is again a constant whose value depends on the experimental conditions. Comparing this relation with equation 4.2, it will be seen that the Cranberg and Slivkov gap dependencies of $V_b \propto d^{\frac{1}{2}}$ and $V_b \propto d$ respectively, are very similar and consequently difficult to discriminate between experimentally. The available experimental evidence does however generally support the above theoretical prediction that V_b should show a power law gap dependence of the form $V_b \propto d^{\alpha}$, although there is a very considerable scatter in the values found for the power α. From a review of typical experimental data [see Section 2.5(iii)] it is found that in most cases α lies in the range 0.4-0.7, so that a mean practical formulation of the Cranberg-Slivkov breakdown criterion would be

$$V_b = C_{cs} d^{0.55} \qquad (4.4)$$

Although the formulation of these early theories of micro-particle initiated breakdown was subject to some criticism, the existance of the physical phenomenon became widely accepted. It was not surprising therefore that a second generation of more refined theories evolved that considered in very much more detail the three main aspects of the mechanism, viz, the origin of micro-particles, their in-flight behaviour and their subsequent impact properties.

4.3. "Primary" and "Secondary" Microparticles

In the context of the present discussion on the initiation of breakdown by naturally occurring microparticles (i.e. as opposed to those artificially introduced into a gap for experimental purposes), the term "primary" refers to those isolated microparticles that initiate the chain of events that culminates in breakdown: they are in fact the same loosely attached microstructures or embedded impurity granules referred to earlier in this chapter that are inevitably present on a virgin electrode surface. "Secondary" microparticles on the other hand are those that are created as a consequence of a micro-discharge or breakdown event involving the local fusion of electrode material such as occurs in the electron emission-based initiating mechanisms discussed in chapter 3, or from a Cranberg type of explosive impact of a "primary" microparticle in which a shower of molten droplets are produced by the "coronet" effect (see Figure 4.2b) and solidify to become "secondary" microparticles. It follows that once a population of secondary microparticles has been generated in the gap they will subsequently represent a serious hazard to its stability since each of them is potentially capable of initiating a secondary breakdown. The following sections of this chapter are devoted to an analysis of the physical properties of microparticles.

4.4. Microparticle Charge Aquisition and Electromechanical Detachment Criteria

The charge carried by a free microparticle is derived from the field-induced surface charge existing on the original microfeature immediately before its detachment from the parent electrode. Now since the surface charge density σ at any given point is directly proportional to the local microscopic field acting at that point, i.e. $\sigma = \varepsilon_0 E$, it follows that at a protruding microstructure where the surface field is locally enhanced, there will be a correspondingly enhanced surface charge density. This observation implies that the charge acquired by a particle originating from such a feature will be strongly dependent on its shape, with rounded structures having generally lower charge-to-mass ratios than elongated structures. Equally, the electromechanical forces tending to detach such surface structures F_d will induce varying internal elastic stresses that will again depend on their shape, with the most vulnerable structures being those that are only attached to the parent electrode by a constricted stalk so that there is a stress enhancement.

These conclusions can be quantitatively illustrated with reference to a detailed theoretical analysis by Rohrbach [3] of the charge acquisition and detachment processes as applied to the idealised geometries of Figure 4.1, i.e. similar to those used for microemitter models in chapter 3. Thus, for spherically based structures such as Figs 4.1c and d, where γ (= h/r) $\gtrsim 5$,

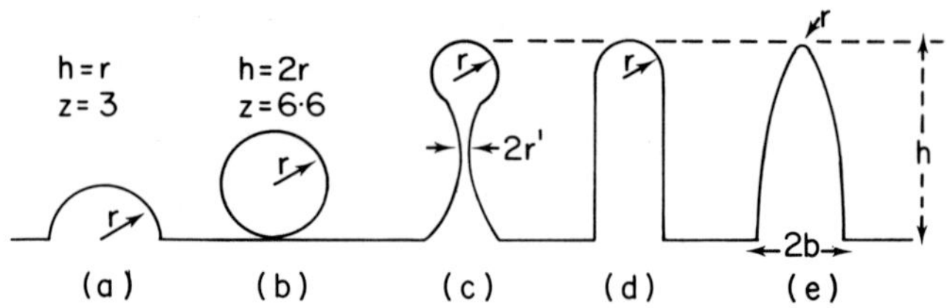

Fig. 4.1 A selection of idealised electrode surface microstructures that have been analysed as potential microparticles[3].

we can use the approximation of equation 3.18, viz. $\beta(\gamma) = 2 + h/r$, in which case the charge acquired by the resulting microparticle would be

$$Q_p(\gamma) = 4\pi\varepsilon_o h^2 \frac{(\beta-3)}{(\beta-2)^2}.E \tag{4.5}$$

where, as usual, E is the uniform macroscopic field in a plane-parallel gap. For geometries where $h \sim r$, such as for the cases illustrated in Fig. 4.1a and b of a spherical particle that is either half-embedded or resting on the electrode surface, the particle charge would be given by

$$Q_p(\gamma) = Z\pi\varepsilon_o r^2 E \tag{4.6}$$

where Z is a numerical factor that has to be computed for individual values of h/r [4,5], taking the respective values of 3 and 6.6 for the geometries of Figs. 4.1a and b.

In the case of the semi-ellipsoidal microfeature of Fig. 4.1e, whose geometry is defined by the ratio $\lambda = h/b$, and for which the field enhancement $\beta(\lambda)$ is given by equation 3.15, the resulting particle will acquire a charge of

$$Q_p(\lambda) = \frac{\pi\varepsilon_o h^2 \beta}{\lambda^2}.E \tag{4.7}$$

The corresponding expressions for the electromechanical detachment forces F_d acting on these two types of microgeometry are given by [3]

$$F_d(\gamma) = \frac{4\pi\varepsilon_o h^2(\gamma-1)}{\gamma^2}.E^2 \tag{4.8}$$

for the spherically-based geometries and

$$F_d(\lambda) = \frac{\pi\varepsilon_o h^2 f(\lambda)}{\lambda^2}.E^2 \tag{4.9}$$

for the ellipsoidal geometry, where

$$f(\lambda) = \frac{\beta^2(\lambda)}{2(\lambda^2-1)}\left[\frac{\lambda^2}{\lambda^2-1}\log\lambda^2 - 1\right]$$

To establish the critical conditions for microparticle detachment, the electromechanical stress imparted to the attachment cross-section of the microstructure is equated with the yield stress σ_y of the electrode material. Thus, for geometries (a) and (d) of Fig. 4.1, the required condition will be $F_d(\gamma)/\pi r^2 \gtrsim \sigma_y$ or,

$$4\varepsilon_o(\gamma-1)E^2 \gtrsim \sigma_y \tag{4.10}$$

and for the more vulnerable structure (c) $F_d(\gamma)/\pi r^2 \gtrsim \sigma_y$ or

$$4\varepsilon_o(r/r')(\gamma - 1)E^2 \gtrsim \sigma_y \tag{4.11}$$

For the ellipsoidal feature (f) of Fig. 4.1, the corresponding condition will be $F_d(\lambda)/\pi b^2 \gtrsim \sigma_y$ or from equation 4.9

$$\varepsilon_o f(\lambda)E^2 \gtrsim \sigma_y \tag{4.12}$$

However, in this last case, it has to be noted that because of its changing cross-sectional area, there is a considerable variation in the stress along the length of the protrusion, reaching a maximum value at its apex where the detachment criterion is

$$\frac{1}{2}\varepsilon_o\beta^2(\lambda)E^2 \gtrsim \sigma_y \tag{4.13}$$

To illustrate the practical implications of these expressions, we can take the example [3] of a 1 cm plane-parallel gap formed by titanium electrodes and supporting a voltage of 600kV, i.e. $E = 6 \times 10^7 Vm^{-1}$, and assume there to be a fairly blunt microfeature present on one of the electrodes whose β-value is 6. From equations 3.15 to 3.18, this could correspond either to the hemispherically capped cylindrical geometry of Fig. 4.1(d) with $h = 0.4\mu m$ and $r = 0.1\mu m$ (i.e. $\gamma = 4$), or to the semi-ellipsoidal geometry of Fig. 4.1(e) also with $h = 0.4\mu m$ and $r = 0.1$ (i.e. $\lambda = 2.0$). It then follows from equations 4.5 and 4.7 that the surface charges concentrated on these alternative structures, i.e. those that would be carried away by them if they became detached, are respectively 2.0×10^{-16} and 4.4×10^{-16}C. From volume of revolution calculations and a knowledge of their density, the respective masses of these potential microparticles would be 1.9×10^{-17} and 1.8×10^{-16}kg, so that their corresponding Q/M values would be 10 and 2.0 $C.kg^{-1}$; i.e. higher for the narrower cylindrical geometry as would be expected from qualitative reasoning. However, from equations 4.10 and 4.12, the corresponding mechanical stresses existing in the base cross-section of the protrusions are $3.8 \times 10^5\ Nm^{-2}$ and $1.6 \times 10^5\ Nm^{-2}$ respectively for the cylindrical and ellipsoidal geometries. If these values are then compared with the yield strength of titanium at room temperature, viz. $4.4 \times 10^8\ Nm^{-2}$, it clearly follows that such microstructures would be mechanically stable under these field conditions. In fact, it is only with more needle-like geometries ($\beta \gtrsim 100$) or the lower-β "necked" type of structure of Fig. 4.1(c) where there is an internal stress amplification of r/r' that internal stresses approach the yield strength of typical electrode materials and provide the possibility of microparticles being launched into the gap. It also follows that such an extrusion process would give rise to the filamentary structures illustrated in Fig. 4.2, and hence the possibility of a potentially unstable field emitting microprotrusions if the particle originates from the cathode. This reasoning also provides strong grounds for assuming that naturally occurring microparticles can have tail-like structures (see sections 4.6(i) and 4.9(ii)).

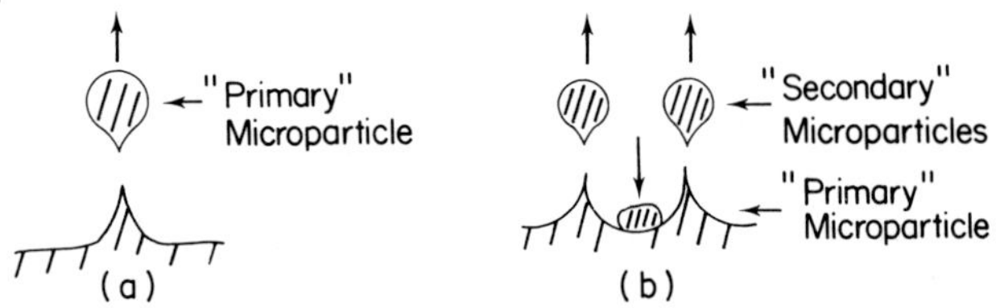

Fig. 4.2. A schematic representation of the creation of (a) a "primary" microparticle by the field-stripping of a protruding microfeature, and (b) a shower of "secondary" microparticles resulting from a high-velocity impact of a primary microparticle.

It will be appreciated that the above analysis only applies to one possible source of microparticles, viz. those that originate from microfeatures that are physical extensions of the bulk parent electrode. An equally important source is that arising from partly embedded impurity granules or dust particles that are attached to an electrode surface through adhesive forces. Boulloud [6] for example has considered the effects of Van der Waals forces and shown that, for large particles, they can be very considerable. For the simple case of a sphere of radius R_p resting on a planar electrode surface, the Van der Waals force F_{vw} is given by

$$F_{vw} = 2A_{vw}R_p \tag{4.14}$$

where A_{vw} is a constant of value $\sim 0.2\ \mathrm{Nm}^{-1}$. This implies that only particles having dimensions $\lesssim 0.5\mu m$ will be lifted from the surface of an electrode by the electrostatic force of equation 4.8 for the typical operational field of $E \sim 6 \times 10^7\ \mathrm{Vm}^{-1}$ considered in the previous example. The importance of surface adhesion forces on the microscopic scale is also highlighted by the recent detailed studies of Pollock [7,8] using a micropoint surface probe technique, where it was established that the mean adhesive pressure acting across the contact area can approach $\sim 10^8\ \mathrm{Nm}^{-2}$; i.e. comparable with the compressional yield stress of many common electrode materials. It should be noted however that these adhesive forces can be significantly reduced by the presence of surface contamination, as for example is commonly associated with poor vacuum conditions.

Apart therefore from thermally activated microparticles, such as may be released from anode "hot spots", or those that originate from "necked" microstructures, it can be concluded from this discussion of particle detachment that the majority of "primary" microparticles are likely to have sub-micron dimensions. In addition, the contamination of electrode surfaces by adsorbed gas under poor vacuum conditions will tend to lower surface adhesive forces, which suggests that the potential number of microparticles per unit electrode area is likely to be significantly higher with "commercial" vacuum gaps ($p \sim 10^{-6}$mbar) than with UHV regimes.

4.5 In-flight Phenomena

Having discussed the origin of naturally-occurring microparticles, it is now necessary to enquire whether their subsequent acceleration across the gap by the applied field is a "passive" or "active" event: i.e. whether or not the particle can act as an agent for the initiation of breakdown. In physical terms this therefore points to a consideration of possible in-flight mechanisms that would destroy the conservation of particle charge and mass, since all breakdown mechanisms are initiated by some form of charge exchange process (i.e. a discharge) with associated material vaporisation. It must also be appreciated that even if such processes do not actually initiate a discharge, they will still have an important influence on events through their control over the final impact velocity v_i acquired by a particle, and hence the nature of its interaction with the target electrode surface (see Section 4.7).

4.5.(i) Particle charge modification by electron emission

Here, the basic question to ask is whether the initial charge acquired by a particle at detachment Q_p will be conserved during its flight between the electrodes, or whether the local electric field on its surface can reach a sufficiently high value (i.e. $\gtrsim 3 \times 10^9$Vm^{-1}) for there to be in-flight charge exchange between the particle and electrode by field electron emission (FEE). The possibility that such a mechanism might indeed occur was first suggested from the findings of experiments by Udris [9], Rosanova [10] and Olendzkaya [11] where, by introducing artificial particles into the vacuum gap, it was demonstrated that in-flight microdischarges could occur between a particle and electrode. The mechanism was subsequently formalised as the "trigger discharge" and will be discussed in detail in the following section. However, it has to be stated at this stage that the experiments indicated that the mechanism only operates for relatively large particles (> 100μm diameter) and then only at very close distances of approach to an electrode. This observation was subsequently explained by the theoretical analysis of Martynov [12], which showed that it was only when the particle was one-diameter from the electrode that the microscopic field associated with a charged particle can approach the threshold of $\sim 3 \times 10^9 Vm^{-1}$ necessary for field electron emission to occur.

Consideration must also be given to the alternative analysis of Hurley and Parnell [13]whose presentation was contemporary with that cited above. Although the approach of these authors was less rigorous, in that they ignored the positional dependence of the particle in the gap, they introduced the important new concept that the microscopic field between a particle and electrode could be additionally enhanced by a factor β due to the presence of microasperities on the particle surface such as would result from the extrusion process illustrated in Fig. 4.2.

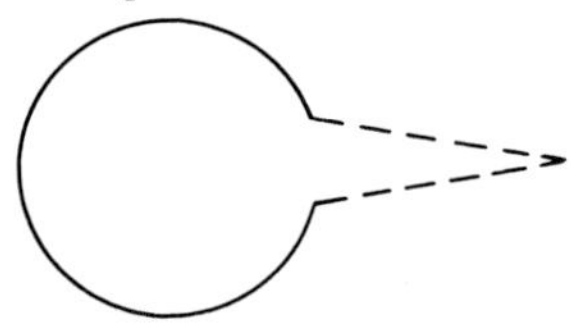

Fig. 4.3. An idealised spherical microparticle having a subsidiary conical protrusion that gives rise to a greatly enhanced electric field at its tip and the possibility of in-flight field emission [13].

According to this model, the microscopic field E_m acting at the tip of the approximately conical asperity attached to the spherical particle of radius R_p shown in Fig. 4.3 would be given by

$$E_m = \beta \; (3E - Q_p/4\pi\varepsilon_o R_p^2) \tag{4.15}$$

where E is the macroscopic gap field. This expression illustrates how E_m is the resultant of a component 3E arising from the enhancement of E by an uncharged conducting sphere and a second component $Q_p / 4\pi\varepsilon_o R_p^2$ arising from the actual charge carried by the particle: it should however be compared with equation 4.17 which gives the more exact expression for E_m at close distances of approach. Computations based on equation 4.15 above show that such surface features can have a dramatic influence on the mechanism and could therefore be an important consideration in practical situations where particles are likely to acquire a "necked" structure during their detachment such as in Fig. 4.2. Attention was also drawn by this analysis to the fact that a positively charged cathode-bound particle which does not field emit will acquire a higher single-transit impact velocity than a similar particle originating from the cathode that loses charge by in-flight FEE: indeed, computations showed that micron-sized anode-bound particles with field enhancing asperities could even have their velocity reversed by this mechanism. The polarity discrimination implied by these observations will be referred to again in Section 4.7 when considering the initiation of breakdown by the impact of naturally occurring high velocity microparticles.

However, in the absence of any direct experimental evidence confirming the predictions of this approximate theory it has to be concluded from the more exact calculations of Martynov [12] that in-flight FEE is unlikely to play a significant role with naturally occurring micron and sub-micron particles found in typical high voltage gaps. This therefore implies that the initial charge Q_p can be tentatively assumed to be conserved in the calculations of final impact velocities given in Section 4.7.

4.5.(ii) The "Trigger Discharge" breakdown mechanism

As indicated in the last section, this breakdown-initiating mechanism was originally proposed by Udris[9] and Olendzkaya [11] following their experiments with mm-sized ion spheres that had been artificially introduced into a test high voltage gap. The mechanism is based on the concept that as a charged particle approaches an electrode, the localised electric field associated with it can reach a sufficiently high value to cause field electron emission and hence the possibility of a "cathode" or "anode" initiated discharge (see Chapter 3) being struck between the particle and electrode; i.e. involving the vaporisation of either particle or electrode material. A particularly attractive feature of this mechanism is that it provides an explanation for the type of microparticle-based electrode damage and breakdown events described, for example, by Slivkov [2], where it is positively known that the terminal velocity of particles is too low ($< 200\ ms^{-1}$) to give rise to the impact-initiated breakdown mechanism discussed in Section 4.7. In fact, it was concluded by Olendzkaya [11] from her experiments with mm-sized spheres that with such a mechanism it is the gap field rather than the kinetic energy acquired by a particle that determines the breakdown condition.

The trigger-discharge hypothesis was first treated analytically by Martynov [12] for the idealised geometry of a charged sphere approaching a planar anode such as shown in Fig. 4.4(a): subsequently, Chatterton et al. [14], following a similar approach to that used earlier by Hurley and Parnell [13], extended the model to the geometry of Fig. 4.4(b) where a positively charged sphere is approaching a field-enhancing boss or asperity on an otherwise planar cathode; i.e. an attempt to more closely approximate the real microtopography of an electrode surface. In both analyses, the central aim was to determine the microscopic field E_g existing in the gap between the particle and electrode at close distances of approach. Thus, recalling from the previous section that E_g will be the resultant of a component E_1 arising from the enhancement of E by the particle and a component E_2 arising from the charge Q_p on the particle, Martynov [12]

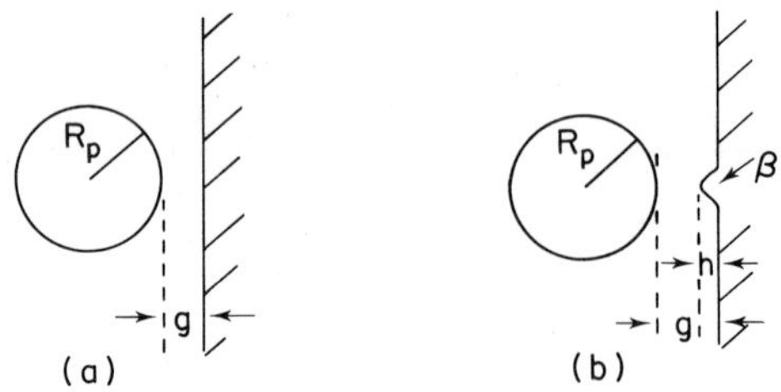

Fig. 4.4. The pre-impact particle-electrode regimes used by (a) Martynov [12] and (b) Chatterton et al [14] in their analyses of the trigger discharge mechanism.

obtained the following relation for the variation of E_g with gap separation g

$$E_g = E_1 + E_2$$

$$= Ef_1(g/R_p) + E_s f_2(g/R_p) \qquad (4.16)$$

Here, E is again the uniform macroscopic gap field and E_s is the field on the surface of the charged particle in the absence of E and the conducting electrode, viz. $E_s = Q_p/4\pi\varepsilon_o R_p{}^2$: f_1 and f_2 are geometric functions that determine how the proximity of a conducting electrode influences E_1 and E_2. At close distances of approach ($g \sim R_p$) they increase rapidly and, for $g/R_p < 0.3$, can can be approximated by $f_1 \simeq (\pi^2/6) f_2 \simeq 1.29(R_p/g)^{0.8}$ so that equation 4.16 becomes

$$E_g = 1.29(R_p/g)^{0.8}(E + 3Q_p/2\pi^3\varepsilon_o R_p^2) \qquad (4.17)$$

In this treatment by Martynov, no account was taken of the curvature of the particle and it was assumed that when $g \sim 0.3R$ a uniform field existed in the particle-electrode interspace. The corresponding expression for E_g in the regime of Fig. 4.4(b), where the boss is characterised by a field enhancement factor β and g<<R, is given by Chatterton et al [14] as

$$E_g = \beta/g \left[(R_p + g)E + Q_p/4\pi\varepsilon_o R_p \right] \qquad (4.18)$$

where Q_p was taken as the charge acquired by a spherical particle in contact with a plane electrode (Fig. 4.1), which from equation 4.6 is $Q_p = (2\pi^3/3)\varepsilon_o R_p{}^2 E = 6.58\pi\varepsilon_o R_p E$. Also, the field enhancement factor β will clearly vary with g for the geometry being considered and therefore has to be represented by the Miller expression [15] $\beta = \beta_\infty(1-h/g)$, where β_∞ is the value of β for g>>h.

From numerical evaluations of equations 4.17 and 4.18, it becomes evident that the implicit supposition of the trigger hypothesis, viz. that a discharge is struck between the particle and electrode, can only occur at close distances of approach when E_g exceeds a value of $\sim 3 \times 10^9 Vm^{-1}$ when significant field emission can occur. It also follows that the critical gap separation at which this occurs will increase with increasing particle radius through the dependence of E_g on both the ratio R_p/g and $Q_p(\propto R_p^2)$. In the case of the Martynov model [12], computations confirm the associated experimental observations [16, 17] that particles have to be $\gtrsim$ 100μm in diameter for the phenomena to occur: however, with the modification introduced by the theoretical model of Chatterton et al. [14], it would appear that the mechanism can operate with ∿20μm diameter particles if the microasperity is assumed to have a β-value of ∿ 5-10.

This more recent analysis of Chatterton et al. [14] contained two further important developments in the theory of this discharge model. Firstly, by taking account of the diminishing value of Q_p in equation 4.18 that follows the onset of field emission, it has been shown by computation for a given particle radius that there is a particular gap separation g at which the microscopic gap field E_g passes through a maximum: for example, in the case of 40 and 80 μm radius particles moving in a macroscopic field $E = 2 \times 10^7 Vm^{-1}$ and approaching a boss with a β-factor of 7, E_g reaches maximum values of ∿ 6.5 and $7.0 \times 10^9 Vm^{-1}$at g ∿ 1 and 2 μm respectively. Secondly, the "anode" versus "cathode" breakdown criteria discussed in Chapter 3 were applied to the micro-regime of Fig. 4.4(b) in an attempt to establish more precisely how the discharge is initiated. It was generally concluded from these computations that whereas "cathode" initiated breakdown, i.e. the vaporisation of the field emitting microasperity, was unlikely except for large particles of radius >500μm, the necessary condition for "anode" initiated breakdown, i.e. the vaporisation by electron bombardment of material (either gas or metal) from the surface of the incident particle, appears to be satisfied for particle diameters > 20μm. This analysis, in common with that of Martynov [12], highlights how sensitive this breakdown initiating mechanism is to the particle radius R_p: thus, for say aluminium particles in a 1 cm gap, the breakdown voltage is only ∿ 40kV for R_p = 80μm but increases to ∿ 200kV for R_p = 20μm. It should be added that this prediction provides one explanation of why arced electrodes, with their profusion of large microparticles formed from droplets of molten metal, have generally lower breakdown voltages.

Although the above analyses of the in-flight electron bombardment process indicate that the local temperature rise of small microparticles with radii $\lesssim$ 10μm is too low for the initiation of breakdown by the trigger discharge mechanism, it was nevertheless recognised by Beukema [18] that there is an alternative mechanism whereby even a sub-critical heating of a particle could create the necessary conditions for a subsequent breakdown event. This assumed that the local temperature of the electron-bombarded surface region of a positively-charged, cathode-bound microparticle could be raised sufficiently to cause melting and and the consequent welding of the particle to the electrode on impact. Under these circumstances, it follows that such a feature would give rise to a local enhancement of the surface field with the associated possibility of it becoming a new emission site that could subsequently initiate a breakdown if the microscopic field exceeded the critical value of $\sim 7 \times 10^9 Vm^{-1}$discussed in Section 3.3.(i). It was also pointed out that the creation of such a site would be even more likely if the impacting microparticle had a surface asperity that further enhanced the field. From a practical standpoint, such a mechanism would clearly play an important role in determining the voltage hold-off properties of real gaps, since it applies to particles having micron-size dimensions that are thought to be typical of those occurring naturally.

The validity of this concept was investigated by Beukema from both a theoretical and experimental point of view [18]. In the first place, he set up a theoretical model based on a sphere-plane impact regime and showed that the predicted local temperature rise for the range of gap fields and particle geometries appropriate to practical systems were sufficient to promote particle welding. On the experimental level he developed an ingeneous technique involving the use of various combinations of conditioned and unconditioned electrodes that provided convincing corroberative evidence for the existance of this microparticle process. Thus, it was demonstrated for example that the emitting properties of a fully conditioned cathode, as measured by its β-factor defined in Section 3.1.(i), could change dramatically when it was used in conjunction with an unconditional anode; typically, the application of a relatively low gap field could result in an increase of β from say ~ 40 to 100. From other supportive evidence, such as obtained from SEM studies of electrode surfaces and the observation that there is frequently a correlation between the occurrence of current pulses and the changes in β, it was also possible to infer that material in the form of microparticles is transferred from an unconditioned to a conditioned electrode on the first application of a gap field; a conclusion that was subsequently to be confirmed by the direct experimental techniques described later in Section 7.2(ii).

4.5.*(iii) The "Particle Vaporisation" breakdown mechanism*

From a theoretical consideration of the anode processes resulting from localised electron bombardment [19] and the subsequent experimental observation described in Section 7.2(ii) that neutral electrode vapour originating from the anode is liberated in a gap a few microseconds before its breakdown [20], Davies and Biondi developed their "heated-anode-particle" model [20,21] illustrated schematically in Fig. 4.5. In this a field emitting microprotrusion on the cathode, characterised by an enhancement factor β and emitting radius r, gives rise to an anode hot spot as described

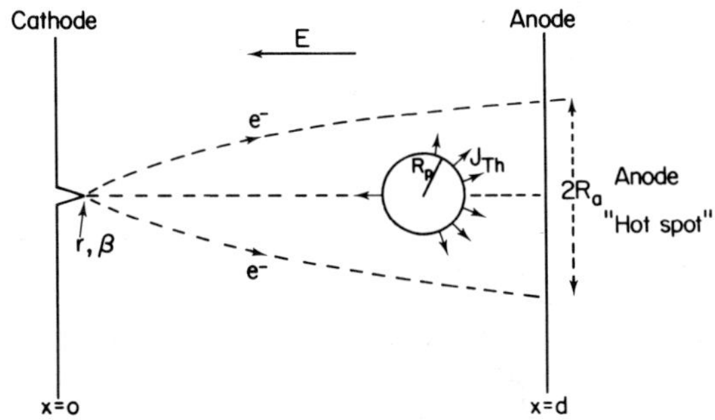

Fig. 4.5 A schematic illustration of the "heated-anode-particle" breakdown initiating model; the idealised spherical microparticle is created at the anode hot-spot formed by the electron emission from a cathode microprotrusion having a geometrical field enhancement factor β.
(From Davies and Biondi [21,22], with permission).

in Chapter 3; it is then assumed that thermal instability occurs first at the anode, such that a semi-molten droplet is extruded from its surface by the applied field and in passing through the "necked" structure shown in Figs. 4.1 and 4.2 will acquire a high initial positive charge Q_p that will cause it to be accelerated towards the cathode. Since however this microparticle will be moving in the path of the on-coming electron beam it will simultaneously experience a progressive charge neutralisation (which will have the effect of prolonging its transit time) and a rapid increase in temperature as a result of electron bombardment heating. In the limit, this latter process could lead to the mid-gap vaporisation of the particle with an associated increase in the local vapour density that is sufficiently high for the onset of regenerative electron-atom ionisation processes and the consequent breakdown of the gap. It follows therefore that the mechanism is really a development of the "anode" initiated breakdown process described in Section 3.3(ii), where the microparticle is behaving as an anode.

A complete theoretical analysis of this model [22] involves the solution of the following set of six inter-related time-dependent differential equations. The first accounts for the thermal energy exchange processes at the particle, in which the heat gained by electron bombardment is equated with that lost by surface evaporation, radiation and the well known thermionic emission cooling U_{Th} [23],

$$\frac{dT}{dt} = \frac{1}{M_p C}\left[F_1F_2V_p i_F - 4\pi R_p^2 G\left(L - \frac{6kT}{\rho R_p}\right) - 4\pi R_p^2 \sigma_s T^4 - U_{Th}\right] \qquad (4.19)$$

where T is the temperature of the particle; t is its flight time after leaving the anode; F_1 and F_2 are respectively the fraction of the total cathode field emission current i_F intercepted by the particle and the fraction of the incident bombardment energy retained by the particle after back-scattered and secondary emission losses (largely determined by the electron range in the particle as given by the Widdington Law [24]; G is the rate of loss of mass per unit area; V_p is the potential of the particle relative to the cathode; k and σ_s are the Boltzmann and Stephan constants; C, L and ρ are respectively the specific heat, latent heat of vaporisation and density of the particle material, and $M_p(=4\pi\rho R_p{}^3/3)$ is the particle mass: it follows therefore from the definition of G that

$$\frac{dR_p}{dt} = -\frac{G}{\rho} \tag{4.20}$$

Next, if i_{Th} is the current emitted thermionically from the particle determined by the Richardson-Schottky relation [25], and if i_c is defined as the fraction of the intercepted field emission current that is actually collected after secondary electron emission, the net rate of accumulation of negative charge will be given by

$$\frac{dQ_-}{dt} - \frac{dQ_+}{dt} = i_c - i_{Th} \tag{4.21}$$

Finally, the velocity and acceleration of the particle will be respectively

$$\frac{dx}{dt} = v_p \tag{4.22}$$

and

$$\frac{dv_p}{dt} = E.\frac{Q_p(t)}{M_p} \tag{4.23}$$

where $Q_p(t) = Q_p - Q_-(t) + Q_+(t)$, being the particle charge at any given instant after detachment.

After making appropriate substitutions for V_p, F_1, F_2, i_F, i_c, i_{Th} and U_{Th} in equations 4.19 to 4.23, they have been solved numerically for the contrasting cases of a non-refractory copper particle of radius 0.5μm and a similar sized refractory molybdenum particle [22]. The findings are illustrated in Fig. 4.6 where it has been assumed that at t = 0, $T = T_o = T$, the boiling point of the particle material. These computations were also specially chosen to fit some previous experimental breakdown measurements [19, 26] where, for Cu, the microscopic breakdown field was calculated from a measured β value of 130 to be E_b = 7 x $10^9 Vm^{-1}$, whilst for Mo, where β = 100, E_b = 6.8 x $10^9 Vm^{-1}$. When interpreting the data presented in this figure it should be noted that we are dealing with a cathode-bound particle where

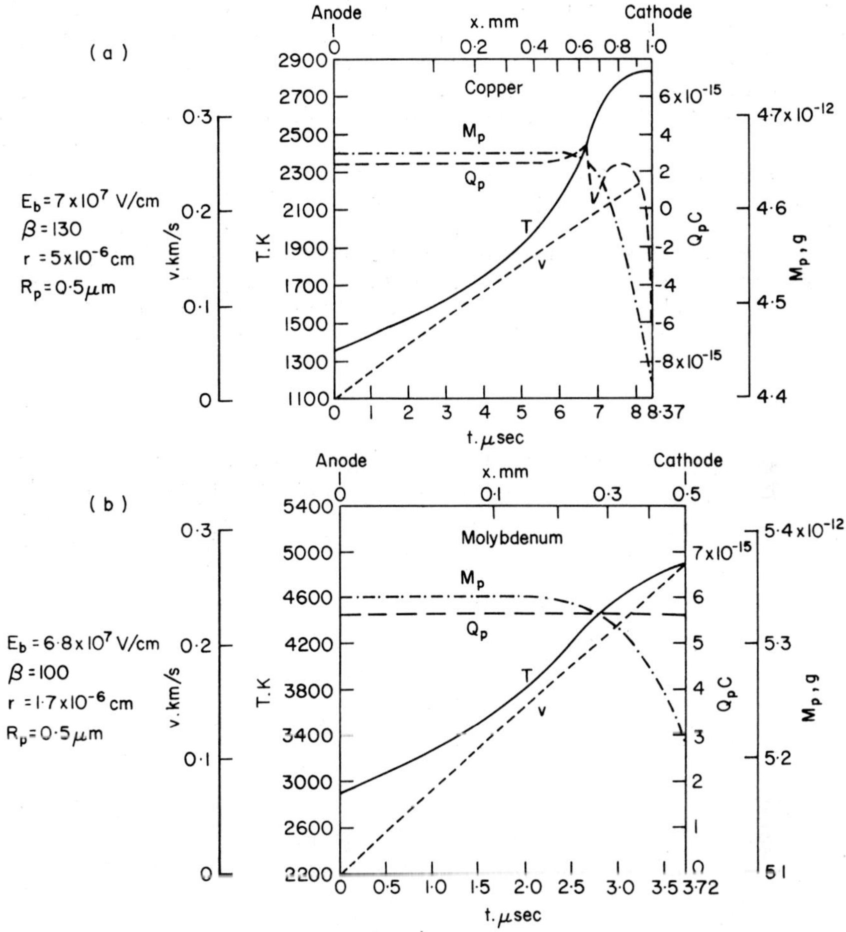

Fig. 4.6 Collated data showing how the mass M_p, charge Q_p, velocity v and temperature T of the microparticle involved in the "heated-anode particle" model vary as it crosses the gap from anode to cathode: (a) corresponds to the case of a copper particle, and (b) to a molybdenum particle [22]. (From Davies and Biondi [22], with permission).

the conventional positions of the cathode and anode shown in Fig. 4.5 have been transposed in order to have a left-to-right reading. Thus, for both materials, these plots clearly show that after a few microseconds, as the particle approaches the cathode, M_p begins to fall off steeply as $T \rightarrow T_{max}$, indicating a rapid vaporisation process and a consequent pressure rise in the gap that would create the necessary condition for an arc to be initiated. The more rapid increase of T with the Mo particle can be attributed to its lower thermal capacity.

From an extensive analysis of this model covering a wide range of values of the variable parameters, it has been concluded that breakdown can be initiated by this mechanism for particle sizes of $R_p \lesssim 3\mu m$. With larger particles i_o always exceeds i_{Th} so that they become negatively charged and return to the anode before their temperature reaches a high enough value for significant vaporisation to occur.

4.6. Single-Transit Impact Phenomena

The physical nature of the interaction between a microparticle and an electrode surface is principally determined by the impact or terminal velocity v_i of the particle which, from equation 4.1, is given by $v_i = \sqrt{2Q_pV/M_p}$ where Q_p and M_p are respectively its initial charge (assumed conserved) and mass of the particle, with V being the gap voltage. To gain some insight into the range of impact velocities likely to be encountered in practice, the above equation may be evaluated for the idealised particle geometries analysed in Section 4.4. Thus, considering for example the case of a semi-ellipsoidal microstructure, the particle charge will be given by equation 4.7, its mass by $M_p = 2\pi h^3\rho/3\lambda^2$ (ρ being the density of the particle material), so that

$$v_i = \left(\frac{3\varepsilon_o\beta(\lambda)}{h\rho d}\right)^{\frac{1}{2}}.V = \left(\frac{3\varepsilon_o\beta(\lambda)}{r\lambda^2\rho d}\right)^{\frac{1}{2}}.V \qquad (4.24)$$

since the radius of curvature of the tip $r = b/\lambda$ or $h = r\lambda^2$. The practical implication of this equation can be illustrated [3] by considering the three typical high voltage gap regimes of d = 1, 10 and 100 mm with V = 20, 100 and 1000 kV respectively, where in all cases the electrode material is titanium ($\rho = 4.5 \times 10^3 kg.m^{-1}$) and the vulnerable surface microstructure is characterised by $\beta(\lambda) = 6$ and $r = 0.1\mu m$. We find that v_i increases from 180 ms^{-1} for the 30 kV low voltage gap ($E = 2 \times 10^7 Vm^{-1}$) through 280 ms^{-1} for the intermediate voltage 100 kV gap ($E = 10^7\ Vm^{-1}$) to $v_i = 900\ ms^{-1}$ with the 1 MV high voltage gap ($E = 10^7\ Vm^{-1}$). A similar range of impact velocities are obtained from estimates based on a spherical microparticle geometry [27]. It must however be pointed out that this type of estimate is very sensitive to the β and r values chosen for the initial microfeature: sharper structures will be more highly charged and hence acquire very much higher impact velocities. This therefore implies that there is likely to be a large variety in the types of particle/electrode interaction in most practical situations.

4.6(i) Low Impact Velocities ($v_i \lesssim v_c$)

These are defined as the range for which permanent plastic deformation of either projectile or target is absent, so that there will be a semi-elastic non-destructive bouncing impact. The limiting value of v_i for this type of event, defined as the critical impact velocity v_c, will depend on the material constants of the colliding surfaces; for the case of similar materials, which is likely to be appropriate to most high voltage gap situations, its value has been given by Cook [28] from a hydrodynamically-based theory as

$$v_c \simeq \left(\frac{8\sigma_y}{\rho}\right)^{\frac{1}{2}} \qquad (4.25)$$

where σ_y is the yield strength of the colliding materials and ρ their density. Introducing appropriate material constants into this equation [29] predicts values of v_c ranging from $\sim$ 200 ms^{-1} for a "soft" material such as copper ($\sigma_y = 5.5 \times 10^7 Nm^{-2}$) through $\sim$ 500 ms^{-1} for stainless steel ($\sigma_y = 2.8 \times 10^8 Nm^{-2}$) to as high as $\sim$ 1 kms^{-1} for titanium ($\sigma_y = 8 \times 10^8 Nm^{-2}$), a material commonly used for high voltage electrodes. Whilst these predictions appear to be in reasonably good general agreement with the findings of the controlled microparticle impact studies described in Chapter 6, it should be pointed out that they differ by over three orders of magnitude both from the values of v_c predicted by classical elastic impact theory [30] and those found from the corresponding macroscopic sphere-plane impact experiments [31] where typically $v_c \sim 0.05 - 0.1$ ms^{-1}. This discrepancy, which is discussed in greater detail in Chapter 6, can however be explained on the basis that impact events on the microscopic scale have to be thought of as single crystal collisions, whereas on the macroscopic scale collisions will be between poly-crystalline systems whose elastic modulii have been found by Gane [32] to be significantly lower.

It has also been pointed out by Menon and Srivastava [29] that for any given operating gap where V is constant, particles will have to be smaller than some critical dimensions if their impact velocities are to exceed v_c. Thus, for the ideal case of a spherical particle resting on a plane electrode, we have from equation 4.6, $Q_p = 6.6\pi\varepsilon_o ER_p^2$ which, when substituted into equation 4.1, gives $R_p \simeq (10\varepsilon_o/v_i^2\rho d)V^2$. This therefore implies that there will be a critical particle radius $(R_p)_c \propto V^2/d$ below which $v_i > v_c$. For a 1 cm gap supporting 200 kV one finds $(R_p)_c$ varies from 0.7 μm for copper electrodes through 0.14 μm for stainless steel to 0.05 μm for titanium.

In the absence therefore of any direct impact damage, and excluding the possibility of the conventional trigger discharge mechanism described in Section 4.6(ii) operating for the anticipated particle dimensions of < 5 μm, there remains only one other mechanism by which a low-velocity microparticle ($v_i < v_c$) could directly initiate a breakdown. This is by the "hot-welding" model of Beukema [18] , also described in Section 4.6(ii), in which a positively charged particle is heated in-flight by electron bombardment and, as a result, sticks to the cathode to form a potentially unstable field emitting site. Apart from this, there is however another indirect mechanism to be discussed in Section 4.8, whereby a particle undergoing a semi-elastic bouncing impact could initiate a breakdown following a subsequent transit of the gap.

4.6(ii) Intermediate Impact Velocities ($v_c \lesssim v_i \lesssim 5v_i$)

In this velocity range, it is assumed that most of the incident kinetic energy of the particle will be dissipated irreversibly in the permanent mechanical deformation of the colliding surfaces. This type of particle impact event will therefore be highly inelastic, giving rise either to identation microcraters in the surface of the target electrode, or a protruding microfeature if a particle becomes impacted or welded to the surface. A direct experimental demonstration of these processes may be obtained from the controlled laboratory studies of microparticle impact phenomena described in Chapter 6. In both cases, if such a particle impacts on the cathode electrode, there is the possibility of creating an "instantaneous" electron emission site, as would be evidenced by an abrupt change in the I-V characteristic of the gap [18]. It follows that if this were to occur it would bring with it the subsequent risk of breakdown being initiated by any of the mechanisms discussed in Chapter 3. In the case of target indentation, such emission sites will tend to be located around the rim of the microcrater where the electrode surface is most distorted; for the embedded microparticle situation, any electron emission will occur at the sharpest point of the newly formed protruding microfeature.

Whilst corresponding impact events on the anode electrode will cause similar surface damage, they cannot of course give rise to electron emission processes: accordingly anode-bound microparticles must be regarded as less dangerous from a breakdown point of view. This discrimination is also reinforced by the in-flight field emission considerations of Section 4.6(i), where it was pointed out that anode-bound particles are more susceptable to charge loss and will hence have lower impact velocities for a given gap voltage. For these reasons, it could be anticipated that with gaps having non-uniform geometries, there would be a polarity effect in their voltage hold-off capability, with the more stable regime being that where the higher surface field is arranged to act on the cathode, since this would favour the detachment of anode-bound particles (see Section 4.5). It must also be pointed out however, that as with low-velocity impacts, there remains the possibility of particles undergoing inelastic "reflections" and multiple transits of the gap (see Section 4.7), thus masking the polarity effect just outlined.

4.6(iii) High Impact Velocities ($v \gtrsim 5v_c$)

At these high velocities, corresponding to the conditions covered by the Cranberg hypothesis, an ever increasing fraction of the incident kinetic energy of the particle will be dissipated irreversibly in thermal processes, particularly the vaporisation of particle or electrode material. In this connection, Cook [28] has shown that the extreme situation of complete vaporisation of the particle will occur when

$$v_i \gtrsim 4(L_v)^{\frac{1}{2}} \tag{4.26}$$

where L_V is the latent heat of vaporisation of the colliding materials. For titanium, as an example, where $L_V \simeq 7MJ.kg^{-1}$, this would correspond to an impact velocity of $\sim$ 10 kms^{-1}. It must be emphasized however, that experimental evidence from simulation studies (see Chapter 6) strongly suggests that the necessary local rise in vapour pressure for initiating breakdown can occur for particle impact velocities significantly lower than 10 kms^{-1}. For refractory metals such as molybdenum the critical velocity is probably $\sim$ 5 kms^{-1}, but could be as low as 1.5 kms^{-1} for non refractory metals such as copper. Sub-critical impact events are assumed to be observed as microdischarges as opposed to complete breakdown. Direct confirmation of this vaporisation of particle or electrode material has been provided by mass spectrometry analyses of the species of metallic ions (both charged and neutral) that are present in the gas burst that accompanies a simulated high-velocity microparticle impact (see Chapter 6).

On this picture, the localised cloud of metal vapour resulting from a high velocity impact event will be rapidly ionised by a combination of thermal and field-based mechanisms so that a microplasma is formed in the vicinity of the impact zone. At this stage regenerative processes come into play that allow the microplasma to expand under the applied field to fill the gap and so initiate breakdown by the formation of an arc between the electrodes. In fact, the latter stages of this mechanism closely resemble the sequence of events operating in the electron emission induced breakdown mechanism discussed in Chapters 3 and 5. As with "intermediate velocity" impact events, it is important to note that cathode-bound particles will again have a greater probability of initiating breakdown by this mechanism since the the regenerative ionisation processes that sustain the growth of the microplasma are likely to be considerably enhanced by electron emission from cathode sites created by the impact. An impressive experimental demonstration of this selectivity was obtained by Slattery et al. using artificially generated charged microspheres [33]. This and other simulation studies of the impact ionisation and electrode microcratering processes will be fully described in Chapter 6.

Before concluding this discussion, the reader should be reminded that the critical condition of this type of microparticle initiated breakdown is determined by the voltage across the gap rather than the field, i.e. as required by the Cranberg hypothesis of equation 4.2. Experimental details of this type of behaviour are given in Section 2.5(iii).

4.7. Multi-Transit Impact Phenomena

4.7(i) Particle bouncing

The phenomenon of particle bouncing between the high voltage electrodes of a vacuum gap was first demonstrated experimentally by Olendzkaya [11] using mm-sized steel spheres that had been artificially introduced into the gap. She showed that below the breakdown voltage of such a gap these particles would oscillate between the electrodes and give rise to a measurable current in the external circuit, although no details were given of how its magnitude was related to the particle charge, velocity, or its oscillation frequency. However, the potential importance of the contribution from such a charge transfer mechanism to the total prebreakdown current was subsequently considered by Boulloud [6] and shown to be far too small to account for the magnitude of typical prebreakdown currents. The experiments of Olendzkaya [11] also showed that whilst the breakdown of the gap is prematurely initiated by the presence of these particles, it was by a trigger discharge mechanism rather than by a "total voltage" effect as would be required by the Cranberg impact hypothesis.

4.7(ii) Particle kinetic energy enhancement

The concept that particle bouncing could also provide the basis of a mechanism for enhancing the kinetic energy of a microparticle once released in a vacuum gap was first formulated by Latham [34] as a model for explaining how a Cranberg type of impact- initiated breakdown mechanism could operate in low voltage ($\lesssim$ 15 kV) gaps where single transit impact velocities are well below the threshold for generating adequate impact ionisation (see Section 4.6). An important feature of such a mechanism is that it would be particularly relevant for micron and submicron sized particles where breakdown could not be prematurely initiated by the trigger discharge mechanism of Section 4.5(ii): in fact, this observation is strongly supported by microcratering evidence discussed in Chapter 7.

The two basic requirements of this energy enhancing model are that during a bouncing impact there is an efficient reversal of both the particle momentum and particle charge. This ensures firstly, that a particle is launched into a second transit of the gap with a high initial velocity and secondly, that such a "reflected" particle will be re-accelerated by the applied field. Thus, referring to Fig. 4.7, which illustrates the principle of the model, it will be seen that a particle of initial charge Q_{p_1} and mass M_p acquires an initial single-transit impact velocity $v_1 = (2Q_{p1}V/M_p)^{\frac{1}{2}}$, a rebound velocity of ev_1 (where e is the coefficient of restitution between the particle and electrode) and, assuming conservation of particle mass, a second-transit impact velocity of $v_2 = [(ev_1)^2 + 2VQ_{p2}/M_p]^{\frac{1}{2}}$ where Q_{p2} is the magnitude of the"reversed" charge acquired by the particle during its con-

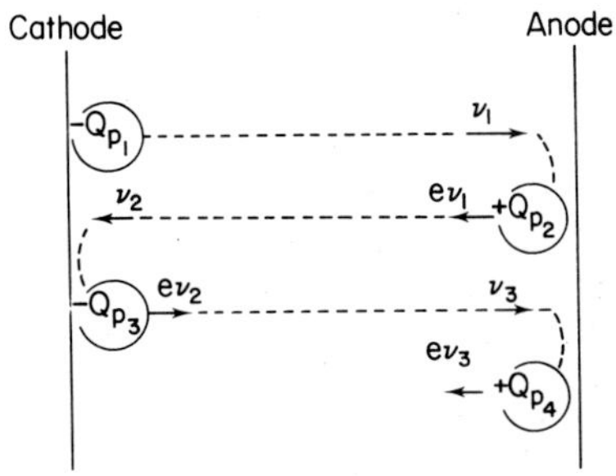

Fig. 4.7. An illustration of the progressive kinetic energy enhancement model of Latham [34], in which a microparticle undergoes successive bouncing impacts with associated momentum and charge reversal.

tact with the oppositely charged electrode. For energy enhancement at this second impact we evidently require $|v_2|>|v_1|$ which reduces to the condition

$$e^2 + \left|\frac{Q_{p2}}{Q_{p1}}\right| > 1 \tag{4.27}$$

It follows that if v_2 is still less than the critical impact velocity v_c, defined by equation 4.25, there can be further bouncing impacts until the particle velocity builds up to a value in excess of v_c, when one of the previously discussed breakdown mechanisms can be initiated.

The criterion defined by equation 4.27, which is a general relation applying to any of the subsequent bouncing events illustrated in Fig. 4.7, highlights how this energy-enhancing mechanism depends firstly on the mechanical properties of the electrodes through e, and secondly, on the electrical properties of their surfaces through the ratio Q_{p2}/Q_{p1} which is a useful measure of their control over the charge reversal process. An attractive feature therefore of this model is that it provides a physical explanation of why certain materials provide more stable electrode pairs than others. For example, the well established technological practice of using stainless steel rather than say copper electrodes, could be anticipated on the basis of the present model since these materials are characterised by having surface oxide films that are respectively insulating and semiconducting [34]; i.e. the contact charge exchange process and hence the energy enhancing mechanism would tend to be more inhibited with stainless steel than copper. In a later chapter (6), laboratory simulation experiments with artificially generated charged microspheres will be described that provide an impressive confirmation not only of the energy enhancing mechanism itself, but also of the importance of the atomic state of an electrode surface in controlling the charge exchange process.

4.7(iii) Theoretical basis of charge exchange

To gain further insight into the fundamental physical processes that occur during a semi elastic particle impact event, we shall now analyse the mechanical and electrical impact response of the idealised sphere-plane geometry shown in Fig. 4.8(a): in fact, as will be seen from Fig. 6.16, this is a good approximation of the microregime associated with the simulation studies of this phenomenon (see Section 6.6). As a further simplification of the model, it will also be assumed that the particle and electrode are the same material and hence covered by identical semiconducting or insulating surface oxide films of thickness s, which is typically 30-50Å (i.e. $s \ll R_p$).

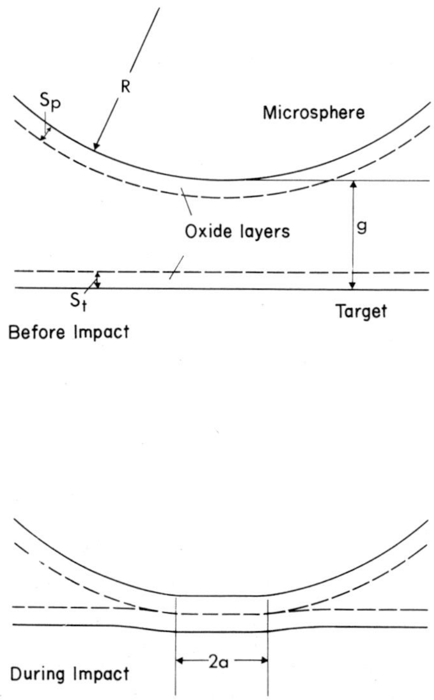

Fig. 4.8. The idealised model used for analysing the mechanical and electrical interaction between a metallic microsphere and a planar target having respectively surface oxide layers of thickness s_p and s_T: (a) before impact ($t < 0$), (b) during contact ($t \sim t_c/2$). (From Latham and Brah [37], with permission).

Mechanical considerations: At the instant of maximum depression during a semi-elastic impact, i.e. when the particle is momentarily at rest, the contact surfaces will be reversibly deformed as shown schematically in Fig. 4.8(b), where $\Delta z \ll R_p$. This regime is described by the well established equations of classical impact theory, as originally derived for macro systems by Hertz (see Andrews [35]). Thus, if Y is Young's modulus of the impacting material and $\bar{F}$ is the mean force transmitted to the target during its elastic deceleration, the radius of the circle of contact will be

$$a \simeq (FR_p/Y)^{1/3} \tag{4.28}$$

Now for an initial impact velocity v_i and total contact time t_c, the mean force F acting during a uniform deceleration period $(t_c/2)$ will be approximated by

$$\bar{F} \simeq M_p v_i/(t_c/2) \tag{4.29}$$

where $v_i = (2Q_p V/M_p)^{\frac{1}{2}}$ and, from the analysis of Hertz

$$t_c \simeq 4.5(5M_p/\pi Y R_p^{\frac{1}{2}})^{0.4} v_i^{-0.2} \tag{4.30}$$

From discussions in Chapter 6 and by Latham et al. [36] elsewhere it emerges that when these equations are applied to microsystems where impact events are likely to be between single grains, it is more appropriate to use "single crystal" values for the elastic constants which can exceed the corresponding "bulk" (i.e. macroscopic) values by factors $\sim$ 25. Hence for the example of a 1μm copper microsphere impacting on a copper electrode with a velocity of 50 ms^{-1}, one finds $t_c \sim 10^{-9}$s and $a \sim 3 \times 10^{-8}$m. It should however be added that the recent micro-contact experiments of Pollock et al. [7] indicate that the above estimate of a is probably too low, since no account was taken of possible plastic deformation arising from the additional compression of the surfaces caused by contact adhesive forces: for similar reasons, the estimate of t_c is also likely to be too low.

Electrical considerations: For the ideal case of Fig. 4.8, where both the spherical particle and planar electrodes are atomically clean, charge exchange during contact would only be limited by the relaxation time τ of the metal which is typically $\sim 10^{-14}$s. Since therefore, $\tau \ll t_c$, it follows that $Q_{p1} = Q_{p2} = Q_{p3}$ etc. in Fig. 4.7 and will be equal to the equilibrium charge Q_o acquired by a spherical particle resting on a planar electrode; i.e. $Q_o = 2\pi^3 R_p^2 \varepsilon_o E/3 = 6.6\ R_p^2 \varepsilon_o E$ as given by equation 4.6. However, referring to Fig. 4.8(b), it will be seen that, in practice, transitory electrical contact is established between the particle and electrode via an oxide junction whose surface area will vary continuously between zero and a maximum of πa^2 during the compression and recovery stages of the impact. To a first order of approximation therefore the mean area of the junction during the time of contact t_c can be taken as $\pi a^2/2$ and, if the oxide films are assumed to be incompressible, the junction thickness can be taken as 2s. For a regime such as this, charge may be exchanged between the particle and electrode by either direct ohmic conduction through the composite film or quantum mechanical electron tunnelling across the junction. However, from a detailed consideration of the electrical properties of surface oxide films and the relative efficiencies of these alternative mechanisms, it was shown by Latham and Brah [37] that the process is dominated by the tunnelling mechanism: it follows therefore that we are dealing with a metal-oxide-metal (MOM) tunnel junction situation whose d-c properties have been thoroughly analysed for example by Simmons [38-40].

The electrical behaviour of this type of tunnel junction is conventionally described in terms of its d-c tunnel resistivity $\rho_t(\Omega m^2)$ defined as

$$\rho_t = V_p/j_t \tag{4.31}$$

where V_p is the potential of the particle relative to the planar electrode, i.e. the bias voltage existing across the junction, and j_t is the tunnel current density: it follows therefore that the instantaneous current flowing across this junction will be

$$i_t = \pi a^2 j_t = \pi a^2 V_p/\rho_t \tag{4.32}$$

Although ρ_t is a complicated function of the thickness and electrical properties of the oxide [38-40], it may be approximated for the present purposes by the exponential dependence [37]

$$\rho_t = \rho_{ot} \exp.(-KV_p) \tag{4.33}$$

where K is a constant ($\sim 2\Omega m^2 V^{-1}$) that can be taken as independent of the oxide material, and ρ_{ot} is another constant that depends on the thickness, band-gap and dielectric properties of the oxide film [38-40]. In applying this steady-state model to estimate the total charge Q_T transferred by the transient tunnelling current flowing during a bouncing impact, it is necessary to integrate equation 4.32 over the interval t = 0 to t = t_c, i.e.

$$Q_T = \int_o^{t_c} i_t dt = \pi \int_o^{t_c} (aV_p(t)/\rho_t) dt \tag{4.34}$$

$$\equiv |Q_{p1}| + |Q_{p2}|$$

at the first bouncing impact of Fig. 4.7. If now $V_p(t)$ is assumed to decay according to an exponential relaxation law, we shall have

$$V_p(t) = V_{op} \exp(-t/\tau_t) \tag{4.35}$$

where V_{op} is the initial potential of the particle at the instant of contact and τ_t is the time constant associated with the tunnelling charge exchange process: the value of τ_t can be assumed to be $\lesssim t_c$ since it has been shown from controlled laboratory studies of this phenomenon (Chapter 6) that the charge reversal process approaches completion during such a bouncing impact. Hence, assuming a mean contact area $\pi a^2/2$ and substituting for ρ_t and $V_p(t)$ in equation 4.34 from equation 4.33 and 4.35, and integrating we find

$$Q_T \simeq [\pi a^2 \tau_t \exp (KV_{op})]/2\rho_{ot}K \tag{4.36}$$

Finally, the field calculations described earlier in section 4.6 (ii) in connection with the impact trigger discharge mechanism may be used to evaluate V_{op}. Thus, from equation 4.17, which gives the axial field E_g in a vacuum gap between a particle and electrode, we have for the present oxide gap of dielectric constant ε.

$$V_{op} = 2s.E_g = 2.58s(R_p/g)^{0.8}(E + 3Q_p/2\pi^3\varepsilon_o\varepsilon R_p^2) \tag{4.37}$$

From an inspection of these last two equations, it will be apparent that the efficiency of this charge reversal process, as measured by Q_T, will be determined by the properties of the oxide film through the inverse dependence of Q_T on ρ_{ot} and ε. Thus an insulating film (large band gap and hence a large ρ_{ot}) having a high dielectric constant ε can be anticipated to promote the process much less efficiently than say a low bandgap semiconducting film. It follows therefore that the likelihood of breakdown being initiated as a result of successive energy-enhancing transits of a gap will be much higher for electrode pairs having semiconducting oxide films (eg. copper) than for those having insulating films (eg. stainless steel).

As a specific example of the application of this theory, consider a 1μm diameter microsphere moving in a 1 mm electrode gap across which there is a potential of 10 kV (or $E = 10^7 Vm^{-1}$) and assume that its initial detachment charge $Q_{p1} \equiv Q_o = 2.5 \times 10^{-16}C$ as calculated from equation 4.6. If the thickness s of the oxide films on the particle and the electrode surfaces are taken as 30Å, their dielectric constant as 3, their band gap as $\sim$ 1 eV (i.e. semiconducting), and the tunnelling resistivity ρ_{ot} is approximated from the published data of Simmons [38-40] as $\sim 5 \times 10^{-2}\Omega.m^2$, computations using equation 4.37 then show [37] that $V_{op} \sim 7V$. Substituting finally these values into equation 4.36 with $\tau_t \simeq t_c \simeq 3 \times 10^{-9}s$ (from equation 4.30) we find $Q_T \simeq 3.5 \times 10^{-16}C$. If this value is now compared with that associated with an "ideal" impact between atomically clean surfaces where $Q_T \simeq 2Q_o = 5 \times 10^{-16}C$ it follows that the charge reversal process will be $\sim$ 70% completed during a "real" impact with such an oxidised surface: under these circumstances, it can also be inferred from equation 4.27 that there will be a high probability of the kinetic energy of the particle being enhanced during its "return" transit of the gap. As will be described in Chapter 6, these predictions are in good agreement with the direct findings of laboratory simulation studies [37] with charged microspheres impacting on copper electrodes whose ambient oxide is known to be semiconducting: on the other hand, comparable studies with stainless steel electrodes whose ambient oxide film is insulating, have confirmed that both the charge exchange process and energy enhancement mechanism are significantly inhibited. This type of evidence is therefore taken as lending strong support to this tunnelling explanation of how charge is exchanged during the bouncing impact of a microparticle and how the electrode surface properties play a vital role in controlling the process.

4.8. Microparticle Behaviour with Impulse Voltages

Before concluding this review of microparticle initiated breakdown mechanisms, it is necessary to consider what additional factors have to be taken into account when, instead of d-c voltages, fast and linearly rising impulse over-voltages, such as illustrated in Fig. 4.9, are applied across large gaps ($\gtrsim$ 2mm) where microparticles are thought to play a dominant role.

4.8(i) Impact-initiated Breakdown

Following the analysis of Farrall [41], a particle is assumed to become detached from an electrode at some time t_d on the rising edge of the pulse, where t_d is small compared with the rise time t_r of the pulse: the voltage V_d corresponding to $t = t_d$ is also identified with the Cranberg d-c breakdown voltage given by equation 4.2. Because of the finite transit time t_t of the particle, the impulse breakdown event will be delayed by this time interval and be experimentally observed at a time t_b, where $t_b = t_d + t_t$. This reasoning therefore explains how the impulse breakdown voltage V_b' of a given gap can be higher than its corresponding d-c value. It also follows from this model that if the duration of the pulse is less than the transit time of the particle, breakdown cannot occur by this mechanism since the impact event will occur under zero-field conditions where any resulting microplasma will expand "passively" without any possibility of an arc being struck between the electrodes.

Since the Cranberg relation has been shown to provide a useful guide for predicting the breakdown behaviour of d-c gaps, it is important to enquire how its form has to be modified when using impulsed over-voltages. Accordingly, Farrall [41] has analysed the cases of pulses having either a *constant rise rate* dV/dt or *constant rise time* t_r, where it is assumed that breakdown is initiated by single transit impacts. Under these circumstances therefore, Fig. 4.9 indicates that the impulse breakdown voltage

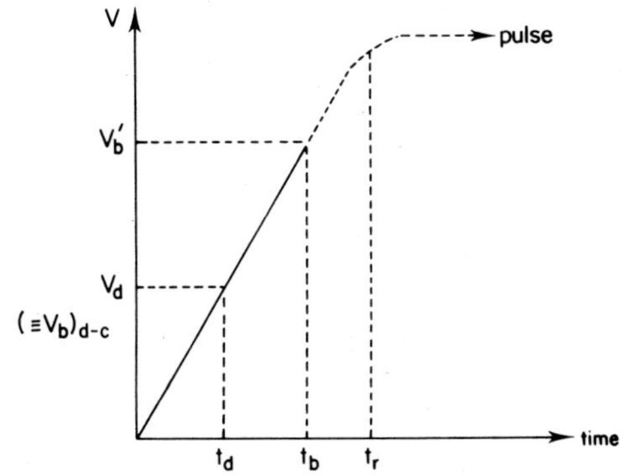

Fig. 4.9. Impulse voltage waveform, showing the typical relation between the d-c and impulse breakdown voltages, V_b and V_b' respectively, for a given gap regime.

V_b' will be given by

$$V_b' = V_d + t_t \frac{dV}{dt} \tag{4.39}$$

In this equation, dV/dt is a known experimental variable and the transit time t_t is determined from the equation of motion of the particle across the gap, viz.

$$M_p \frac{d^2x}{dt^2} = \frac{Q_p}{d}\left(V_c + t\frac{dV}{dt}\right) \tag{4.40}$$

where for a spherical particle initially in contact with a planar electrode $Q_p = \frac{2}{3}\pi^3 R_p^2 \varepsilon_o E$ (see equation 4.6) and $M_p = \frac{4}{3}\pi\rho R_p^3$. To obtain the theoretical dependence of V_b on d and other experimental parameters, these last two equations may now be independently solved for the two impulse regimes referred to above. For "typical" experimental conditions, such an analysis[41] shows that to a good approximation, *constant rise rate* pulses result in

$$V_b' \propto R_p^{1/3} d^{5/6} \tag{4.41}$$

and for *constant rise time* pulses

$$V_b' \propto R_p d^{5/2} \tag{4.42}$$

It will be seen that the gap dependence in both of these expressions differs significantly from Cranberg's d-c relation $V_b \propto d^{\frac{1}{2}}$; they also indicate a size-dependence which was not accounted for in the original Cranberg hypothesis. Since the examples of complementary experimental impulse data are very limited, it is difficult to give a reliable appraisal of the validity of this theory. However, from a review of impulse breakdown data covering a range of ill-defined operating conditions, Farrall [41] concluded that the gap-dependence of V_b' does in fact show a variation from $d^{0.4}$ to $d^{1.9}$ which is in reasonably good agreement with the maximum predicted theoretical range of $d^{0.5}$ to $d^{2.5}$.

4.8(ii) The "detachment" trigger discharge

Another important phenomenon that can only occur with impulse voltages is the initiation of breakdown by a trigger-like discharge that is struck between a negatively charged particle and its parent cathode-electrode almost immediately after detachment. The phenomenon was demonstrated experimentally by Poshekhonov and Solov'yev [42] by introducing artificial microparticles into a gap and observing the delay in the incidences of breakdown associated with both cathode and anode-launched particles. Apart from typical delay times of 0.5-2 msec found for both polarity particles, which can be satisfactorily explained in terms of particle transit times, there was also a very high incidence of breakdown events associated with cathode-launched particles that had delay times of only 1-3 μsec after the onset of the voltage pulse; such events were therefore identified as being initiated by this alternative type of trigger discharge.

These same authors [42] were able to provide a physical explanation for this detachment trigger mechanism in terms of the local microscopic field E_g existing in the gap between the particle and its parent electrode immediately following separation. The microgeometry of this ideal sphere-plane regime will be identical to that shown in Fig. 4.4(a), so that the resultant field E_g will again be given by the sum of the two components E_1 and E_2 of equation 4.16, defined for the analysis of the "impact" trigger discharge given in section 4.5(ii). However, in the present case, where the particle is leaving the electrode, these two components will be oppositely directed so that

$$E_g = E_1 - E_2$$

$$= 1.29(R_p/g)^{0.8}(E - 3Q_p/2\pi^3\varepsilon_o R_p^2) \qquad (4.43)$$

where Q_p is the particle charge and E is the macroscopic gap field. In the absence of any in-flight charge exchange, Q_p will be the charge acquired by the spherical particles in contact with the planar electrode, viz. $Q_p = \frac{2}{3}\pi^3\varepsilon_o R_p^2$, so that in a d-c situation where E is constant, the above equation indicates that $E_g = 0$, i.e. no discharge can occur. However, for fast-rise impulse voltages, E will no longer be constant with time, being now defined by $E(t) = (1/d)(dV/dt)$, and consequently $E_g \neq 0$. It follows therefore that if $E_g \rightarrow 10^9 Vm^{-1}$, electron emission will occur between the cathode and particle, thus providing the possibility of the same breakdown-initiating vaporisation processes discussed in section 4.5(ii) for the impact trigger mechanism.

An obvious consequence of this electron emission mechanism is that the negative charge on the particle will increase during its flight from the cathode, thereby promoting an associated increase of E_2. It therefore follows from equation 4.43 that this effect will exert a controlling influence on E_g, limiting it to some maximum value $(E_g)_m \sim 10^9 Vm^{-1}$ set by the field emission threshold. The actual charge carried by the particle will in fact increase from its initial detachment value $Q_p = \frac{2}{3}\pi^3 \varepsilon R_p^2 E$ at $t = t_c$ to a maximum value $(Q_p)_m$ at a time t_o after detachment when the charging current (i.e. the electron emission) ceases to flow. The value of t_o can be determined from the condition $dQ/dt = 0$ whilst $(Q_p)_m$ will be given to a good approximation by

$$(Q_p)_m = \frac{2}{3}\pi^3 \varepsilon_o R_p^2 \left[\frac{1}{d}\left(\frac{dV}{dt}\right)(t_d + t_o) - \frac{E_m}{1.29(R_p/g)^{0.8}}\right] \quad (4.44)$$

As would be expected from the time-dependence of E, viz. $E(t) = 1/d\ (dV/dt)$, experiments confirm [42] that the probability of breakdown being initiated by this mechanism increases rapidly with the rate of rise of the impulse voltage(dV/dt). In addition it was found that the present "detachment" trigger discharge mechanism, like the "impact" mechanism, only plays a significant role in the initiation of breakdown where particle diameters are in excess of 100μm. An explanation for this observation has been provided by computations of the duration t_o of the charging current. These show that this parameter falls off rapidly with decreasing particle diameter so that below some limiting value of $t_o \sim 3\mu s$ the trigger discharge cannot be sustained for a sufficient time to initiate an arc across the main gap. For the typical pulse rise rates of $(dV/dt) \sim 10^{10} Vs^{-1}$ used in the experiments cited [42], calculations have confirmed the experimental finding that this limit can only be exceeded for particle diameters $\gtrsim$ 100μm.

It should be finally noted that in a "real" gap situation, microparticles are likely to have been torn from an electrode surface with the associated formation of the field-enhancing filamentary structures illustrated in Fig. 4.2. Therefore, since such a microgeometry represents a more favourable field emitting regime, and since also both the emitter and effective anode have very much lower thermal capacities and consequently more liable to vaporisation, it follows that the threshold conditions for this type of trigger mechanism to operate are likely to be significantly lower than for the artificial sphere-plane regime.

4.9 References

1. Cranberg, L., *J. Appl. Phys.* **23**, 518-22, (1952).
2. Slivkov, I.N., *Sov. Phys-Tech Phys.* **2**, 1928-34, (1957).
3. Rohrbach, F., *Rpt. CERN*, **71-38** *(NTIS)*, (1971).
4. Jeans, J.H., *In* "The Mathematical Theory of Electricity and Magnetism", 5th Edn., Cambridge University Press, (1958).
5. Lobedov, N.N. and Skal'skaya, I.P., *Sov. Phys.-Tech. Phys.*, **7**, 268-71, (1962).
6. Boulloud, A., *Le Vide*, **99**, 240-3, (1962).
7. Pollock, H.M., Shufflebottom, P. and Skinner, J., *J.Phys.D: Appl. Phys.*, **10**. 127-38, (1977).
8. Pollock, H.M., *J.Phys. D : Appl.Phys.*, **11**, 39-54, (1978).
9. Udris, Ya. Ya., *Radio Engng. Electron Phys.*, **5**, 226-37, (1960).
10. Rosanova, N.B., *Bull. Acad. Sci. USSR*, **11**, 1262-4, (1962).
11. Olendzkaya, N.F., *Radio Engng. Electron Phys.*, **8**, 423-9, (1963).
12. Martynov, Ye.P., *Elektronnaya Tekhnika*, Ser.**10**,3-10, (1968).
13. Hurley, R.E. and Parnell, T.M., *J.Phys. D: Appl.Phys.*, **2**, 881-88, (1969).
14. Chatterton, P.A., Menon, M.M. and Srivastava, K.D., *J.Appl. Phys.*, **43**, 4536-42, (1972).
15. Miller, H.C., *J.Appl. Phys.*, **38**, 4501-4, (1967).
16. Martynov, Ye.P. and Ivanov, V.A., *Radio Eng. Electron Phys.*, **14**, 1732-7, (1969).
17. Martynov, Ye.P., *Sov. Phys-Tech. Phys.*, **16**, 1364-8, (1972).
18. Beukema, G.P., *J.Phys. D: Appl. Phys.*, **7**, 1740-55, (1974).
19. Davies, D.K. and Biondi, M.A., *J.Appl. Phys.*, **39**, 2979-90, (1968).
20. Davies, D.K. and Biondi, M.A., *J.Appl. Phys.*, **41**, 88-93, (1970).
21. Davies, D.K. and Biondi, M.A., *J.Appl. Phys.*, **42**, 3089-3107, (1971)
22. Davies, D.K. and Biondi, M.A., *Proc. VII DEIV (Novosibirsk)*, 121-9,(1976).
23. Nottingham, W.B., *Phys. Rev.* **59**, 907-10, (1941).
24. Widdington, R., *Proc. Roy. Soc.* **A89**, 554-60, (1914).
25. Schottky, W., *Z. Phys.*, **14**, 63-106, (1923).
26. Williams, D.W. and Williams, W.T., *J.Phys. D:Appl. Phys.*, **5**, 1845-54, (1972).
27. Latham, R.V. and Braun, E., *J.Phys. D: Appl. Phys.*, **3**, 1663-70, (1970).
28. Cook, M.A., *In* "The Science of High Explosives", Reinhold, New York, (1958).
29. Menon, M.M. and Srivastava, K.D., *Proc. VI DEIV (Swansea)*, 3-10, (1974).
30. Davies, R.M., *Proc. Roy. Soc.* **A317**, 367, (1970).
31. Tabor, D., *Proc. Roy. Soc.* **A192**, 247-74, (1948).

32. Gane, N., *Proc. Roy. Soc.* **A317**, 367-91, (1970).
33. Slattery, J.C., Friichtenicht, J.F. and Hanson, D.O., *Appl. Phys. Letters*, **7**, 23-5, (1965).
34. Latham, R.V., *J.Phys. D:Appl. Phys.* **5**, 2044-54, (1972).
35. Andrews, J.P., *Phil. Mag.*, **9**, 593-610, (1930).
36. Latham, R.V., Brah, A.S., Fok, K. and Woods, M.O., *J.Phys.D: Appl. Phys.*, **10**, 139-151, (1977).
37. Latham, R.V. and Brah, A.S., *J.Phys. D:Appl. Phys.*, **10**, 151-167, (1977).
38. Simmons, J.G., *J.Appl. Phys.* **34**, 2581-90, (1963).
39. Simmons, J.G., *Trans. Met. Soc. AIME*, **233**, 485-496, (1965).
40. Simmons, J.G., *J.Phys. D:Appl. Phys.*, **4**, 613-57, (1971).
41. Farrall, G.A., *J.Appl. Phys.*, **33**, 96-99, (1962).
42. Poshekhonov, P.V. and Solov'yev, V.I., *Radio Enging. Electron Phys.*, **16**, 1545-49, (1972).

5 Simulation Studies I – The Point-to-Plane Field Emitting Diode

5.1 DC Measurements
(i) Experimental regime
(ii) DC emission characteristics
5.2 Microsecond Pulse Measurements
(i) Experimental regime
(ii) Pulse emission characteristics
5.3 Nanosecond Pulse Studies of Arc Initiation
(i) Optical measurements of cathode flare velocities
(ii) Electronic measurements of explosive emission currents
(iii) Rate of vaporisation of emitter material
(iv) Oscillatory instabilities with high over-voltage pulses
5.4 References

The evident importance of the microprotrusion model for breakdown initiation discussed in Chapter 3 stimulated a vigorous research investigation into the electron emission properties of the type of metallic microemitters that can exist on broad-area high voltage electrodes. Since, however, such naturally occurring emitters are generally found in groups at random and ill-defined locations on an electrode surface (see Chapter 7), it is not possible to use the broad-area electrode regime for making detailed in-situ measurements on a given isolated emitter of known geometry. In addition, the microscopic complexity of such a regime allows the possibility of simultaneous cooperative phenomena occurring that would greatly complicate the interpretation of experimental data. Accordingly, the approach adopted in these investigations was to artificially fabricate individual emitters having a similar geometry to those found naturally and then to study their properties under controlled laboratory conditions.

5.1 DC Emission Measurements

5.1(i) Experimental regime

It is fortuitous that the technology for manufacturing such tips had previously been developed for the well known research techniques of field electron emission microscopy, pioneered by Müller [1], and later field ion microscopy. A wide range of metals have been studied using these techniques, and details of the various tip preparation procedures can be found in standard works on these subjects [2,3]. In the case of tungsten for example [4], which is one of the most widely studied materials, tips are electrochemically etched from a fine wire (typically ∿ 0.1mm diameter) in a 2M solution of sodium hydroxide using the arrangement of Fig. 5.1. As illustrated by the inset, the etching process takes place at the meniscus, and as soon as

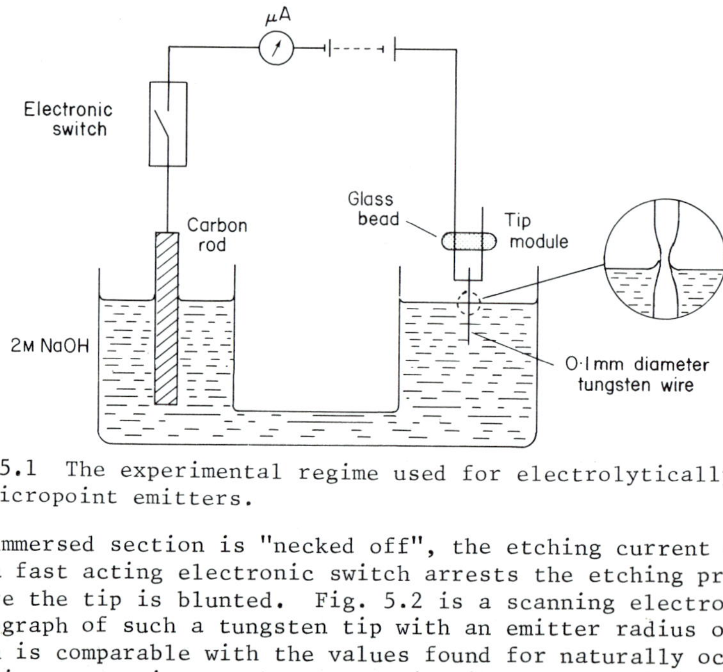

Fig. 5.1 The experimental regime used for electrolytically etching micropoint emitters.

the immersed section is "necked off", the etching current drops and a fast acting electronic switch arrests the etching process before the tip is blunted. Fig. 5.2 is a scanning electron micrograph of such a tungsten tip with an emitter radius of ∿50nm, which is comparable with the values found for naturally occurring microprotrusions such as shown in Fig. 7.6(b). Since these tips are extremely fragile and hence difficult to handle, the short wire specimen is normally spot welded to the tungsten "cross-bar" of a standard specimen mount before etching.

The basic experimental regime required for studying the emission characteristics of these microtips is illustrated schematically in Fig. 5.3. It is seen to consist of a point-to-plane diode configuration, where both the microtip cathode C and metallic anode disc A can be heated in situ to high temperatures for their initial out-gassing treatment; the cathode by passing an electric current through the "cross-bar", and the anode by electron bombardment using the thermionic filament TF. This elec-

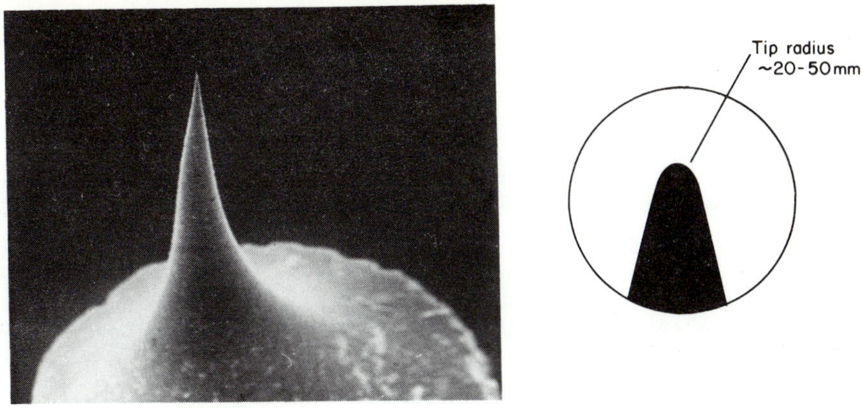

Fig. 5.2 A scanning electron micrograph of a micropoint emitter that has been etched from a 0.1mm diameter tungsten wire.

trode assembly has to be mounted in either a glass or metal UHV chamber capable of reaching pressures $\lesssim 10^{-10}$mbar, with the electrical feed-through to A insulated up to $\sim$ 10kV.

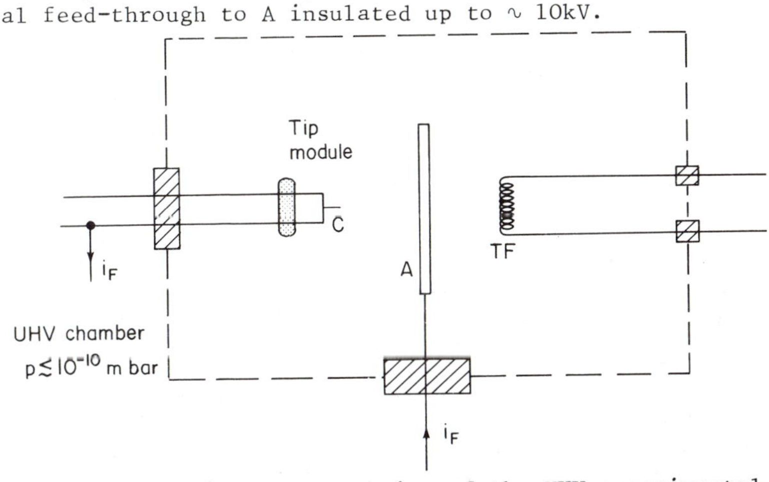

Fig. 5.3 A schematic representation of the UHV experimental facility required for studying the field emitting properties of the micropoint emitter C: A is a planar anode and TF is a thermionic filament used for out-gassing A.

In order to give a quantitative interpretation of the data obtained from this experimental regime, it is essential to measure the radius r of the micro-emitter before its assembly in the specimen chamber. This is normally done by mounting the tip module in a suitably modified specimen holder of a transmission electron microscope so that a high resolution profile image of the emitting surface can be obtained. Typically such a micrograph appears as in the inset to Fig. 5.2, from which it is seen that the tip profile closely approximates to a section through a spherically-capped cone. However, the tip radius can also be estimated from empirical relations based on the operating characteristics of the emitter: for example, that of Drechsler and Henkel [15] takes the form

$$r = 0.015\ \phi^{-2} V_{10}\ \text{(nm)} \tag{5.1}$$

where ϕ is the work function of the emitter measured in electron volts and V_{10} is the voltage that has to be applied across the diode to give an emission current of 10μA. For this type of emitter, the enhanced electric field E acting at the spherical apex of the tip can then be closely approximated by the relation

$$E = V/fr \tag{5.2}$$

where V is the voltage applied across the diode and f is a complicated dimensionless geometric function of the tip dimensions and the d-spacing of the diode [6]: however, in cases where d>>r, such as in the field emission microscope, f can be taken as a constant having a value of $\sim$ 5 [2]. It must also be recognised that as one moves over the surface away from the apex of the emitter, the surface field E will fall-off rapidly from the maximum value defined by equation 5.2. As will be described in the following section, the actual surface distribution of E for a given emitter can be obtained from its profile electron micrograph (such as the inset of Fig. 5.2) by firstly constructing the equipotentials in the immediate vicinity of the emitting surface and then using standard field plotting techniques to determine the local values of E [6].

Historically, the first quantitative investigation using this type of regime was due to Haefer [7] in 1940 with his classic experimental verification of the Fowler-Nordheim theory of field electron emission. However, with the growing interest in both the potential practical application of micropoint field emission electron sources, and their important role in limiting the insulating capability of high voltage vacuum gaps, Dyke and his co-workers published the first series of important papers describing their detailed fundamental studies on the properties of laboratory-etched micropoint emitters [8,9].With the advantage of improved vacuum conditions ($\sim 10^{-12}$mbar), and the introduction of sophisticated ancilliary experimental techniques for comparing the d-c and pulsed field operational behaviour of such emitters, this work represented a major advance on earlier investigations.

5.1(ii) DC emission characteristics

The electrical circuitry required for studying the d-c current-voltage characteristic of the point-plane regime illustrated in Fig. 5.3 needs to be no more complicated than that shown in Fig. 5.4. In this, a regulated EHT supply provides a variable d-c

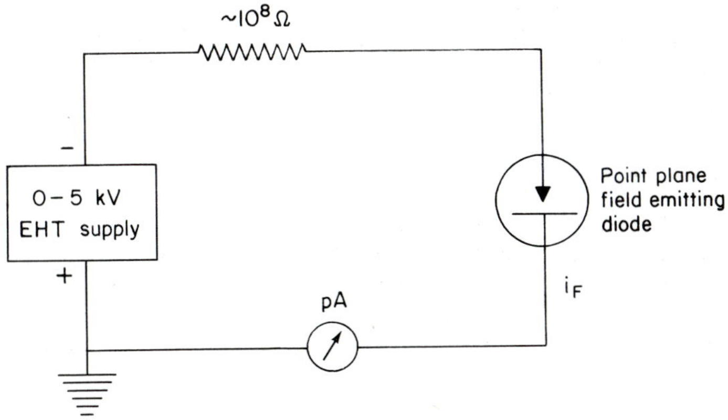

Fig. 5.4 The electrical circuit for measuring the current-voltage characteristic of the point-plane diode shown in Fig. 5.3.

voltage source and a picoammeter measures the total field emission current i: a high series-resistance is also included to limit the circuit current should a micro-discharge occur. In practice, it is usual to cautiously "build-up" the characteristic by progressively cycling the applied voltage V through an increasing range until the diode begins to show signs of instability. However, in order to obtain a stable and reversible current-voltage characteristic from the diode assembly shown in Fig. 5.3, it is essential to follow an in situ cleaning procedure *before* applying a high voltage. That used by Dyke and Trolan [9] involved thoroughly out-gassing both electrodes by heating them simultaneously to temperatures in excess of 1300 K until all desorbed gas has been re-absorbed by a tantalum gathering agent, and then to "flash" the emitter by heating it to ∿ 2500 K under zero field conditions in order to remove all remaining surface contamination. With a field emission microscopic regime, such as would exist if the metal anode A in Fig. 5.3 was replaced by a phosphor screen, the effectiveness of this procedure can be directly assessed from the appearance of the emission image. For example, an atomically clean, [110] orientated single crystal tungsten emitter would give the characteristic four-lobed image shown in Fig. 5.5(i); i.e. reflecting the small variation in work function associated with the specific crystallographic planes that intersect the emitting surface. With clean emitters, it is typically possible to draw stable emission currents of ∿ 8μA and 20μA from tips having radii of ∿ 30nm and ∿ 230nm respectively.

Two alternative approaches have been used for presenting the stable current-voltage data obtained from such emitters. The first, which takes historical precedence, is based on the empirical relation

$$i_F = A \exp(-B/V) \tag{5.3}$$

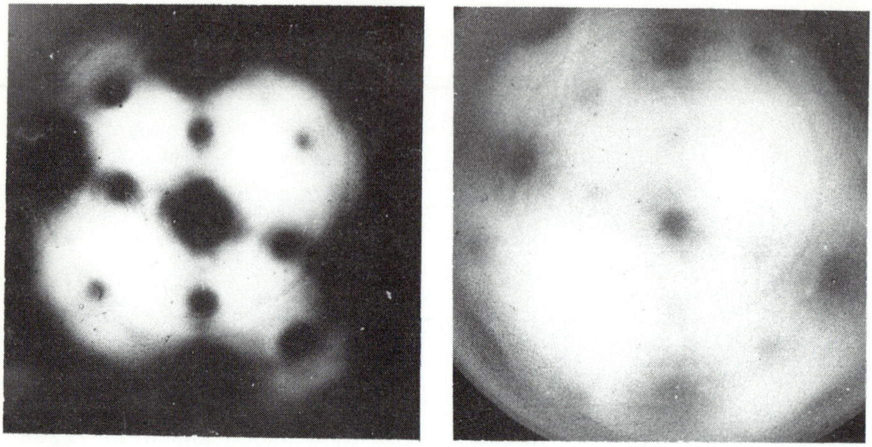

Fig. 5.5 (i) The field emission image of an atomically clean tungsten micropoint emitter orientated with the [110] crystal direction parallel to the axis of the wire. (ii) The image of the same emitter, but at higher emission current densities where space-charge blurring is occurring.
(From unpublished results of B. Juttner).

where A and B are constants. This formulation was originally due to Millikan and Lauritsen [10] and, because of the excellent linearity of the experimental plots of log i_F against 1/V, has subsequently been used by many authors including Dyke and Trolan [9]. It does however have the serious disadvantage that it has not been possible to satisfactorily relate the constants A and B to the physical parameters of the system. In contrast, the alternative approach has the advantage of being based on the well established Fowler-Nordheim electron emission theory; for this reason it has become more favoured by recent authors and will therefore be used in the present treatment. Thus for the low-temperature emission regime described by equation 3.9 of Section 3.1(i), the total emission current from a micropoint emitter would be given by

$$i_{OF} = A_e j_{OF} = A_e C_1 E^2 \exp(-C_2/E)$$

in which j_{OF} is the emission current density at the tip of the protrusion where the surface field E has the value defined by equation 5.2, and A_e corresponds to some "effective" emitting area.

If however account is taken of the appreciable variation of E, and hence j_{OF}, over the highly curved surface of a micropoint source, i_{OF} should more correctly be expressed in the form

$$i_{OF} = \int_{\substack{\text{emitting}\\ \text{surface}}} j_{OF}\, dA \tag{5.4}$$

To evaluate this integral for the typical microemitter geometry shown in Fig. 5.2, and thereby obtain a more meaningful definition of the "emitting area", Dyke et al. [6] applied field plotting techniques to determine the variation of E over the emitter surface and then, assuming a constant work function, used equation 3.2 to compute the corresponding distribution of the low-temperature emission current density j_{OF}. The general findings of these studies can be illustrated schematically with reference to the ideal spherically-capped conical emitter shown in Fig. 5.6(i).

(i)

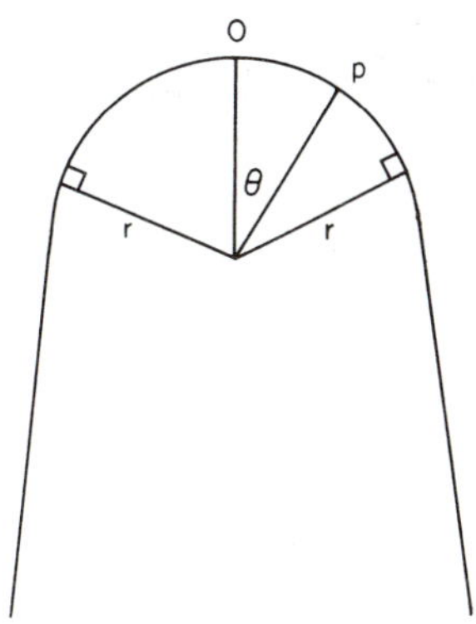

(ii)

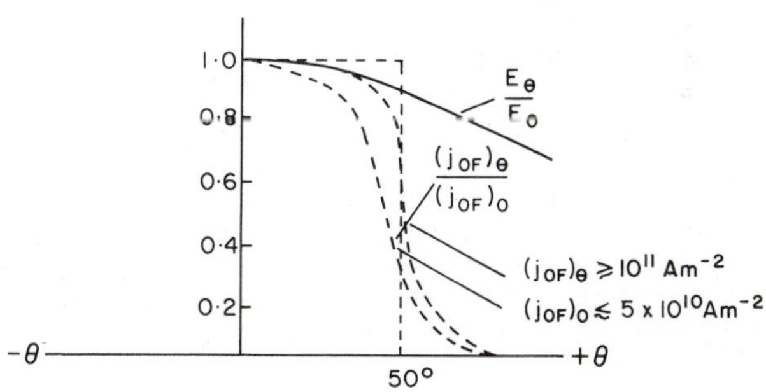

Fig. 5.6 (i) The microgeometry of an idealised spherically-capped conical emitter. (ii) The surface variation of (a) the normalised field distribution E_θ/E_0 and (b) the low and high emission current density distribution $(j_{OF})_\theta/j_{OF})_0$. (From Dyke and Trolan [9], with permission).

Assuming rotational symmetry, all points of constant field on the emitting surface can then be defined in terms of the polar angle θ with an origin of co-ordinates located at the centre of curvature of the spherical cap of the emitter. The normalised field and FEE current density distributions, E_θ and $(j_{OF})_\theta$, then appear as shown in Fig. 5.6(ii), where E_o and $(j_{OF})_o$ are respectively the maximum values of E and j_{OF} at the apex of the emitter where $\theta = 0$. From these plots, it can be seen that for all practical purposes, the emitting area A_e can now be defined as the region bounded by $-50^o \lesssim \theta \lesssim 50^o$ which contributes $\sim$ 85% of the total emission, and over which the surface field E_θ varies by less than 10%, i.e we can take

$$A_e \simeq \pi r^2 \tag{5.5}$$

Fig. 5.6(ii) further indicates that with increasing $(j_{OF})_O$, i.e. at higher fields, the total low-temperature emission current i_{OF} can be closely approximated by the product of the peak FEE current density $(j_{OF})_O$ and this newly defined emitting area A_e viz.

$$i_{OF} = \int_{\substack{\text{Emitting}\\ \text{area}}} j_{OF}\, dA \simeq \pi r^2 (j_{OF})_O \tag{5.6}$$

Substituting for $(j_{OF})_O$ from equation 3.9, and for $E_o \simeq V/kr \simeq V/5r$ from equation 5.2, we obtain finally

$$i_{OF} = 0.04\pi C_1 V^2 \exp(-5C_2 r/V) \tag{5.7}$$

indicating that an F-N plot of the i-V characteristics of such an emitter (i.e. log (i/V^2) versus $(1/V)$ will be linear with a slope of $5C_2r$ and an intercept of $0.04\pi C_1$ which, significantly, is independent of the emitter radius within the limits of the above approximations.

Experimental plots are found to have the general form shown in Fig. 5.7, thus confirming that there is a wide range of fields, viz. $E \lesssim 5 \times 10^9 Vm^{-1}$, for which the characteristic is both linear and reversible [4]. Beyond this limiting field E_ℓ however, the emission ceases to obey the Fowler-Nordheim relation but instead begins to follow the well known diode three-halves power law $i_F = PV^{1.5} \alpha V^{1.5}$, where P is the perveance of the diode; i.e. indicating that at these high fields the emission is being space charge limited. From their experimental plots, Dyke and Trolan [9] showed that the limiting emission current density for the onset of these space charge effects is $(j_F)_\ell \sim 6 \times 10^{10} A.m^{-2}$; they also established by a simple calculation that this controlling action occurs within a distance of 2×10^{-8}m from the surface of the emitter where the current density is highest. Under these conditions, the local crystallographic variations of emitter work function, as highlighted by the characteristic emission image of Fig. 5.5(i), are smoothed out to give the more diffuse

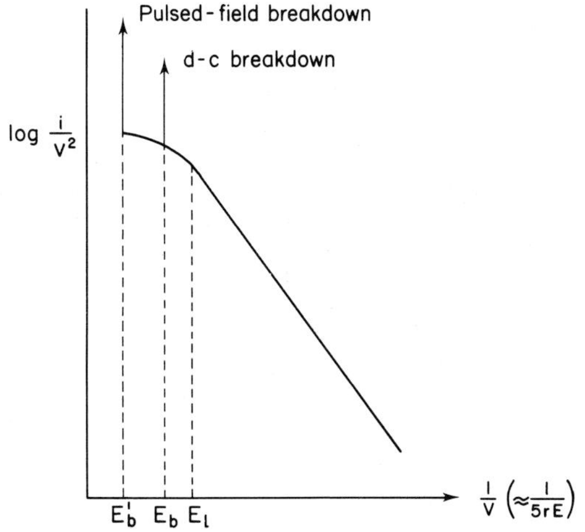

Fig. 5.7 The typical form of the Fowler-Nordheim plot of the current-voltage characteristics of a micropoint field emitting diode.

pattern of Fig. 5.5(ii).

As the field is increased beyond E_ℓ, both the emission current and the associated emission image become progressively unstable until, as shown in Fig. 5.7, a critical field $E_b \sim 8 \times 10^9 Vm^{-1}$ and current density $(j_F)_c \sim 5 \times 10^{11} A.m^{-2}$ is reached when the diode spontaneously breaks down. The instability associated with this high-field regime, which also manifests itself as a significant "scatter" in the measured values of E_b among emitters, is thought to result from the onset of some sort of time-dependent emitter contamination mechanism that locally modifies the effective work function and hence the emitting regime. Two favoured possibilities are the adsorption of contaminant atoms released from the anode by electron bombardment heating, or the field-assisted surface diffusion of contaminant atoms from the shank of the emitter. This latter type of process can also be activated by the bombardment of ions from the anode and has in fact been considered by Cavaille and Drechsler [11] as a means of promoting crystal growth through the self-diffusion of surface metal atoms to form microprotrusions on broad-area HV electrodes.

If the profile of an emitter is re-examined in the electron microscope following a breakdown event, it will be found to have become grossly blunted as shown in Fig. 5.8, with clear evidence of tip melting and vaporisation [12], as would follow an "explosive" surface process. As discussed in section 3.3, the initiation of such an instability will be fundamentally determined by the condition that the emission current density reaches some critical value $(j_F)_c$ where its heating effect (Joulian and Nottingham) is sufficient to cause local vaporisation of the emitter surface and the consequent generation of a microplasma.

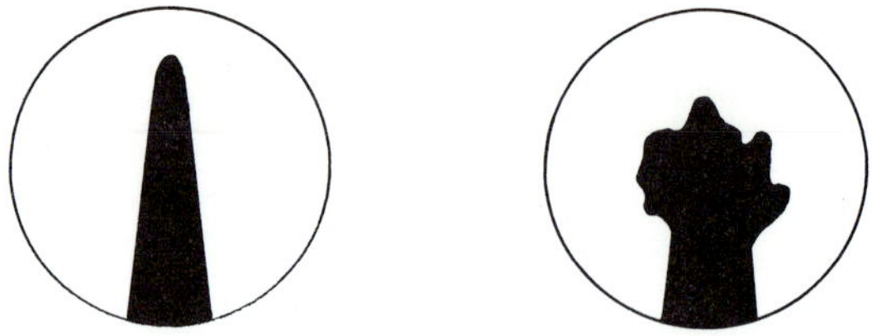

Fig. 5.8 A comparison of the profiles of (i) a virgin micropoint emitter and (ii) one that has suffered a breakdown event.

5.2 Microsecond Pulse Measurements

With the recognition that the electrical breakdown of these micropoint-emitter diodes was a sub-microsecond "explosive" phenomenon involving the thermal response of the emitter, it became evident that high-speed pulse techniques would have to be employed if more detailed information was to be obtained about the evolution of the breakdown mechanism. The early experiments were again pioneered by Dyke and his co-workers in America [9, 12], who used microsecond pulse techniques to study how the growth of the emission current waveform depends on the magnitude and duration of the applied field. More recently, the groups of Fursey and Mesyats [13-18] in the U.S.S.R. have used more refined nanosecond pulse techniques to resolve the sequence of events involved in the breakdown mechanism of these diodes. These investigations also incorporated synchronised high-speed optical recording techniques to study the development of the microplasma or "cathode flare" that is a precursor to the actual breakdown of the diode.

5.2(i) Experimental regime

The practical requirements for this type of impulse measurement are principally dictated by the demands of high speed pulse technology. Thus, if nanosecond rise times are to be achieved, it is essential to minimise all stray capacitances, and to ensure that the external drive and detection circuitry are impedance-matched throughout. In the type of system developed initially by Mesyats et al. [14] and later by Fursey and Zhukov [15], which is illustrated schematically in Fig. 5.9, these conditions have been satisfied in part by generally reducing the dimensions of the electrode assembly. More important however, the planar anode of the d-c experimental regime (Fig. 5.3) has been replaced by a "transparent" earthed grid G, whilst an additional "collector" electrode C has been introduced immediately behind G. This new triode arrangement has the important advantage of reducing the anode-to-cathode capacitance and thereby minimising the interference from the displacement currents that must inevitably flow following the application of a voltage pulse and that would

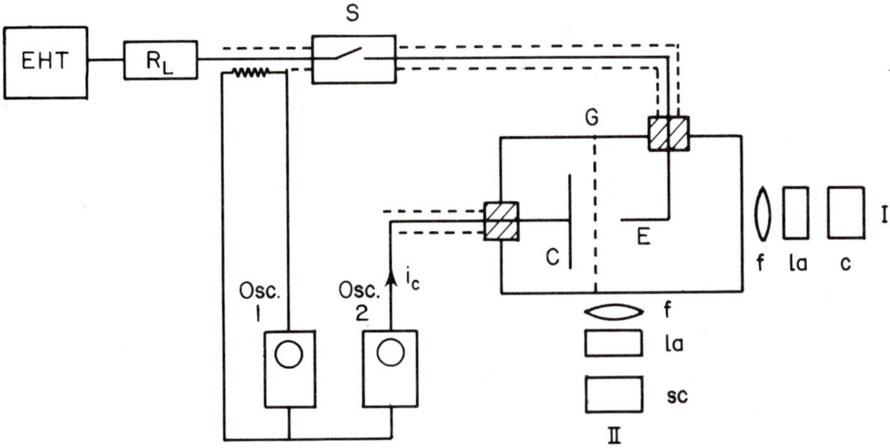

Fig. 5.9 The experimental regime used for studying the electronic and optical processes associated with the pulsed-field breakdown of micropoint emitters.
(From Fursey and Zhukov [15], with permission).

otherwise mask the true electron current. The omission of an electron bombardment anode heating facility is acceptable for these fast impulse experiments provided the system receives a thorough external bake-out before sealing off the test diode. This is because the thermal response time of the anode is very much longer than the rise time of the emission current so that its surface processes can have no influence on the emitter behaviour. It was also found possible to eliminate the cathode heating arrangement of Fig. 5.3, since emitters can be satisfactorily cleaned by a reverse-polarity field-desorption procedure. The orthogonally orientated optical monitoring systems I and II shown in Fig. 5.9, incorporating focussing f, light-amplifying la and camera c modules, are used respectively for studying the reference electron emission image displayed on C (i.e. if phosphor-coated), and the photon emission from interelectrode microplasma processes. Referring finally to the associated electrical circuitry, the negative-going high voltage pulses that are applied to the micropoint emitter are derived from an EHT supply that is electronically switched by a fast acting three electrode switch S that is filled with nitrogen at a pressure of 15 atm. Oscilloscopes 1 and 2, that are synchronously triggered from the initial fast pulse resulting from the charging of the transmission line, record respectively the total emission current and the collector current. For minimal pulse distortion, it is vital to impedance-match the transmission lines to the test diode assembly.

5.2(ii) Pulse emission characteristics

We shall consider first the earlier experiments pioneered by Dyke and his collaborators [9,12], and later developed by Fursey [19], that used μ-second pulse techniques to investigate the thermal response of micro-emitters. These showed that for emission current densities $j_F \lesssim (j_F)_L$ (see Fig. 5.7), the total current transient had the type of waveform illustrated in Fig. 5.10(i), where the initial spike is due to the displacement current associated with the charging of the inter-electrode capacitance and the following constant-current plateau region is indicative of stable emission conditions.

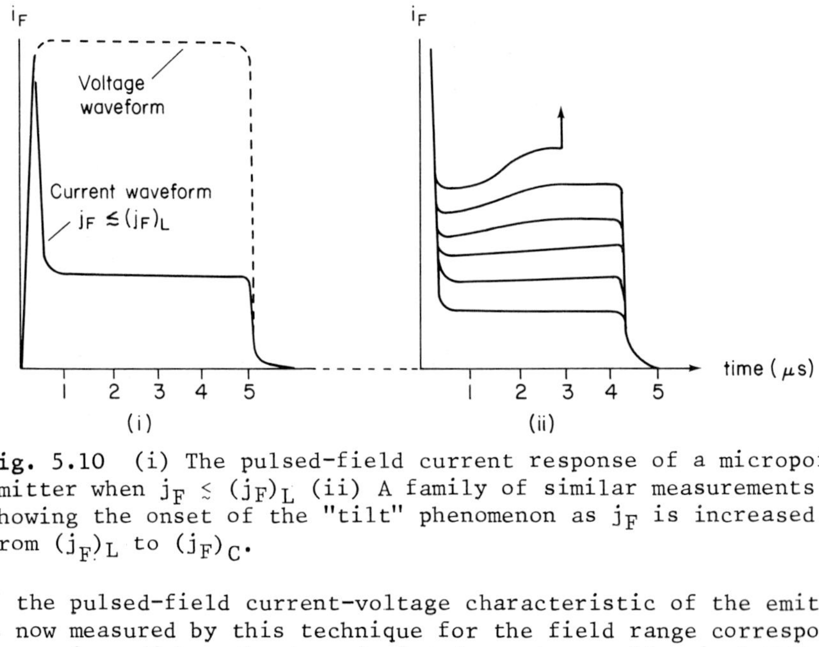

Fig. 5.10 (i) The pulsed-field current response of a micropoint emitter when $j_F \lesssim (j_F)_L$ (ii) A family of similar measurements showing the onset of the "tilt" phenomenon as j_F is increased from $(j_F)_L$ to $(j_F)_C$.

If the pulsed-field current-voltage characteristic of the emitter is now measured by this technique for the field range corresponding to $j_F \lesssim (j_F)_L$, the data is found to give an identical F-N plot to the d-c behaviour shown in Fig. 5.7. When these pulse measurements are extended to higher fields, where the d-c emission current density would exceed $(j_F)_L$, the current waveform begins to develop an upward "tilt" as illustrated in the traces of Fig. 5.10(ii); i.e. the current exhibits a spontaneous growth at constant field, approaching a saturated equilibrium value with a time constant $\tau \sim$ 1-2μs. Provided these saturated emission current values are used, the F-N plot of the emitter continues to closely follow the d-c behaviour of Fig. 5.7 into the non-linear region. However, with pulse experiments, breakdown is more predictable and generally occurrs at somewhat higher field E_b' corresponding to a pulsed-field critical emission current density $(j_F)_c' \sim 7.8 \times 10^{11} A.m^{-2}$. The associated emission image, as recorded by the open-shutter camera of optical system I in Fig. 5.9, is found to have the same general form as found with d-c experiments, including the space charge "blurring" effect of Fig. 5.5(ii) that occurs when $j_F \gtrsim (j_F)_L$. There is however an additional feature that develops at the highest pulse fields used, i.e. just prior to breakdown and coincident with the onset of current "tilt". As illustrated in Fig. 5.11(i) this takes the form of a bright ring structure or halo that skirts the emission image and can reach intensities considerably in excess of the rest of the image [12]. Subsequently, Fursey [19] showed that this halo could in fact be resolved into several well-defined concentric rings.

(i)

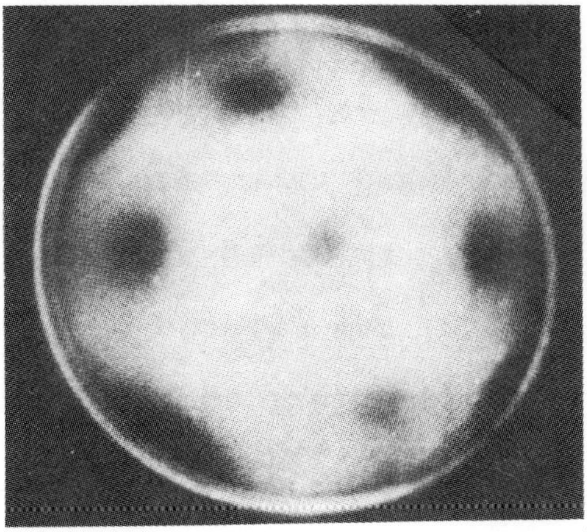

(ii)

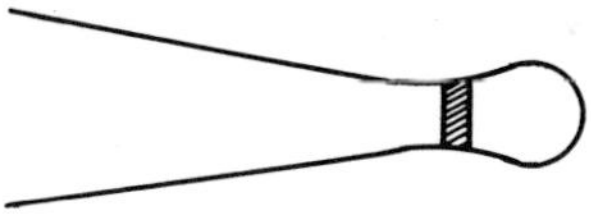

Fig. 5.11 (i) The space-charge blurred emission image with associated "ring" phenomenon that occurs when $j_F \to (j_F)_c$, and is coincident with the onset of the "tilt" phenomenon illustrated in Fig. 5.10(ii).
(From Fursey [19], with permission).
(ii) The characteristic "necked" structure of an emitter that has been overloaded and become thermally unstable.
(From Dyke, Trolan, Martin and Barbour [12], with permission).

The evident correlation between these "tilt" and "ring" phenomena led Dyke et al. [12] to attribute them to a thermally enhanced field electron emission mechanism, viz. T-F emission as discussed in section 5.2(ii), which begins to contribute significantly to the total emission current as local regions of an emitter reach temperatures $\gtrsim 2000^{\circ}$K. This explanation was supported by the observations that the profile of emitters that had previously exhibited these effects were characterised by having a "necked" structure as shown in Fig. 5.11(ii), and that the electrons forming the ring came from the relatively low-field shaded region situated very near the neck of the emitter where the internal current density, and hence the Joulian heating effect, will be a maximum; i.e. creating a particularly favourable location for the onset of T-F emission. However, more recent scanning electron micrographs of tips that have become thermally unstable, i.e. such as shown in Fig. 7.13(iii), have indicated rather that the surface of the shaded neck region of Fig. 5.11(ii) acquires a corrugated or "bellows-like" structure whose periodic field enhancing properties could well account for the multiplicity of the rings forming the halo surrounding the emission image shown in Fig. 5.11(i). It also follows from this model that the characteristic 1-2μs rise time τ_t of the "tilt" current must be related to the establishment of a thermal equilibrium in the emitter. An impressive check on this assumption can be made by observing how the maximum stable emission current density depends on the duration t_p of the applied voltage pulse, particularly when the pulse length is reduced to the situation where $t_p \lesssim 0.2\tau_t \lesssim 0.5\mu s$, so that the temperature increase of an emitter will be limited to well below its maximum equilibrium value. The earliest experiments of this kind using microsecond pulse techniques [12] confirmed that $(j_F)_c$ could be increased by an order of magnitude to $\sim 5 \times 10^{12} A.m^{-2}$: however, the more recent nanosecond experiments to be discussed in the following section showed even more dramatic increases of $(j_F)_c$ approaching $\sim 10^{15} A.m^{-2}$.

5.3 Nanosecond Pulse Studies of Arc Initiation

Although the above microsecond pulsed field investigations had shown that the vacuum arc is established within a time of $\lesssim 10^{-8}$s, they were unable to provide information about the final stages of the physical mechanism that leads to the arc. In particular, it was not possible to resolve the time-dependence of the "explosive" growth of the emission current through two to three orders of magnitude, such as occurs from the plateau region on the highest current trace of Fig. 5.10(ii) to breakdown. It is not surprising therefore that a fundamental misconception arose in the early understanding of the phenomena; viz. that the arc stemmed from a regenerative T-F emission process that led to a rapid vaporisation of emitter material which, after being ionised, progressively neutralised the electronic space charge that had previously limited the emission current and so created the conditions for a *smooth* but rapid avalanche build-up of the diode current to breakdown. However, with the introduction of pulse techniques having a nanosecond resolution, it was soon shown that the current waveform accompanying arc formation had a quite different form from that predicted by the above model. This finding therefore stimulated the development of new diagnostic techniques for obtaining more information about the physical processes involved and hence a revised explanation of the arc initiation mechanism.

5.3(i) Optical measurement of cathode flare velocities

The "cathode flare" model, which has now become widely accepted, was based on complementary measurements of the light emission and current growth accompanying the establishment of an arc across an electrode regime such as shown in Fig. 5.9. Thus the optical system II, incorporating an open-shutter high speed streak camera SC, records the temporal evolution of all pre-arc optical processes occurring in the gap, whilst oscilloscopes 1 and 2 record respectively the associated emitter and collector currents. The amplitude of the arc-inducing over-voltage pulses used in these experiments is carefully chosen so that "explosive" emission will be initiated just as the pulse reaches its maximum value. From this type of optical observation, Mesyats et al. [20] were able to establish that an arc is initiated from a pinpoint of light that appears at the tip of the microemitter and then, as shown in the sequence of Fig. 5.12, rapidly develops into a luminous spherically-shaped flare that grows across the gap to establish an arc. The underlying physical mechanism that is now thought to be responsible for this process in the case of an isolated micropoint emitter [13,19] is as illustrated in the more detailed sequence of Fig. 5.13.

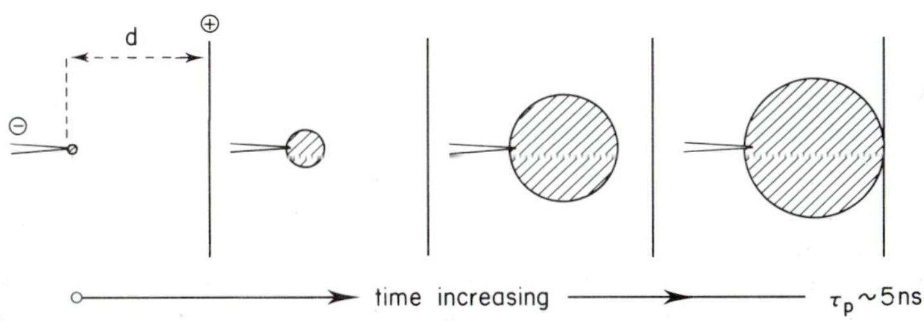

Fig. 5.12 A schematic illustration of the initiation and growth of a "cathode flare" until it bridges the electrode gap.

A breakdown event starts with the generation of a localised microplasma (electrons and positive ions) that surrounds the microemitter following the ionisation of cathode material that has been thermally vaporised as a result of a high T-F electron emission current density. This microplasma then begins to spontaneously expand, but because its constituent electrons have very much higher thermal velocities than the heavy metallic ions, its envelope will rapidly become populated predominantly by electrons. These outer electrons now come under the influence of the gap

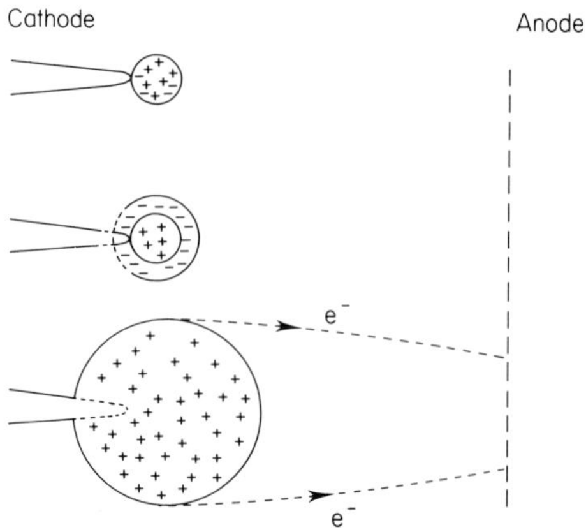

Fig. 5.13 An illustration of how it is possible for a charge separation to occur in the expanding microplasma, and hence an enhanced cathode field due to the accumulation of positive space charge.

field and so break away from the plasma sphere to be collected by the anode. As a result of this charge separation, the emitter will experience a greatly enhanced field due to the uncompensated positive space charge remaining in the expanding flare, and this, in turn, will lead to an increase in both the emission current density and rate of evaporation of emitter material to levels that are more than adequate for sustaining the growth of the flare until it reaches the anode and establishes an arc across the diode. From a knowledge of the d-spacing of the diode and the photographically measured time for the flare to cross the electrode gap, it was estimated that the expansion velocity of the flare envelope was $\sim 10^4 m.s^{-1}$. It should also be noted that the value of this parameter is determined almost entirely by the space charge density; i.e. the externally applied field has very little influence.

5.3(ii) Electronic measurements of explosive emission currents

According to the model illustrated in Fig. 5.13, an electron current would be recorded at the collector of the experimental regime shown in Fig. 5.9 both before and during the time that the flare is crossing the gap: in fact, with a grid that is effectively transparent to electrons, this current could be identified with the total emitter current. However, with the establishment of an arc between the emitter and grid, the gap field would collapse and with it the collector current $i_c(\simeq i_F)$; the grid current on the other hand, which would previously have been minimal, will now increase by several orders of magnitude. This behaviour has indeed been confirmed experimentally by complementary electrical studies of the flare phenomenon, where Fig. 5.14

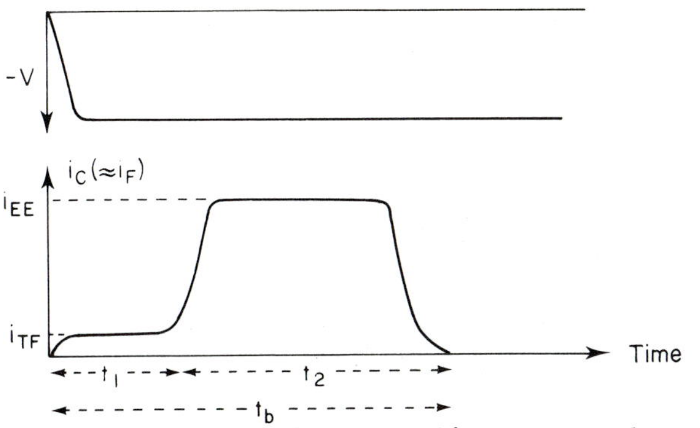

Fig. 5.14 The general form of the applied over-voltage waveform and the resulting "explosive emission" current transient, showing the emitter heating time t_1 and the commutation time t_2.

illustrates the typical relation between i_c and the applied voltage V. The characteristic initial plateau of the i_c waveform corresponds to a quasi-stable temperature-assisted FEE regime whose duration t_1 is very sensitive to the over-voltage coefficient of the applied pulse α_V, defined as the ratio of the amplitude of the pulse being used to the slow-rise d-c voltage that would just maintain stable emission. This regime is terminated at $t = t_1$ by the onset of explosive emission where the current rapidly increased by two or more orders in a time $\sim$1 ns to a new value i_{EE} whose magnitude is also very sensitive to α_V. There then follows a second plateau region of duration t_2, the "commutation time", that can be identified as the time during which the cathode flare is expanding across the gap. Hence, from a knowledge of the emitter-to-grid separation, these measurements were able to confirm that cathode flare velocities are in the range 2-3 x $10^4 ms^{-1}$ and, as anticipated, are almost independent of the gap field.

As already illustrated in Fig. 5.8, this type of event inevitably leads to severe and irreversible damage to the emitter. It follows therefore that if quantifiable information is to be obtained about the dependence of t_1 and i_{EE} on the over-voltage coefficient α_V and the applied field E, it is necessary to conduct single-shot experiments on a series of similar emitters whose initial tip profiles have been electron optically recorded for subsequently calculating E as described in section 5.1(ii). To minimise space charge effects, it is also desirable to use the sharpest possible emitters with tip radii $\lesssim$ 100nm. With this technique, Fursey and Zhukov [15-17] were able to compile families of explosive emission characteristics such as illustrated in Fig. 5.15. As will be seen, these transients correspond to only a limited range of α_V from $\sim$ 1.2 to 1.4 and therefore clearly highlight how very sensitive both t_1 and i_{EE} are to E; for example, i_{EE} can readily increase from $\sim$ 0.5A to $\sim$ 100A for

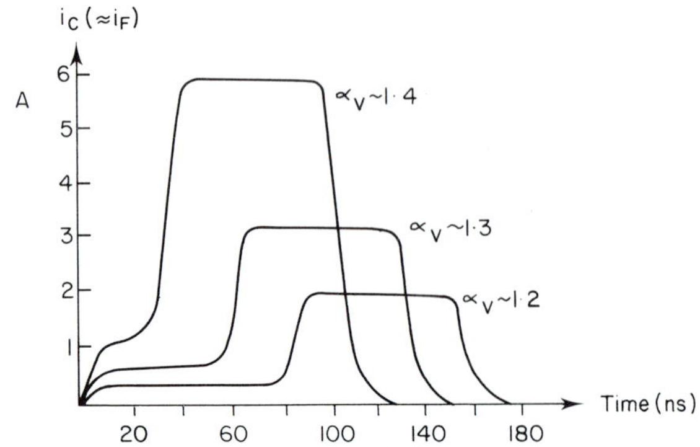

Fig. 5.15 A family of idealised "explosive emission" current transients illustrating the strong influence of the over-voltage coefficient α_V of the applied pulse.

a 20% increase in E. It must however be re-emphasized that this sort of dramatic response can only be obtained when fast-rise pulses are used; i.e. indicating that the explosive electron emission mechanism (EEE) must depend on the rate at which energy can be supplied to the system, or more specifically to the flare plasma, since it has proved impossible to explain this finding in terms of the emitter behaviour alone.

This dependence of i_{EE} on E also implies that there should be a corresponding relationship between i_{EE} and j_F; indeed a similar indication follows from a consideration of the important ionising role played by the electron emission in initiating the formation of a microplasma. Accordingly, Fursey and Zhukov [15] were able to show that a plot of log i_{EE} against the emission current density j_F, as calculated from the Fowler-Nordheim theory (equation 3.2) using values of E_m computed from the initial emitter profiles and applied voltage, yielded the good straight line of Fig. 5.16 within the measured range $10^{12} \lesssim j_F \lesssim 10^{13} Am^{-2}$ i.e. indicating an empirical relation of the form

$$i_{EE} \propto \exp(kj_F) \qquad (5.7)$$

where k is a constant. From a knowledge of i_{EE} and the dimensions of the enlarged emitting area, as given by the exploded tip profile of Fig. 5.8(ii), it can further be shown that the mean explosive emission current density j_{EE} is typically $\sim 10^{11}$-10^{12} Am^{-2}, which is an order of magnitude lower than the corresponding FEE current densities drawn initially from undamaged emitters. This rather surprising finding can however be plausibly explained on the basis that i_{EE} is not in fact uniform over the surface of an exploded emitter, but rather reaches very high values at a multiplicity of sub-sites where the tip profile locally enhances the surface field.

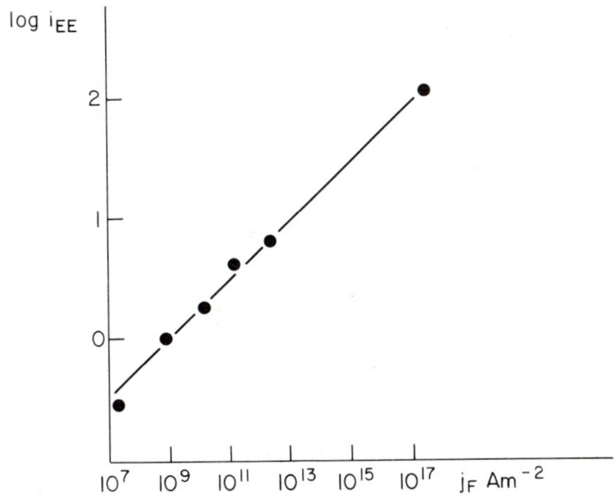

Fig. 5.16 Illustrating the exponential dependence of the explosive emission current i_{EE} on the electron emission current j_F. (From Fursey and Zhukov [15], with permission).

Although this detailed discussion of the breakdown processes that occur in a point-plane diode was justified on the grounds that it provided a valuable insight into the mechanisms occurring in the more complicated regime of a broad-area gap, there is one important respect in which the model developed in these last two sections has to be qualified. It will be recalled from the discussion in Section 3.4(i) that, with broad-area electrodes, the explosive emission current during the commutation period is space-charge limited and given by equation 3.47. This therefore implies that the degree of charge separation, and hence cathode field enhancement, envisaged by Fig. 5.13 cannot occur with this type of regime: indeed, as already pointed out in this section, it is only with the sharpest emitters ($r \lesssim 100$nm) that space charge effects can be neglected. The absence of an excessive positive space charge field in the vicinity of an emitter on a broad-area electrode has also been verified experimentally by Proskurovsky and Pucharov [21] by showing that the sheath voltage between the cathode and plasma flare is only $\sim$ 50 volts, i.e. of the same order as in d-c arcs.

5.3(iii) Rate of vaporisation of emitter material

From pairs of micrographs such as shown in Fig. 5.8, it is clear that cathode material has been vaporised to "feed" the cathode flare of an explosive emission event. The question however arises as to how the rate of vaporisation of emitter material varies with the evolution of the flare. To obtain this sort of detailed information, and thereby gain further insight into the explosive emission mechanism, a special pulse-arrest technique was developed by Bazhenov et al. [22] and later extended by Proskurovsky et al. [24] and Fursey and Zhukov [16,17]. Starting with a series of freshly prepared emitters having similar initial profiles, each of them was then subjected to progressively longer over-voltage pulses of constant amplitude so that the explosive emission mechanism was arrested at various stages in the i_{EE} current transient of Fig. 5.14. These "partially exploded" emitters were then re-examined in an electron microscope and from the change in their profiles it was possible to estimate the mass of material vapourised at each stage. A typical sequence of superimposed profiles might appear as illustrated in Fig. 5.17, from which it may be concluded that the highest rate of vaporisation of emitter material occurs during the initial rapid increase of the explosive emission current; thereafter, although the micro-profile may change in detail, with the appearance of numerous sub-micron protrusions extruded from the molten surface of the emitter by the applied field, the macro-profile becomes relatively stabilised with material vaporisation falling off rapidly to a very much lower and nearly constant rate. It should be added that the formation of these sub-micron protrusions and their subsequent role in initiating emitter "side flares" is a very important mechanism in the successful operation of commercial devices such as portable "flash" X-ray tubes and electron accelerators that use explosive emission cathodes.

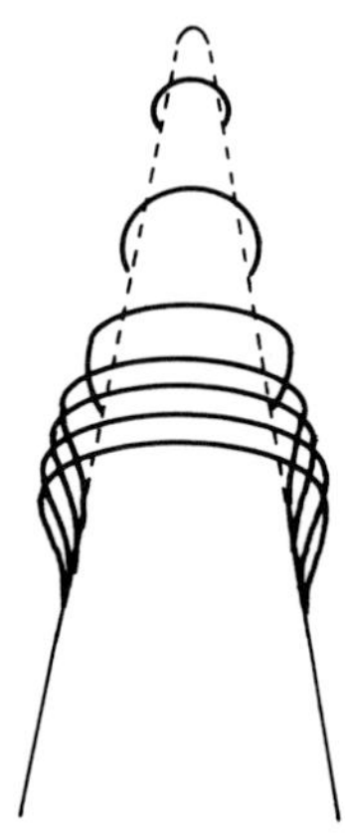

Fig. 5.17 A schematic illustration of how the end-profile of a tip is progressively blunted following a succession of over-voltage pulses. (After Fursey and Zhukov [15-17].

5.3(iv) Oscillatory instabilities with high over-voltage pulses

If the amplitude of the over-voltage pulse being applied across a diode is increased beyond the level discussed in the previous section, there is a further dramatic rise in the explosive emission current. This therefore leads to an inevitable increase in the physical complexity of the processes occurring in the gap: this is particularly true with broad-area electrode configurations such as exist, for example, in a practical device like a power X-ray tube, where the current levels can temporarily approach the kA or MA range. A characteristic feature of this type of regime is the occurrence of a wide variety of effects associated with the onset of plasma instabilities. Although this topic is of considerable technological importance, an adequate review of its extensive literature is beyond the scope of this book: accordingly, the interested reader must again be referred to such introductory texts on arc phenomena as those cited under references 37 and 38 of chapter 1.

It is however relevant to refer briefly to one type of investigation which is a direct extension of the experiments described in the previous sections. Thus, if the explosive emission current transient measurements of Fig. 5.15 are extended to even higher over-voltage pulses [23-25], perhaps $\gtrsim$ 100kV for micron-radius tips, a new mechanism comes into operation that gives rise to an oscillatory instability in the current transient. This is illustrated in Fig. 5.18, where the amplitude of the superimposed 30-60 nanosecond current spikes can be typically 2-5 times greater than the level of the "plateau" current shown dotted in Fig. 5.18. It was also established by mass spectrometry techniques that these current spikes coincide in time with intense bursts of high-energy ionic bombardment of the emitter. More

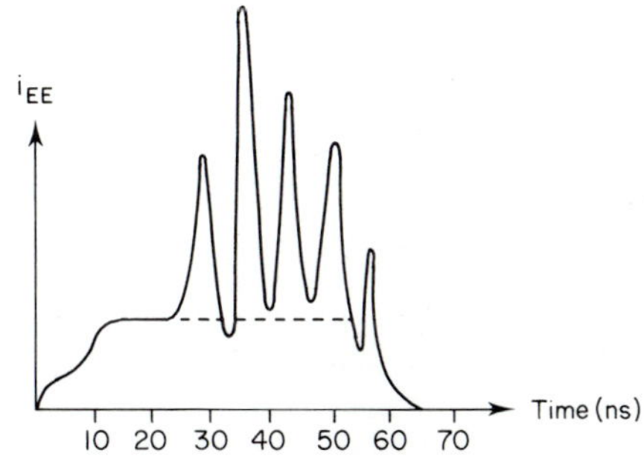

Fig. 5.18 A schematic illustration of the oscillations that can appear on the "explosive emission" current transient at high over-voltages. (After Korop and Plyutto [23,24] and Proskurovsky et al. [25]).

specifically, these ions were also identified as having originated from the vaporisation of emitter material, and that they had subsequently been re-accelerated back towards the cathode to acquire energies comparable with the gap potential. To account for these new experimental observations, it was necessary to revise the simple cathode-flare model of the explosive emission mechanism. Thus, recognising that the expanding flare plasma is electrically neutral and represents an equi-potential volume at virtually cathode potential, it follows that the external voltage V applied across the diode will be dropped across a diminishing "effective" gap bounded by the advancing flare envelope and the anode. This means that by the time the flare has half crossed the "real" gap, a very high field will be acting at its surface; sufficiently high in fact for it to penetrate the plasma and create a flux of "hot" electrons that further depletes the envelope region of negative charge and thereby greatly enhances the charge separation mechanism existing with the simple flare model. This process will therefore leave a highly localised positive space charge density in the vicinity of the plasma envelope and a consequent re-distribution of the gap potential as shown in Fig. 5.19(i) and (ii). The resulting positive potential peak, which can approach $\sim$ 0.8 of the voltage applied across the gap, therefore gives rise to a strong electric field that will

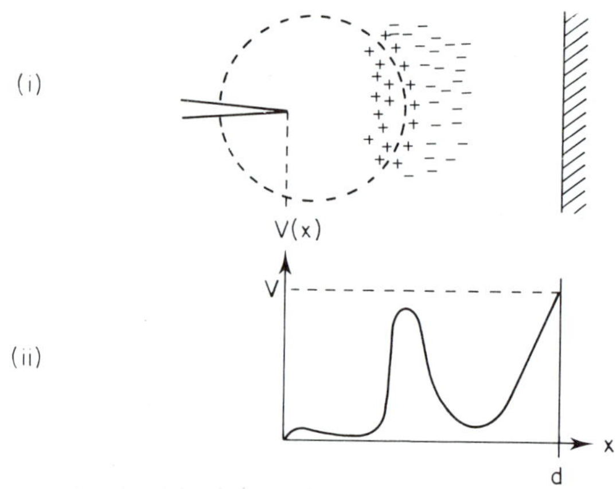

Fig. 5.19 To illustrate how a potential "peak" can form at the envelope of the expanding plasma flare where charge separation has occurred. (After Korop and Plyutto [23,24]).

accelerate the positive ions in its vicinity back to the cathode with energies approaching the maximum they could require from the total gap voltage. This flow of energetic ions then heats the emitting surface to a very high temperature and so gives rise to the initial current peak observed in Fig. 5.18. However, at this stage, the thermally enhanced electron flux is sufficient to neutralise the positive space charge, so that the potential hump of Fig. 5.19(ii) collapses and, with it, the heating effect of the positive ions. The emission current therefore falls until it reaches a value where the potential build-up for the next current peak can again be initiated. It follows that these oscillations will continue until the flare has crossed the gap.

5.4 References

1. Müller, E.W., *Z.Physik*, **106**, 541-50, (1937).
2. Gomer, R., *In* "Field Emission and Field Ionisation", Oxford University Press, Oxford, (1961).
3. Dobretsov, L.N. and Gomoyunova, M.V., *In* "Emission Electronics", Kater Press Binding, Israel, (1971).
4. Van Oostrom, A.G.S., *Philips Res.Rep. Suppl.* No.1, (1966).
5. Drechsler, M and Henkel, E., *Z.angew. Phys.*, **6**, 341-6, (1954).
6. Dyke, W.P., Trolan, J.K., Dolan, W.W. and Barnes, G. *J.Appl. Phys.*, **24**, 570-6, (1953).
7. Haefer, R.H., *Z.Physik*, **116**, 604-22, (1940).
8. Dyke, W.P. and Dolan, W.W., *Adv. Electronics Electron Phys.*, **8**, 89-185, (1956).
9. Dyke, W.P. and Trolan, J.K., *Phys. Rev.* **89**, 799-808, (1953).
10. Millikin, R.A. and Lauritsen, C.C., *Proc. Nat. Acad. Sci. U.S.*, **14**, 45-9, (1928).
11. Cavaille, J.V. and Drechsler, M., *Proc. VII-DEIV.* 217-221, (1976).
12. Dyke, W.P., Trolan, J.K., Martin, E.E. and Barbour, J.P. *Phys. Rev.* **91**, 1043-54, (1953).
13. Fursey, G.N. and Vorontsov-Vel'yeminov, P.N., *Sov. Phys. - Tech. Phys.* **12**, 1377-82, (1968).
14. Mesyats, G.A., Rotshteyn, V.P., Fursey, G.N. and Kartsev, G.K., *Sov. Phys.-Tech.Phys.*, **15**, 1202-4, (1971).
15. Fursey, G.N. and Zhukov, V.M., *Sov.Phys.-Tech.Phys.* **21**, 176-81, (1976).
16. Zhukov, V.M. and Fursey, G.N., *Sov.Phys.-Tech.Phys.* **21**, 182-6, (1976).
17. Zhukov, V.M. and Fursey, G.N., *Sov.Phys.-Tech.Phys.*, **21**, 1112-17, (1976).
18. Bougaev, S.P., Lopatin, V.V., Litvinov, E.A. and Mesyats, G.A., *Proc. V-DEIV*, 37-41, (1972).
19. Fursey, G.N., *Proc. III-DIEV*, 113-118, (1968).
20. Mesyats, G.A., Bougaev, S.P., Proskurovsky, D.I., Eshkenazy, V.I. and Urike, Ya.Ya. *Proc. III-DIEV*, 212-17, (1968).
21. Proskurovsky, D.I. and Puchkarov, V.F., *Zhurn. Tekhn. Fiz.* **49**, 2611-18, (1979).
22. Bazhenov, G.P., Litvinov, E.A., Mesyats, G.A., Proskurovsky, D.I,, Shubin, A.F. and Yankelevich, E.P., *Sov.Phys.-Tech. Phys.* **18**, 795-9, (1973).
23. Korop, E.D. and Plyutto, A.A., *Sov.Phys.-Tech.Phys.*, **15**, 1986-9, (1970).
24. Korop, E.D. and Plyutto, A.A., *Sov.Phys.-Tech.Phys.*, **16**, 830-1, (1971).
25. Proskurovsky, D.I., Rotshteyn, V.P., Shubin, A.F. and Yankelevich, E.B., *Sov.Phys.-Tech.Phys.* **20**, 1342-6, (1975).

6 Simulation Studies II – Microsphere Impact Phenomena

6.1 Introduction
6.2 The dust-source microparticle gun
6.3 Particle injection experiments
6.4 Impact ionisation measurements
6.5 Impact damage
6.6 Particle bouncing
6.7 References

6.1 Introduction

From the discussion of chapter 4, it is clear that microparticle-initiated breakdown is a well established concept. However, for most of the theoretical mechanisms considered, it is very difficult to obtain more than indirect supportive evidence for their occurrence, since the degree of control that can be built into direct measurements made on the complex microscopic system of an extended-area high voltage gap is very restricted. A more profitable approach for verifying the predictions of these theories has been to devise experimental techniques in which microparticle phenomena are studied in isolation under controlled laboratory conditions that simulate those existing in operational high voltage gaps.

The simplest type of experiment merely involves placing micron-sized particles either directly on the surface of pre-assembled electrodes, or in some form of specially prepared reservoir in the surface of an electrode [1-3], and showing that the voltage hold-off capability of such a gap is significantly lower than an identically prepared control gap that is free of artificial microparticles. In a very much more sophisticated version of this approach that was developed for studying the trigger discharge mechanism discussed in Section 4.6(ii), Martynov and Ivanov [4] used single 100μm diameter iron spheres that were electro-magnetically held to an electrode surface until the gap was suitably stressed. Upon release, a charged sphere is accelerated across the gap and, on approaching the opposite electrode, is discharged through a visible microspark or "trigger discharge" that is temporarily correlated with the breakdown of the gap. By reversing its charge during the ensuing impact, the sphere subsequently oscillates between the plane-parallel electrodes, giving rise to a succession of trigger discharge and associated breakdown events. Although this technique provided an impressive demonstration of this breakdown mechanism, its findings are only of limited relevance to most practical gap regimes since, as discussed in section 4.6(ii), the mechanism can only operate with large particles(>100μm diameter) which must be considered to be extremely rare occurrences following modern electrode polishing and cleaning procedures.

An alternative approach, that has subsequently proved to be very much more valuable for studying the impact behaviour of the micron and submicron diameter particles thought to be responsible for initiating breakdown events in operational gaps, employs the concept of using "externally" generated microparticles of known size, charge and velocity, that can be either injected into a high voltage gap or used in other experimental regimes for studying such phenomena as impact ionisation and impact damage. The findings from these and other studies based on this approach will now be reviewed in the following sections of this chapter.

6.2 The dust-source microparticle gun

Since the basic requirement for this type of investigation must clearly be some form of microparticle "gun", it was fortuitous that at about the same time that these microparticle-based breakdown theories were being established, an almost ideal particle source had been independently developed for micrometeorite simulation studies in connection with the American space research programme. The original design of this device, which is so named because the particles are derived from a reservoir of fine powder, was due to Shelton et al. [5], with subsequent developments by Friichtenicht [6]. Its operational principle can be understood with reference to Fig. 6.1, which shows the electrode configuration of the device. The powder, which normally consists of readily available carbonyl-iron microspheres of 0.1-5 micron diameter, with corresponding masses of 10^{-16}-10^{-11}kg, is contained in a re-entrant cup-shaped reservoir electrode R into which projects a bull-nosed snout from the charging electrode C maintained at a fixed positive potential V_1. To "fire" the gun, a negative-going pulse of ∿ 10 kV amplitude and 10-20 ms duration is applied through an external capacitor to R, thereby establishing a temporary electric field within the powder reservoir. As a result, the particles become positively charged by contact with the inner surface of R and, because of the mutually repulsive forces between them, "explode" to fill the reservoir, with a few escaping through the extraction holes H into the high-field gap between C and the accelerating electrode A held at potentials V_1 and V_2 respectively: typically, the "gun voltage" V_g ($\equiv V_2 - V_1$) is ∿ 10-15 kV with V_1 set at earth potential. The "extracted" particles execute bouncing excursions between C and A, and as a result, a few acquire a high positive charge by com-

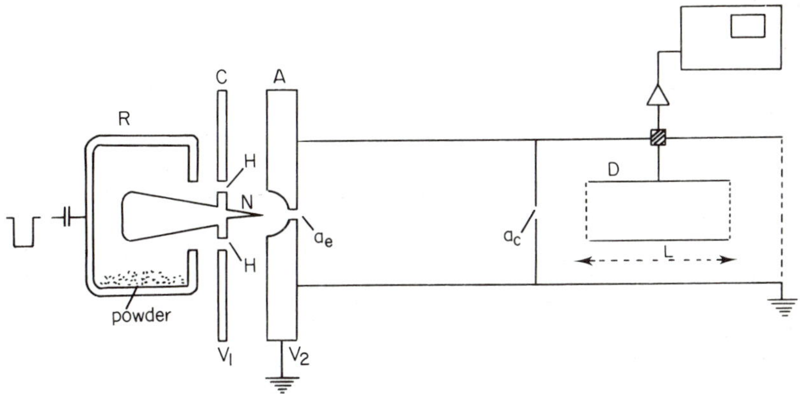

Fig. 6.1 Schematic representation of the dust-source microparticle gun and drift-tube capacitive detecting system as developed by Shelton et al. [5] and Friichtenicht [6].

ing into a glancing contact with the tip of the charging needle N located at the geometrical centre of the hemispherical aperture in A of radius 1-2 mm. These positively charged particles therefore experience a radial accelerating field so that those with approximately paraxial trajectories emerge from the exit aperture a_e of the gun into a field-free space; a supplementary collimating aperture a_c is also included to further select only those particles with axial trajectories. The needle itself is typically etched from a tungsten rod into a conical end profile with an approximately hemispherical tip of radius $R_t \sim 25\mu m$. If, therefore, the charging geometry is taken as a small sphere of radius R_p in contact with a larger sphere of radius R_t, an order of magnitude estimate of the equilibrium charge Q acquired by the microsphere can be made using the relation [5]

$$Q_p = \frac{2\pi^3}{3}\varepsilon_o(V_2 - V_1)\,\frac{R_p^2 R_t}{(R_t + R_p)^2} \qquad (6.1)$$

where for a 1μm diameter microsphere accelerated through 15 kV we find $Q_p \sim 10^{-15}$C; in practice, however, Q will be significantly less than this since, with a glancing contact, the charging process will be incomplete. It should finally be noted that although the device could, in principle, be used for generating negatively charged particles, by simply reversing the polarity of the electrode voltages, this mode of operation is not to be recommended since a negative needle voltage gives rise to high field electron emission currents that rapidly destroy the sharp tip of the needle and cause electrical breakdown of the gun.

The charge and velocity of the axial particles generated by this device are measured by a capacitive detector module [5] consisting of a coaxial drift-tube D faced with transparent metal grids that is connected to an external voltage-sensitive pre-amplifier of gain g followed by a storage oscilloscope. As indicated above, the overall charge sensitivity of this detecting system should be $\lesssim 10^{-16}$C, which nowadays can readily be achieved with a FET input operational amplifier used in the non-inverting mode as illustrated in Fig. 6.2. When a particle of charge Q_p enters the detector an equal charge will be induced on the drift tube, so that if the capacitance of the tube to earth is C_D, the voltage ΔV appearing at the output of the preamplifier is $g.(Q_p/C_D)$. Thus knowing g and C_D, which are constant parameters of the system, and measuring ΔV on the oscilloscope, Q_p may be determined.

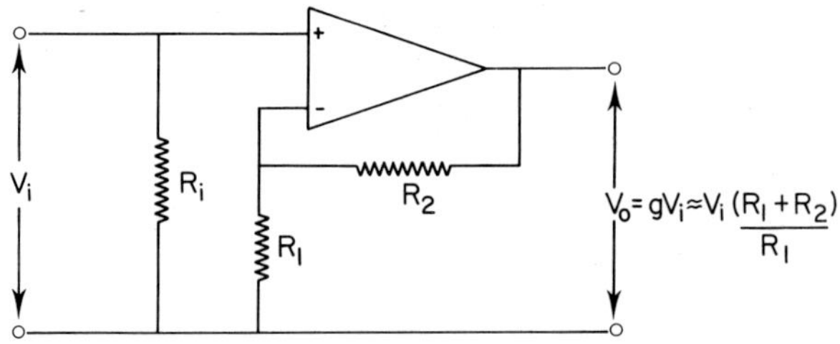

Fig. 6.2 The FET input operational pre-amplifier used for observing the voltage induced on the drift-tube detector by a charged microparticle.

A typical trapezoidal-shaped signal obtained with this arrangement is shown in Fig. 6.3. (Had the facing grids been omitted from the drift tube, the pulse would have been more rounded with less steep leading and trailing edges). The length of the pulse t_t represents the transit time of the particle through the drift tube, so that knowing its length ℓ, the particle velocity v is given by ℓ/t_t.

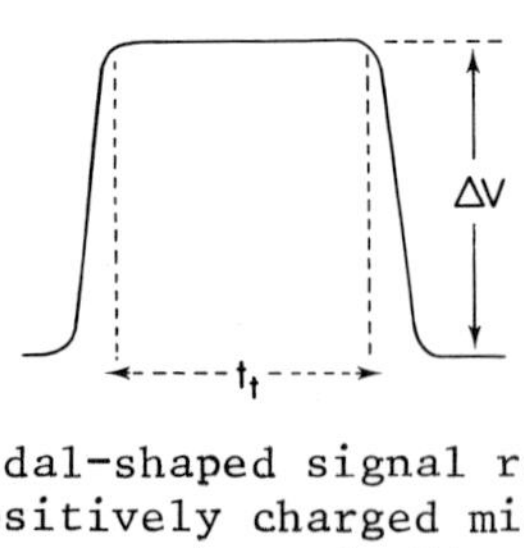

Fig. 6.3 The trapezoidal-shaped signal resulting from the passage of a single positively charged microparticle through the drift tube detecting system shown in Fig. 6.1.

Finally, if the particle charge is assumed to remain constant throughout its passage from the charging needle N, energy conservation requires that

$$\frac{1}{2} M_p v^2 = Q_p V_1 \tag{6.2}$$

from which the particle mass M_p can be calculated. Alternatively, the particle radius R_p can be determined if its density ρ is known, since $M = \frac{4}{3}\pi R_p^3 \rho$ for these spherical particles. From an analysis of a large sample of the type of single particle traces shown in Fig. 6.3, it is found that this type of gun delivers a spectrum of microspheres ranging from those with sub-micron dimensions that have typical charges and velocities of $\sim 10^{-16}$ and 1.5 kms^{-1} to the largest 5μm diameter spheres that can have charges approaching $\sim 5 \times 10^{-13}$C and velocities as low as $\sim 100ms^{-1}$.

In a more recent UHV version of this dust source gun, which was specially developed within the author's research group for obtaining a spectrum of low-velocity particles [7, 8], the needle electrode was replaced by a slightly splayed bunch of 7μm diameter carbon fibres. With this charging system, the operating voltage of the gun can be reduced from the 10 - 15 kV necessary for the needle charging system to only 0.5 - 1 kV for a similar spectrum of particle charges; i.e. representing over an order of magnitude improvement in the charging efficiency of the gun. This therefore has the important consequence that the particle

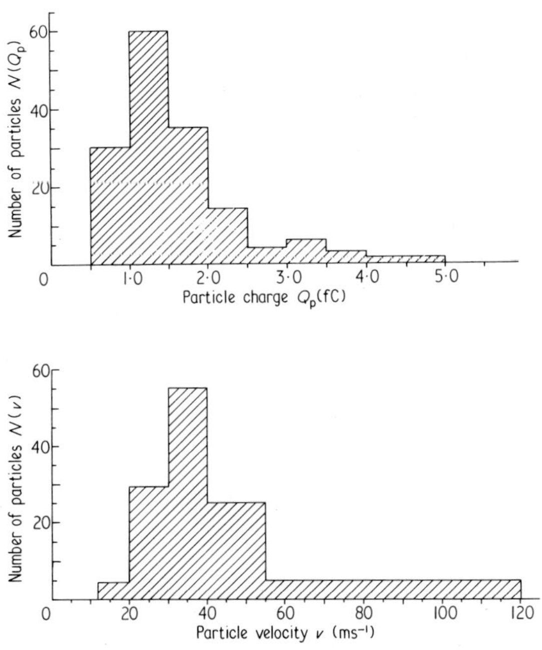

Fig. 6.4 Histograms illustrating the distribution of particle charges $N(Q_p)$ and velocities N(v) delivered by a dust-source gun using a carbon fibre charging arrangement.
(From Brah, A.S. and Latham, R.V. [7], with permission).

velocity spectrum is reduced to a range of $\sim$ 20 - 150 $m.s^{-1}$. Another significant advantage of this fibre charging system is that it provides a much more efficient device in terms of the probability of obtaining a paraxial particle per activating pulse. To illustrate the type of performance characteristics obtained from dust source guns, Figs. 6.4(i) and (ii) give respectively the charge and velocity spectra for a typical sample of 200 consecutive particles produced by this recent low-velocity carbon fibre gun: the spectra obtained for the needle charging guns have a similar form, although the velocity spectrum is naturally shifted to a higher range.

It is also possible to further expand the range of particle velocities obtained from any basic gun module by using either post acceleration or post deceleration facilities. Thus, with a megavolt Van der Graaff powered accelerating and focussing module interposed between a needle-type gun and the drift tube detecting system, as shown schematically in Fig. 6.5(i), hyper-velocity particles may be obtained; e.g., 2 MV acceleration can give particle velocities up to $\sim$ 40 km^{-1} [5, 6, 9-11]. Alternatively, with a two-tube decelerating lens used in conjunction with a carbon fibre based gun as illustrated in Fig. 6.5(ii), it is possible to obtain particle velocities $\sim$ 1 ms^{-1}. To this list of ancilliary facilities, there should also be added the post-gun particle mass and velocity selecting system developed by Rudolph [12].

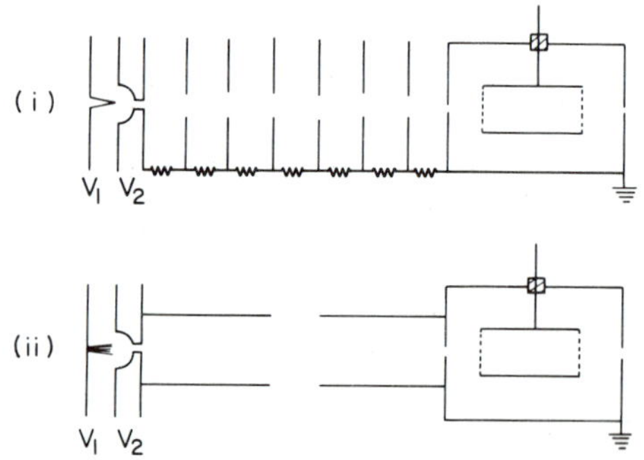

Fig. 6.5 Dust-source microparticle gun systems incorporating (i) post acceleration and (ii) post deceleration.

6.3 Particle injection experiments

The most direct and convincing laboratory demonstration that the breakdown of a stable high voltage gap can be initiated by the impact of a high velocity microparticle was provided by a technique originally developed by Slattery et al. [13]. In this, positively charged microspheres are accelerated to the hyper-velocity range of $\sim$ 2 - 6 kms^{-1} by the type of 2 MV system shown in Fig. 6.5(i) and then injected into the 10 - 30 kV plane-parallel high voltage gap regime illustrated in Fig. 6.6. The stainless steel electrodes of this 2mm gap were inclined at 45° to the incident particle direction in order that their impact zone is shifted from the surface region where the electric field lines are most distorted due to the presence of the 1mm diameter aperture in the low-voltage electrode. Particle-initiated discharges were detected with an oscilloscope by monitoring the current transients flowing in the 0.1Ω resistor connected between the low-voltage electrode and earth.

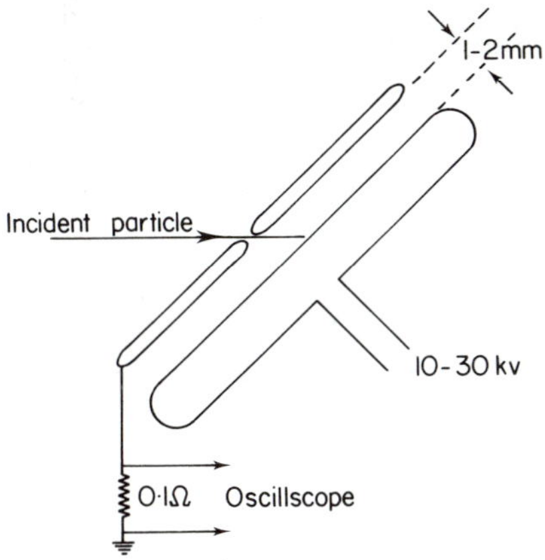

Fig. 6.6 Inclined electrode regime used for studying microparticle initiated breakdown in a plane-parallel high voltage gap. (After Slattery et al. [13]).

The findings of this investigation indicated that for a given gap voltage V there was a minimum particle radius $(R_p)_{min}$ and impact energy U_{min} below which breakdown initiation was very rare. For example, when V = + 15 kV results showed that $(R_p)_{min}$ ∿ 0.9 μm and U_{min} ∿ 0.8 x 10^{-7}J; if, however, V was increased, $(R_p)_{min}$ and U_{min} were significantly lowered, indicating that smaller particles were producing discharge events. It was also found that these thresholds were dramatically lowered if the polarity of the target electrode was reversed: thus, in the above example, if V = −15 kV, both $(R_p)_{min}$ and U_{min} are halved. The authors provided a qualitative interpretation of their data in terms of the Cranberg-Slivkov particle impact model discussed in chapter 4, which imposes the constraint that, before a particle can initiate breakdown, it must have a minimum energy sufficient to produce a gas cloud that is large enough to permit charge multiplication while simultaneously satisfying the conditions at the Paschen minimum. No explanation was proposed at the time for the polarity effect; however, in the light of more recent experimental findings discussed later in this chapter, and the concepts discussed in chapters 3 and 4, three possible mechanisms might be considered. Firstly, the gap field will give rise to a final acceleration or decleration of the particle, so that the impact velocities for a negative high voltage electrode are likely to be significantly higher than when it has a positive polarity. Secondly, the 45° angle between the incident particle direction and gap field means that a particle trajectory will depend on the polarity of the target electrodes so that the final impact angle could be similarly affected and hence the amount of impact ionisation generated [11]. Thirdly, the impacting microparticle could give rise to a new field emitting microprotrusion at which the local microscopic field is enhanced beyond the critical value associated with "cathode" initiated breakdown.

In a more recent experiment of this type, Chakrabarti and Chatterton [14] investigated in more detail how particle-induced discharges and the associated electrode damage are related to the size and velocity of the incident particle, and to the target electrode material. They used the cylindrical electrode geometry shown in Fig. 6.7, in conjunction with a 50 - 60 kV microparticle gun (see Fig. 6.5) that delivered positively-charged iron microspheres with diameters and velocities ranging between 0.5 - 150μm and 600 - 10 ms^{-1} respectively. The 0.05mm diameter central cathode wire, which was the target electrode, was either gold or tungsten and maintained at 0-60 kV with respect to the 3cm diameter concentric stainless steel anode: the cathode wire could also be externally retracted to provide a changing impact region for any given sequence of experiments. A photomultiplier was also included for determining whether specific discharge events gave rise to an emission of light from the gap. For the range of cathode fields used in these experiments, viz. up to around $4 \times 10^{7}\ Vm^{-1}$, it was found that microdischarge and breakdown events with an associated light output were only observed for

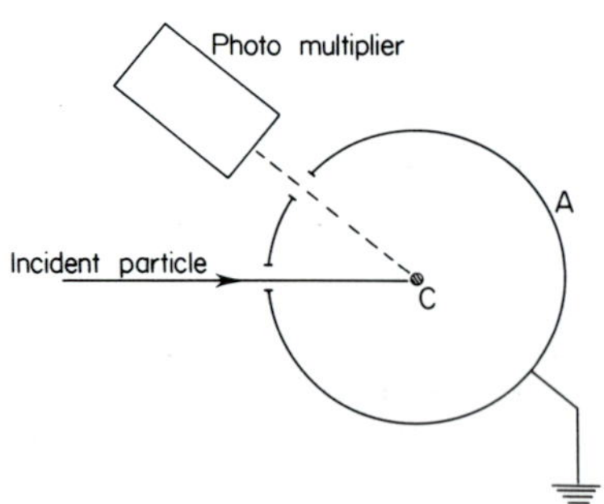

Fig. 6.7 Electrode regime used for studying microparticle initiated breakdown in a cylindrical high voltage gap. (After Chakrabarti and Chatterton [14]).

low-velocity microparticles having diameters ∿ 10 - 25μm: a complementary SEM examination of the relevant impact region of the cathode wire also revealed that such events were linked with the occurrence of fusion induced microcratering. Since however this damage could not be realistically explained on the basis of a Cranberg-Slivkov impact process with such slow particles, the authors concluded that this type of breakdown event was most likely initiated by the trigger discharge mechanism discussed in chapter 4. Although there was considerable evidence of particle melting and/or electrode indentation damage for the smaller particles with higher velocities, no incidence of discharges or breakdowns were recorded. This was a somewhat surprising finding, particularly in the case of the softer gold target wire, where the damage was more pronounced and appeared to include many microfeatures that could give rise to the type of unstable FEE processes discussed in chapter 3.

6.4 Impact ionisation measurements

Although the basic assumptions of the Cranberg-Slivkov particle impact breakdown initiating mechanism discussed in chapter 4 are widely accepted, it is nevertheless clearly desirable to have direct corroborative evidence of the associated phenomena, particularly the ionisation processes. In fact, there have been several major laboratory investigations directed at measuring the transient ionisation that accompanies the impact of high velocity microparticles [6, 9-11, 15, 16]. In all cases, these were conceived as simulation studies of micrometeorite impact phenomena, and used the type of hypervelocity, positively-charged microsphere facility illustrated in Fig. 6.5(i). Most of these measurements were however made with a low-field impact regime, and so it must be recognised at the outset of this discussion that their findings may not be strictly relevant to the high voltage gap situation, where the high electric field and electrode surface charges could well influence both the ionisation mechanisms and the development of the plasma. It is possible, for example, that as a result of charge separation, there could be a build-up of positive space charge in the vicinity of the impact zone which might give rise to a burst of "explosive" electron emission and associated ions, such as occurs during the development of the cathode flare described in section 5.3: i.e. the level of ionisation associated with a "passive" very low field impact event is generally likely to be significantly lower than that associated with an equivalent event in a high-field impact regime.

Our discussion of the main features of this type of investigation will be based on the work of Smith and Adams [16] as providing a recent and representative study of the phenomenon. Their experimental facility is shown schematically in Fig. 6.8, in which, for convenience, the two alternative operational regimes have been combined on the same figure. An incident parcicle with a velocity in the range 0.05 to 10 kms^{-1} is first characterised during its transit through the electrostatic drift tube detector

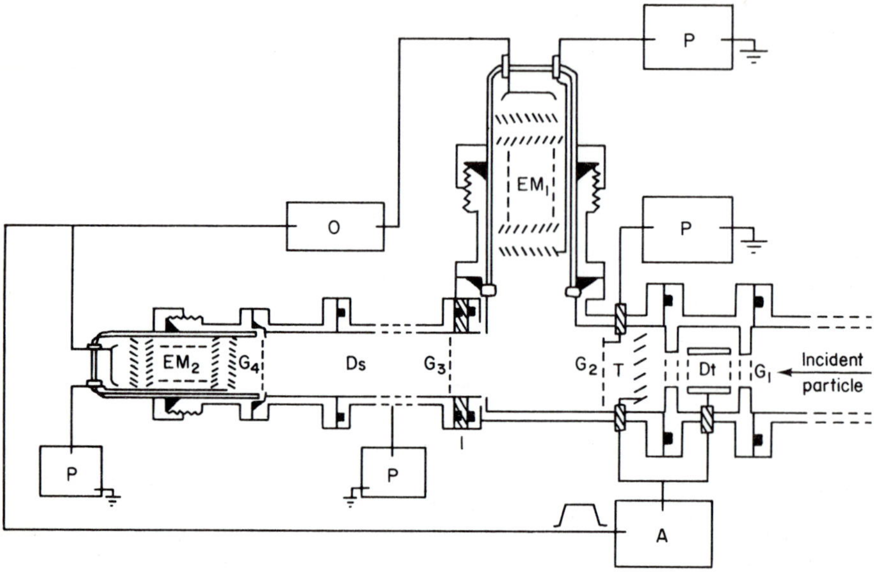

Fig. 6.8 Schematic diagram of a combined apparatus for (a) measurements of the ionisation resulting from the impact of hypervelocity microparticles, and (b) time-of-flight mass spectrometry studies of the ionisation products: G_1 are the screening grids, Dt is the capacitive drift-tube detector, G_2 the charge extraction grid, G_3 the deceleration grid, Ds the drift space, EM_1 and EM_2 the electron multipliers, I an insulating ring, A the amplifier, O the two-channel storage oscilloscope and P are the power supplies.
(From Smith and Adams [16], with permission)

Dt. It then impacts on a slatted molybdenum target T which allows any impact ionisation products to escape in the forward direction through the electrically insulated grid G_2. However, by biassing G_2 either positively or negatively with respect to the target, it is possible to extract either negative or positive ions respectively from the impact-generated plasma. The quantity of charge extracted from the target region is measured in terms of the resulting change in potential of the target as recorded by the amplifier A, which is also used to monitor the potential of the drift tube detector D With this arrangement, the storage oscilloscope O records the sequential signals from Dt and T,which appear as in Fig. 6.9(i) and (ii) for negative and positive ion collection respectively: in both signals, the particle of charge Q_p enters and leaves the drift tube at t_1 and t_2 , and finally impacts on the target at t_3. The liberated charge q_i is then obtained from these oscilloscope traces by subtracting the charge

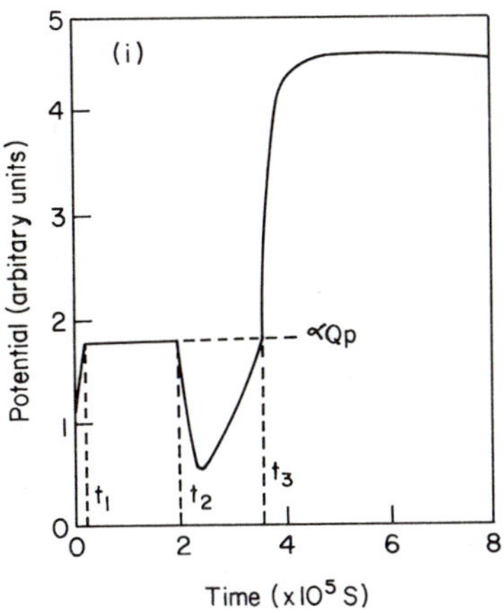

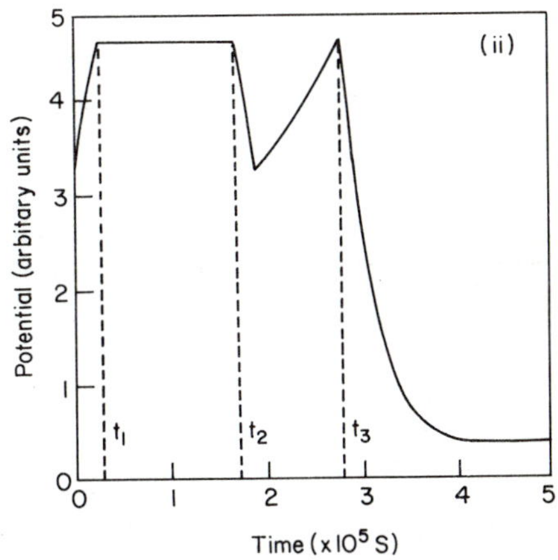

Fig. 6.9 Variation in the potential of the capacitive detector tube and target as a function of time when the potential of grid G_2 (see Fig. 6.8) is (i) positive and (ii) negative with respect to the target. t_1, t_2 and t_3 indicate the times at which the hyper-velocity particles enter and leave the capacitive detector and impact on the target respectively.
(a) $M = 6 \times 10^{-13}$kg, $v = 2.8$ km s^{-1}; (b) $M = 1.6 \times 10^{-13}$kg, $v = 3.4$ km s^{-1}.
(From Smith and Adams [16], with permission).

deposited on the target by the particle (viz. Q_p) from the total target signal. The electron multiplier EM_1 provides an alternative facility for monitoring q_i which, because of its greater sensitivity ($\sim 10^{-17}$C), is particularly valuable for extending the range of measurements to the low levels of ionisation found for low-velocity impacts that are beyond the charge detecting threshold of the target amplifier ($\sim 10^{-15}$C). By reducing the viewing resistor of EM_p so that its response time was $\lesssim 10^{-7}$s, the facility could be put to the further valuable use of measuring the rate at which charge was collected from the impact region.

It was concluded from this [10, 16] and similar types of investigation [11, 15] where refractory metal targets were used, that both the positive and negative charges released by impact ionisation processes follow an empirical relation of the form

$$q_i \propto M_p^{\alpha} v^{\beta} \tag{6.3}$$

where, to a first approximation, α and β can be taken as constants; several investigators [10, 15, 16] have in fact detected a second-order velocity dependence of α. This relation was based on data derived from particles impacting normally on the target; however, if q_i is measured as a function of the angle of particle impact θ , Dietzel et al. [11] found that there is a favoured value of $\sim$ (30-50°) at which q_i can approach four times its value at normal incidence for a given impact velocity. Accordingly, a more correct representation of equation 6.3 would be

$$q_i \propto f(\theta) M_p^{\alpha} v^{\beta} \tag{6.4}$$

The "maximum" associated with this angular effect has been explained qualitatively by these authors in terms of the compromise between the enhanced ionisation to be expected from the increase in contact area that occurs with increasing θ, and the

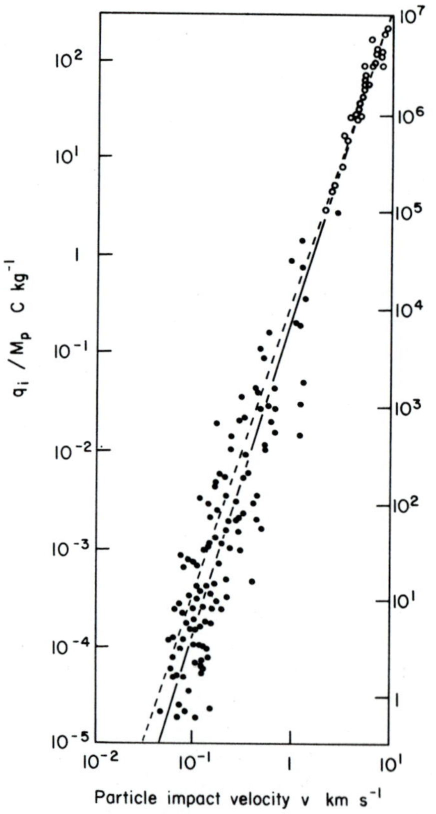

Fig. 6.10 q_i/M_p and q_i/R_p^3 plotted against particle velocity for the impact of spherical iron particles on molybdenum (closed circles). Also included is the data of Auer et al. [15] (dashed line and open circles) and of Friichtenicht [6] (solid line) for the impact of iron particles on W. The solid line also represents a straight line least squares fit to the present data. (From Adams and Smith [10], with permission).

reduction in the normal component of the particle momentum relative to its transverse (i.e. non-destructive) component that also occurs with increasing θ. A quantitative form of equation 6.3, for the case of normal incidence ($f(\theta) = 1$), was determined by Smith and Adams [16] from the type of log-log plot of q_i/M_p or q_i/R_p^3 against v shown in Fig. 6.10 as

$$q_i \propto M_p^{1.33} v^{3.2} \text{ for } 0.5 \lesssim v \lesssim 1 \text{ kms}^{-1}$$
$$q_i \propto M_p^{0.85} v^{3.2} \text{ for } \quad v > 1 \text{ kms}^{-1} \qquad (6.5)$$

where 0.5 kms^{-1} is the velocity threshold below which impact ionisation becomes vanishingly small.

The increased scatter of data points on Fig. 6.10 at lower velocities is a common feature of microsphere impact experiments and will be highlighted again in the following section. In the present context, its origin is discussed in terms of the partition of the incident kinetic energy, typically 10^{-11} to 10^{-7}J (or 10^8 - 10^{12}eV), among the various dissipating mechanisms available at impact, e.g. heat conduction, elastic compression, fusion and vaporisation processes (the latter giving rise to the measured ionisation products). Thus, there are two explanations for this scatter that appear particularly plausible: firstly, at lower velocities, contact times become longer, so that a relatively larger fraction of the incident energy is dissipated irreversibly by thermal conduction processes, and secondly, at lower velocities, certainly below 0.5 kms^{-1}, semi-elastic bouncing impacts begin to occur (see section 6.6) where a large fraction (possibly 30-50%) of the elastic strain energy is recoverable [17] and so is no longer available to "feed" the other dissipating mechanisms that can give rise to ionisation. It is also significant that both of these low-velocity phenomena would tend to produce an increase in the mass power index α, as is in fact found experimentally. The ionisation collection time measurements made by Smith and Adams [16] show that there is a variable build-up time for the ionisation in the range 5-20μs as the potential of the extracting grid G_2 is changed from 300 to 60 volts. Although it is tempting to speculate that the low-field value of 20μs might reflect the duration of the particle impact process, the authors tend to discount this possibility but rather attribute it to the influence of V_{G_2} in controlling the growth and extraction of the plasma.

Referring again to Fig. 6.8, the second type of measurement made with this apparatus [16] used a 3-5 amu resolution time-of-flight mass spectrometry facility to identify the ion species present in the impact generated plasma. In this regime, the grid G_2 has to be maintained at a potential $\sim$ -300v to obtain an efficient extraction of ions. Since, however, this potential gives the ions too high energies for operating the mass spectrometer facility at maximum resolution, a decelerating field is

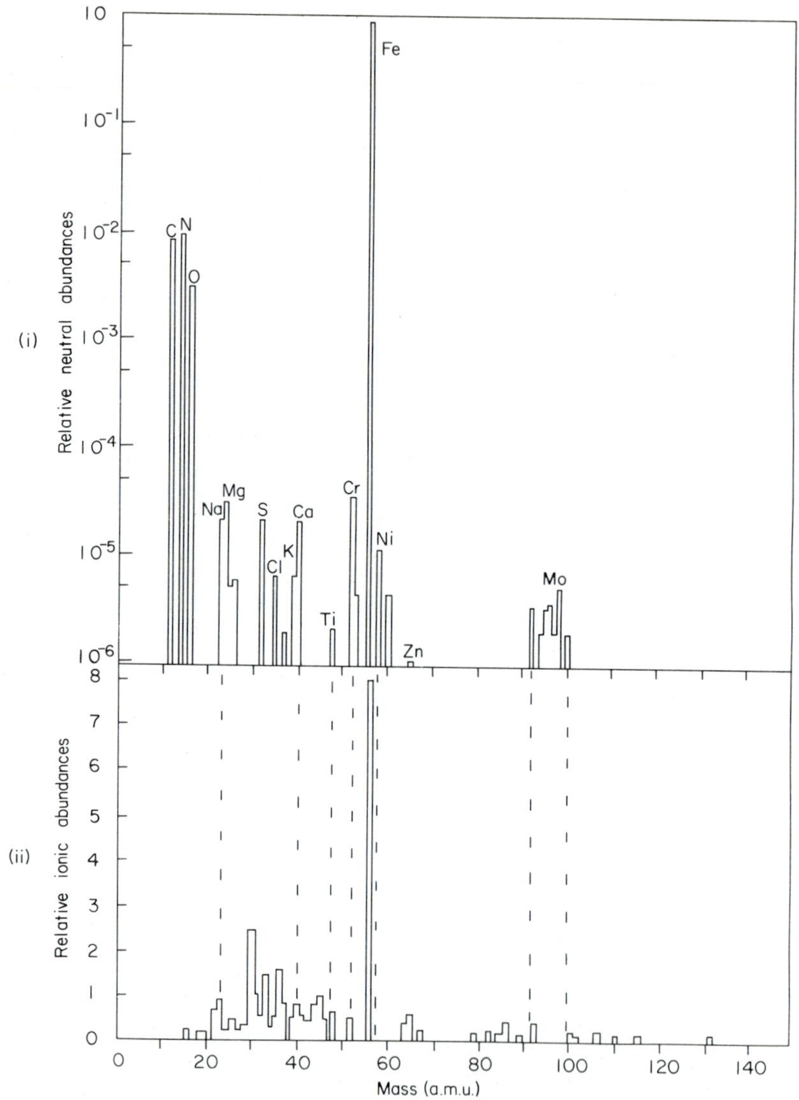

Fig. 6.11 (i) Relative abundances of the elements in the iron projectile material. (ii) A histogram of the relative abundances of ions produced at the impact of eight iron projectiles in the velocity range 2 to 4 km s^{-1} on a molybdenum target. The broken lines connect the two mass scales at some of the important masses. Note that the ordinate in (a) is logarithmic whilst that in (b) is linear.
(From Smith and Adams [16], with permission).

provided between G_2 and G_3 so that they enter the 50cm long field-free drift space between G_3 and G_4 with energies of several tens of electron volts. The distributed ion current, resulting from the separation of the ion species in the drift space, is recorded on the electron multiplier EM_2. A typical spectrum of the relative abundancies of the recorded ion species for a particle velocity range 0.5 - 10 kms^{-1} is shown in the histogram of Fig. 6.11(ii) for comparison, the chemical analysis of the particle material obtained by a spark-source mass spectrometer is shown in Fig. 6.11(i). The important conclusion to be drawn from this result is that the predominant ion species present in the impact plasma is the Fe^+ peak at 56 amu derived from the particle, with a barely significant contribution from the molybdenum target material at 92-100 amu. This type of finding is in agreement with the earlier investigations of Hansen [9] and of Auer and Sitte [15], using similar incident particles, but with tantalum and tungsten targets respectively, who also concluded that the target plays a relatively unimportant role in the impact ionisation processes for velocities $\lesssim$ 10 kms^{-1}. It is only when the incident particle velocity approaches $\sim$ 20 kms^{-1} that the recorded spectra begins to show evidence of target material being ionised: in fact, it is this property that has been exploited in satellite-born detection systems for analysing the elemental composition of micrometeoroids [19,20]. To explain this somewhat unexpected selectivity, it is necessary to refer to hydrodynamic projectile impact theories such as have been discussed by Dietzel et al. [11] and Smith and Adams [16] in connection with hyper-velocity microsphere impacts. This topic will be considered in more detail in the following section, but it can be stated at this stage that for the combination of materials and impact velocities used in all the cited investigations, theory predicts that the impacting particles will be preferentially "shocked" and thus lead to the selective ionisation processes found experimentally. To observe the opposite effect, where the target material is ionised, it would be necessary to use, say, a copper target with the same iron microspheres.

The identification of the subsidiary peaks appearing in the spectra of Fig. 6.11(ii)that dont directly correlate with those in Fig. 6.11(i) has been the subject of considerable qualitative discussion [9,15,16]. However, there is a consensus among these investigators that the two most likely explanations are firstly, the existance of multiply charged ions, and secondly, the general lowering of ionisation potentials due to the action of the strong space-charge based electric field that could exist in the localised impact microplasma (cf.the conditions prevailing in the cathode flare regime discussed in section 5.3). In connection with the quantitative application of the spectroscopic impact ionisation data to the development of a space-launched micrometeoroid detector, there has also been extensive discussion as to whether the ion spectra of Fig. 6.11(ii) are representative of their relative concentration in the initial impact microplasma [9,11,15,16]. This hinges upon the temperature and density of the initial microplasma, since the magnitude of these parameters will determine whether recombination processes are likely to play an important role in degrading the plasma before its composition is measured. In fact, the evidence is somewhat conflicting on this point. On the one hand, estimates of the initial plasma temperature [9], based on measurements of the relative concentrations of the ions ejected from the plasma, are in the range 3-20 x 10^3 ^oK for impact velocities of 1 - 40 kms^{-1} which, if the initial microplasma volume is assumed to be comparable with the indentation volume [20], strongly suggests that recombination effects would be important, particularly at higher impact velocities. On the other hand, there is no evidence to suggest that the collected charge q_i departs significantly from the empirical relation of equation 6.3 at high velocities, as would be expected if recombination processes began to operate. To resolve this contradiction, it has to be assumed that the initial plasma volume is considerably larger than the indentation volume, so that the initial plasma density will be sufficiently low to prohibit significant recombination. Support for this conclusion is provided by the work of Dietzel et al. [11], who developed a scanning X-ray microanalysis technique for a detailed study of how the particle debris is topographically distributed about the impact zone on the target surface. Their results show, for example, that for impact velocities $\gtrsim$ 5 kms^{-1}, particle material is deposited over a surface area that is more than twice the cross-sectional area of the particle.

6.5 Impact damage

From the discussion of chapters 3 and 4 it is clear that any physical process that changes the microtopography of an electrode surface in such a way as to create field enhancing microfeatures must be regarded as a potential agency for initiating one of the main breakdown mechanisms. Thus, microprotrusions formed on the cathode can become unstable field electron emitters and lead to either cathode or anode initiated breakdown (see chapter 3), whilst anode protrusions, for example, can greatly increase the probability of the trigger discharge mechanism occurring if microparticles are present in the gap (see chapter 4). In both cases, such microfeatures are frequently loosely bound to their parent electrode and therefore offer the possibility of being torn off by the electro-mechanical forces of the applied field to become potentially energetic "secondary" microparticles. The detailed nature of this impact damage, and how it depends on the physical parameters of the colliding surfaces has also been the subject of extensive microsphere simulation studies. In fact, this formed an important aspect of several of the investigations cited in the previous section.

The least drastic type of permanent electrode damage is the smooth-profiled indentation microcrater shown schematically in Fig. 6.12(i) that is formed when particle impact velocities only marginally exceed the critical value v_c beyond which elastic recovery of the interacting surfaces is incomplete; i.e. plastic flow takes place. For the experimental regimes studied to date, which mainly consist of iron microspheres impacting on a wide range of mechanically polished electrode materials [11,17,20] it has been generally concluded that $150 \lesssim v_c \lesssim 350\ ms^{-1}$; significantly, a similar order of magnitude is predicted from the theoretical approach of Cook [21] referred to in chapter 4.

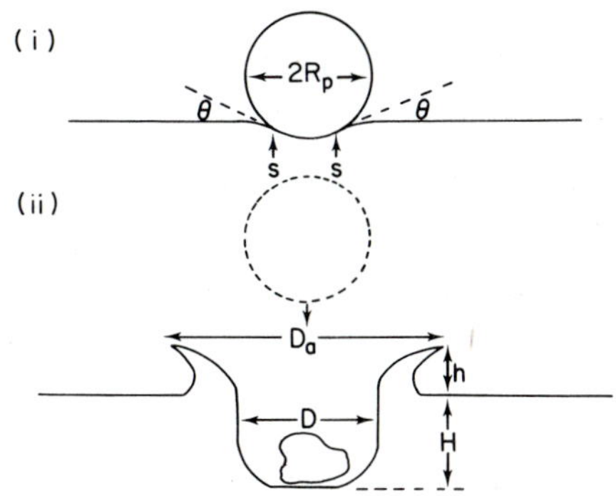

Fig. 6.12 Microcrater regimes produced by microparticles whose impact velocities (i) only marginally exceed the critical value v_c ($\lesssim 300\ m.s^{-1}$), and (ii) are well in excess of v_c, such that there is extensive plastic deformation and progressive melting of the impacting materials.
(After Rudolph [20]).

Apart from the possibility that the microparticle involved in such an impact event might "stick" to an electrode surface by some form of cold-weld process and so create a field enhancing feature, it can otherwise reasonably be assumed that the type of damage associated with this velocity range poses little direct threat to the stability of a high voltage gap. However, at velocities in excess of $\sim 500\ ms^{-1}$, the work of Rudolph [20] and later Dietzel et al. [11] showed that, in addition to severe plastic deformation, with the particle becoming partly or completely embedded in the target, localised melting of the impacting surfaces progressively contributes to the damaging process, so that the crater profile now begins to take the form illustrated in Fig. 6.12(ii). Viewed from above with a scanning electron microscope, these craters appear as shown in the micrograph of Fig. 6.13; i.e. very similar to the familiar "splash" microcraters found on electrode pairs that have broken down (see Figs. 7.9 and 7.22), and whose subsequent high voltage hold-off

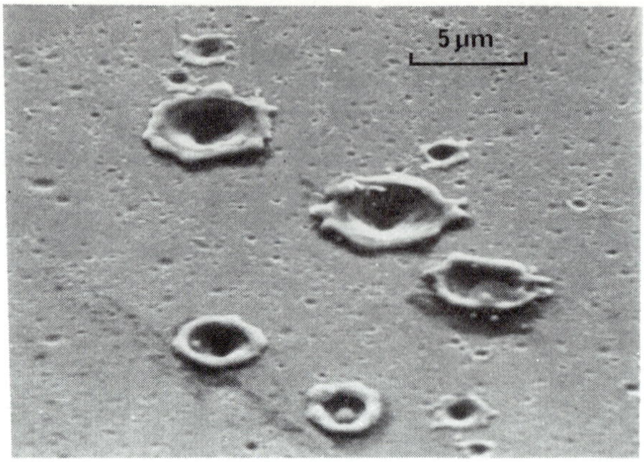

Fig. 6.13 A scanning electron micrograph of the type of high impact velocity microcrater illustrated in Fig. 6.12(ii).

capability is drastically reduced. From a detailed analysis of how the dimensions of the Fig. 6.12(ii) type of crater depend on the incident particle radius R_p, mass M_p and impact velocity v_i for a given target material, Rudolph [20] established the following empirical relations.

For $v_i \lesssim 1\ \text{km.s}^{-1}$

$$D \propto 2R_p \qquad \text{(i)}$$

whilst for $1\ \text{km.s}^{-1} \lesssim v_i \lesssim 10\ \text{km.s}^{-1}$

$$\left.\begin{aligned} D &\propto R_p v_i^{2/3} && \text{(ii)} \\ (\text{or} &\propto M_p^{1/3} v_i^{2/3}) && \\ (H + h) &\propto D && \text{(iii)} \\ D_a &\propto 1.5D && \text{(iv)} \end{aligned}\right\} \qquad (6.6)$$

where the constants of proportionality in 6.6(ii) and 6.6(iii) are functions of the target material, and are tabulated for Pb, Cd, Ag, Cu and Al [20]. The change in the form of these relations at $v_i \sim 1\ \text{km.s}^{-1}$ was identified with the onset of visible deformation of the embedded particle: a conclusion that was also supported by X-ray microanalysis studies of the distribution of projectile material over the target surface [11] and the velocity threshold for the detection of impact ionisation [10].

An understanding of the physical mechanisms that determine the character of microparticle impact damage may be had by considering the well established hydrodynamically-based theories of projectile impact. These broadly deal with how the material constants and velocity of the colliding media determine the partition of the incident kinetic energy between the projectile and the target, and hence their respective shock responses. From a discussion by Dietzel et al. [11], dealing with the impact of iron microspheres on a range of target materials (Fe → Au, W, Cu, Al and basalt), data was presented showing how the immediate post-impact energies of the target and projectile are divided between "kinetic" and "internal" (eg. elastic strain energy) components. Thus, for Fe → Au and Fe → W, the Fe projectile retains ∿ 55% of its initial kinetic energy with ∿ 10% appearing as kinetic and ∿ 45% as internal: for basalt and Al the reverse situation applies, whilst Cu has intermediate properties. In all cases at higher impact velocities, an increasing fraction of the trapped internal energy of the projectile is converted into irreversible heating, where the heating of the projectile is shown to be approximately proportional to its initial kinetic energy. In a complementary discussion, Smith and Adams [16] considered the behaviour of the shock waves that are generated around the perimeter of the contact disc, i.e. at s in figure 6.12(i). These will remain attached to this contact circle whilst its velocity along the interface during the compression process exceeds the velocity of the shock waves in either of the colliding materials. This will generally be true in the initial stages at low contact angles θ, but, for a given impact velocity, a point is reached where this inequality reverses for one of the materials. When this happens, its shock wave will become detached and result in highly shocked, high-energy material being exposed to the surface with the consequent ejection of vaporised and ionised material with accompanying crater formation. Theory shows for example, that for Fe → W or Mo, this detachment first occurs for the Fe-projectile, whilst for a Fe → Cu or Al combination the target shock wave is the first to become detached.

6.6 Particle bouncing

As discussed in section 4.7(ii), Latham has proposed a further development of the original Cranberg-Slivkov single-transit, impact-initiated breakdown mechanism whereby the kinetic energy of a microparticle can be enhanced to a critical value during a multi-transit bouncing sequence between the electrodes of a high voltage gap in which there is a reversal of particle charge and momentum at each impact (see Fig. 4.7). An associated theoretical analysis of the proposed model further showed that the effectiveness of this energy enhancing mechanism would be strongly dependent on the microscopic electrical and mechanical properties of the electrode surfaces. To test the validity of this concept, a laboratory investigation has been in progress to study the bouncing impact behaviour of charged microspheres under controlled experimental conditions that closely simulate those existing in a high-voltage gap.

The basic principle of the experimental technique used for these measurements is shown in Fig. 6.14. A positively charged

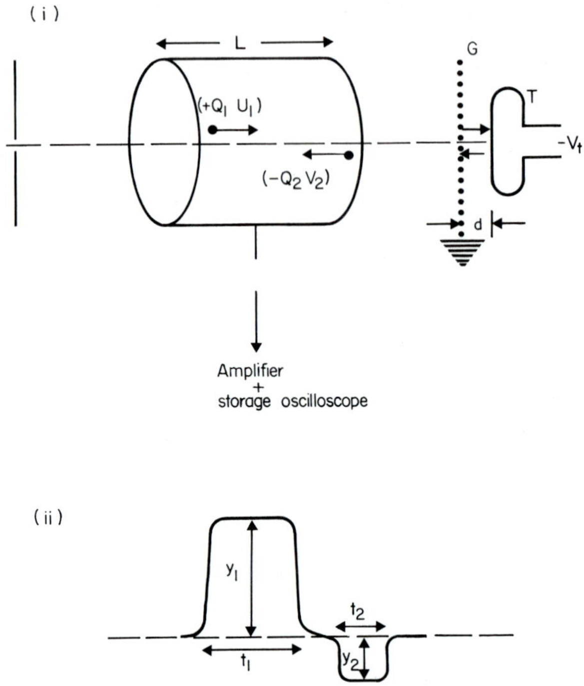

Fig. 6.14 (i) A schematic representation of the experimental regime used for studying the particle bouncing phenomenon: it shows the drift-tube detector, the high-field test gap and the incident and reflected particles (Q_1, u_1) and (Q_2 v_2) respectively. (ii) The sequential trapezoidal signals obtained from such a bouncing event.
(From Latham et al. [17], with permission).

microsphere with an initial charge Q_{p_1} ($\sim 10^{-15}$C) - or Q_1 to simplify the notation in this section - and velocity u_1 ($\sim$ 1-10 ms^{-1}), derived from the low-velocity source illustrated in Fig. 6.5(ii), is recorded on its first transit through the drift tube detector as a trapezoidal pulse of height y_1 and length t_1. It then enters a high field gap d ($\sim$ 1.5mm) formed between a transparent stainless steel earthed grid G and the negatively-charged target electrode T maintained at a negative potential $-V_T$, typically $\sim$ 5-10 kV. If, after being accelerated across the gap to an impact velocity v_1 , the particle then bounces off the target with a reversed negative charge $-Q_2$ and rebound velocity u_2 , it will be re-accelerated by the gap field to acquire a final velocity v_2 and be recorded as a sequential negative-going trapezoidal pulse of height $-v_2$ and length t_2. Since the magnitude of v_2 will depend upon both $|Q_2|$ and u_2, which in turn are

determined by the mechanical and electrical interactions of the impacting surfaces, it is convenient to study the bouncing phenomenon in terms of the two dimensionless parameters:
(i) $|Q_2|/|Q_1|$ - the ratio of reversed to incident charge, which is a measure of the charge exchange during impact, and
(ii) $|v_1|/|u_2|$ - the ratio of the rebound to incident velocities (i.e. the coefficient of restitution e), which is a measure of the momentum exchange during impact. In these experiments, the $|Q_2|/|Q_1|$ value is obtained directly from the detector signal as (y_2/y_1), whilst the e-value has to be computed indirectly. Thus, noting from Fig. 6.14 that $u_1 = L/t_1$ and $v_2 = L/t_2$ one has

$$v_1^2 = u_1^2 + 2Q_1V_T/M_p$$

which after substituting for M_p from equation 6.2 gives

$$v_1 = u_1(1 + V_T/V_1)^{\frac{1}{2}} \tag{6.7}$$

where V_1 is the effective accelerating voltage of the gun (see Figs. 6.1 and 6.5). Similarly

$$v_2^2 = u_2^2 + 2Q_2V_T/M_p$$

which after substituting for M_p from equation 6.2 becomes

$$v_2^2 = u_2^2 + u_1^2(Q_1/Q_2)(V_T/V_1) \tag{6.8}$$

so that finally from equations 6.7 and 6.8

$$e = |u_2|/|v_1|$$

$$= \left\{ \left[(L/t_2)^2-(y_2/y_1)(V_T/V_1)(L/t_1)^2\right] \Big/ \left[(L/t_1)^2\ 1+(V_T/V_1)\right] \right\}^{\frac{1}{2}} \tag{6.9}$$

The UHV experimental facility that was developed by Brah and Latham [7,8,22,23] for this investigation is shown schematically in Fig. 6.15. It is based on the low-velocity microparticle module described in section 6.2, incorporating a carbon fibre dust-source gun M_g, decelerating electrostatic lens El, gravity-correcting deflector plates P_g and drift tube detector Dt with its associated amplifier A. Trace A of Fig. 6.17 shows a typical example of a trapezoidal pulse obtained from this system for the passage of a single positively charged microsphere. After leaving this module, the particle enters a high voltage gap d formed between the earthed grid G and target electrode T which is maintained at a potential $-V_T$ via a spring contact and an insulated lead-through to an external EHT supply; typically d $\sim$ 2mm, $-V_T \sim$ 2-10kV so that the gap fields are in the range (1-5) x $10^6 Vm^{-1}$. There is also an in-situ choice of the pre-selected targets mounted on ceramtic insulating supports C_s that form the

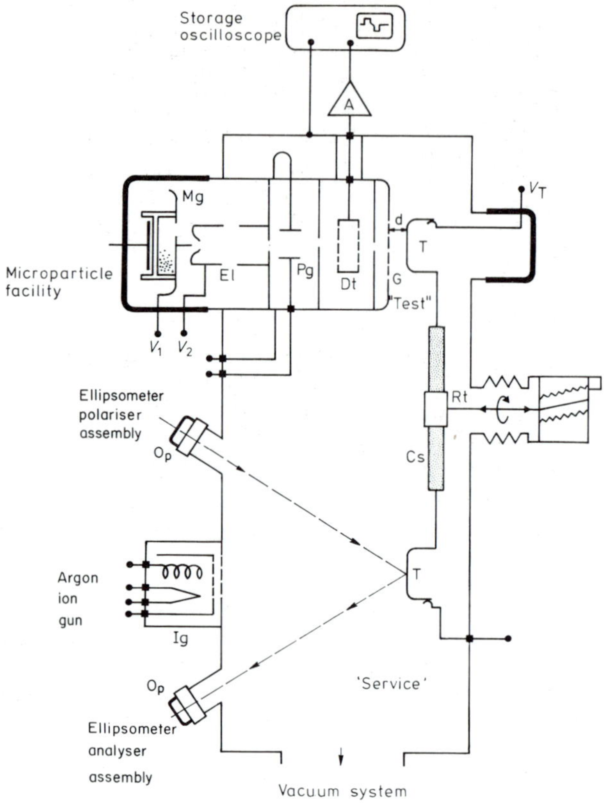

Fig. 6.15 The UHV experimental facility for studying the bouncing impact of positively charged microspheres in a high voltage gap. An argon ion gun I_g provides in situ cleaning of target surfaces, whilst optical ports O_p permit the ellipsometric monitoring of their atomic state.
(From Latham and Brah [23], with permission).

arms of an eight-spoke externally rotatable turret assembly. With this arrangement, a given target can be rotated from a "service" position in the lower part of the vacuum chamber, where an argon ion gun provides an in situ etching facility for cleaning electrode surfaces, to the "test" position in the upper part of the chamber, where it is on the axis of the microparticle source. To give the reader some perspective of the microregime involved in these experiments, Fig. 6.16 shows a 4.2μm diameter microsphere resting on a ¼-micron diamond-polished electrode surface.

The experimental chamber also includes optical ports (Op) for an external ellipsometry assembly [24] that is used to monitor the state of oxidation of a target surface whilst it is in the

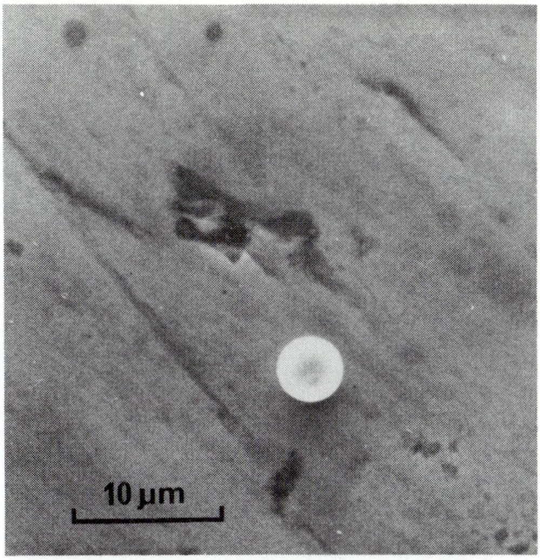

Fig. 6.16 A scanning electron micrograph of a carbonyl-iron microsphere resting on the $\frac{1}{4}$µm diamond-polished surface of a titanium electrode.

"service" position. Full details of this technique are beyond the scope of this text, and can be found in the literature [25, 26]. Very briefly, however, it depends upon the fact that if a beam of plane polarised light from the polariser assembly is incident on a conducting surface, in this case the target T, it will be reflected as elliptically polarised light, where its ellipticity, as measured by the analyser assembly, is determined by the wavelength of the light and the optical constants of the surface, viz. its complex refractive index n. From a knowledge of the n-values for the metal substrate and its surface oxide, it is then possible to determine the thickness of the oxide film: in its most sophisticated form, the technique can be made sensitive to the detection of less than a monolayer coverage. However, for the experiments described here, the facility is only used to measure the thickness of the ambient oxide film present on untreated electrode surfaces, and to determine when it has been removed by the argon ion electrode cleaning facility; viz. as indicated by the ellipticity of the reflected light approaching a constant value with time of etching.

Depending on the potential of the target V_T relative to that of the charging electrode V_1, three types of particle 'reflection' can occur.

(i) For $V_T > V_1$, a particle will be decelerated by the gap field and brought momentarily to rest in mid-gap before being re-accelerated on its return transit. Consequently, there will be complete in-flight momentum reversal with conservation of charge, so that the detector will see two sequential pulses of identical shape as shown in trace B of Fig. 6.17.

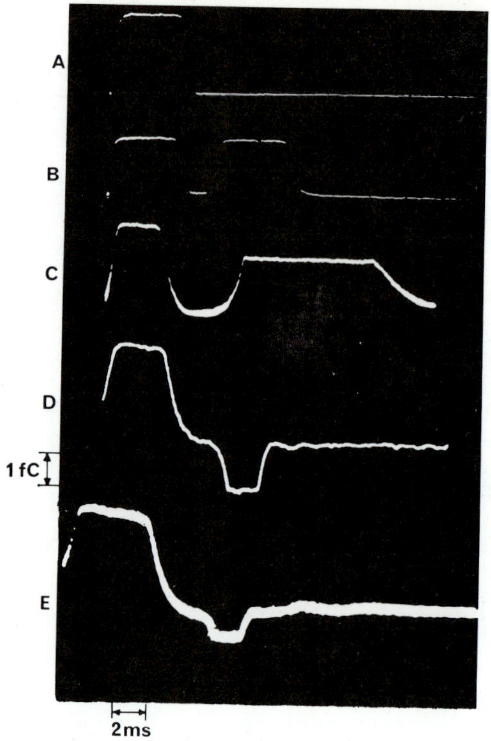

Fig. 6.17 Oscilloscope traces illustrating the important micro-particle events. In each case, positive particles have been used with an oscilloscope time base setting of 2 ms/division and an equivalent charge sensitivity of 1 fC/division. A, a single paraxial particle of velocity 10 ms^{-1} and charge 2.5 fC; B, in-flight momentum reversal $|V_T|>|V_1|$; C, bouncing impact with charge modification $|V_T|<|V_1|$; D and E bouncing impacts with charge reversal and velocity enhancement $|V_T|<0$.
(From Brah and Latham [7], with permission).

(ii) For $0 < V_T < V_1$, the particle will again be decelerated by the gap field but will now impact on the target to loose some of its incident momentum and charge. Thus, although the "return" particle will be re-accelerated across the gap after impact, its final charge and velocity will both be reduced, as indicated by the sequential pulses of trace C of Fig. 6.17.

(iii) For $V_T < 0$, a positively charged particle will be accelerated by the gap field and impact on a negatively charged target, so that there is now the additional possibility of the charge on the particle being wholly or partially reversed during a bouncing impact. If this occurs, it will then again experience an accelerating field for its return transit of the gap with the possibility of its kinetic energy being enhanced as previously hypothesised in section 4.8(ii). Two examples of this type of event, first recorded by Brah and Latham [7,22], are shown in traces D and E of Fig. 6.17, and clearly constitute an experimental demonstration of the proposed model. These traces also illustrate the wide variation in charge reversal efficiency and velocity enhancement that can occur; in trace D, whilst $Q_2/Q_1 \sim 0.5$ the velocity has only been enhanced by a factor of ~ 1.6, whereas in trace E, with $Q_2/Q_1 \sim 0.25$, there has been a threefold velocity enhancement. It is clearly this latter type of event which has a major significance in the discussion of microparticle initiated breakdown, and has therefore been the subject of a detailed study.

To illustrate the important conclusions to emerge from these measurements, we shall compare the bouncing interaction of carbonyl iron microspheres on $\frac{1}{4}$ μm "commercially" polished targets of titanium, stainless steel and copper; the first two of these materials being known to provide stable high voltage electrodes, with the third being acknowledged to be unsuitable for this use. In addition, we shall highlight how the surface state of a target has an important influence on the bouncing mechanism by contrasting the above characteristics with those obtained from the same targets when their ambient oxide coverage has been removed; i.e. where the microspheres are impacting on atomically clean surfaces. Since, as previously explained, the response of a surface is most profitably characterised in terms of the $|Q_2|/|Q_1|$ and e-values of the particle interactions, it is then appropriate in the context of the high voltage vacuum gap to investigate how these parameters depend on the macroscopic electric field acting on each of the target surfaces, which in this case corresponds to the gap field. Accordingly, Fig. 6.18 is a unified presentation of the mean trends of the $|Q_2|/|Q_1|$ and e-values for the "commercially" polished (state A) and atomically clean (state B) surfaces of each target material, as computed from extensive experimental data [8,23,27]. It is however important to emphasize that these measurements are characterised by a very large scatter among the individual bouncing events recorded at a given field [17]. This is not perhaps a surprising finding when it is appreciated how complicated and varied are the local microscopic properties of the type of polycrystalline electrode surface used for targets in the present experiments. For example, there will be a non-uniform oxide coverage that will give rise to a wide variation in the microscopic electrical properties of the surface, an irregular microtopography that will result in complicated particle contact regimes, and varying degrees of work-hardening that will have a large effect on the local mechanical properties of the surface [17]: in addition, there is the spread in particle diameters (0.1 - 5μm) which is likely to compound with these other factors.

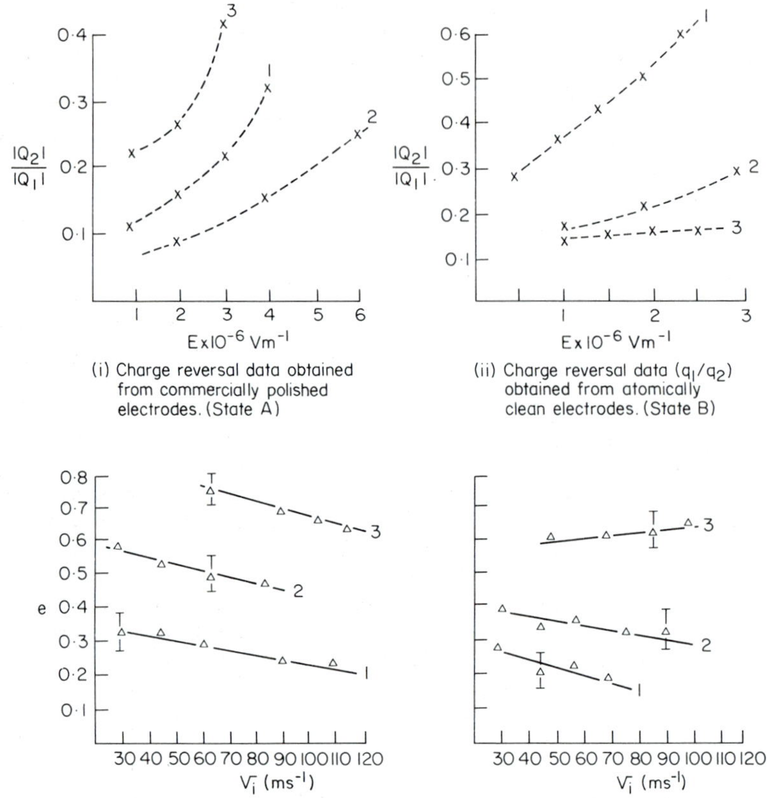

(i) Charge reversal data obtained from commercially polished electrodes. (State A)

(ii) Charge reversal data (q_1/q_2) obtained from atomically clean electrodes. (State B)

(iii) Coefficient of restitution (e) data obtained from commercially polished electrodes. (State A)

(iv) Coefficient of restitution (e) data obtained from atomically clean electrodes. (State B)

Fig. 6.18 The electrical and mechanical impact data obtained from a range of target materials, and showing the influence of the electrode surface preparation: in each case, curves, 1, 2 and 3 correspond respectively to copper, stainless steel and titanium targets. (After Brah, Mohindra and Latham [27]).

The most obvious conclusion to be drawn from the plots of Fig. 6.18(i) and (ii) is that the $|Q_2|/|Q_1|$ values of all surfaces,and hence the charge reversal mechanism, is very sensitive to the macroscopic gap field E. For *low fields* $E \lesssim 5 \times 10^5$ Vm^{-1}, which is a regime where breakdown is not normally encountered and therefore of little significance to the present text, the incidence of charge reversal is generally very rare, although it has been observed for titanium [8] and a limited number of other target materials [28]. For *intermediate fields* $5 \times 10^5 \lesssim E \lesssim 5 \times 10^6 Vm^{-1}$, charge exchange becomes more significant through a complex field-dependent mechanism that is also strongly influenced by the choice of target electrode material and its surface state. At *high fields* $E \gtrsim 6 \times 10^6$ Vm^{-1}, all experimental regimes tend to approach a common charge reversal characteristic that shows only a slow variation with applied field and no longer depends significantly on the physical properties of the target electrode. Under these high field conditions, it has been suggested [23] that the charge acquired by a rebounding particle will approach the equilibrium value it would acquire if it remained in contact with the electrode; i.e. as defined by equation 4.6. It should also be noted that the restricted range of macroscopic E-fields for which measurements are possible with state B surfaces is a consequence of the well known gap instability that results from the ion etching surface cleaning treatment of electrodes. For example, whilst 10 kV can typically be supported across a 1mm gap with a state A target, only ∿ 5 kV can be used for a state B target if breakdown is to be avoided.

A quasi quantitative physical explanation of the main features of such a family of charge reversal characteristics shown in Fig. 6.18(i) and (ii) is provided by the theoretical model of the process developed in chapter 4, where it was shown how the electron tunnelling between target and particle is determined by the local microscopic field E_g and the properties of the intermediate oxide film. In a situation where the particle and target have different work functions, ϕ_p and ϕ_T, as in the present experiments, there will be an additional "internal" contribution to E_g that can either enhance or oppose the "external" contribution to E_g derived from the gap field and charge on the particle. This effect will therefore give rise to either a "forward" or "reverse" biassing of the junction and be most evident in the lower field ranges when the external E_e and E_i contribution to E_g are comparable. On this picture therefore, three types of tunnelling regime are possible:

(i) $E_g = E_e$, corresponding to $\phi_p = \phi_T$ where $E_i = 0$

(ii) $E_g = E_e + E_i$, corresponding to $\phi_p > \phi_T$ so that the junction is "forward-biassed"

(iii) $E_g = E_e - E_i$ corresponding to $\phi_p < \phi_T$ so that the junction is "reverse-biassed".

In considering the interpretation of the data of Fig. 6.18(i) and (ii) it has first to be noted that the mean values of the quoted work function for the three materials under ambient conditions (i.e. equivalent to state A) are

$$\phi_{Cu} \sim 4.45 \text{ eV}, \phi_{Fe} \sim 4.47 \text{ eV}, \phi_{St.St.} \sim 4.5 \text{ eV}, \phi_{Ti} \sim 3.95 \text{ eV}.$$

It therefore follows from the above discussion that since $\phi_{Fe} \sim \phi_{Cu} \sim \phi_{St.St}$, the impact data obtained from the copper and stainless steel targets correspond to tunnelling regime (i) and that the enhanced charge reversal observed for State B targets has to be interpreted in terms of the reduced thickness of the intermediate oxide film as discussed by Latham and Brah [23]. In the case of the State A Ti-target, the tunnelling junction will be "forward biased" since $\phi_{Fe} > \phi_{Ti}$, and this will give rise to an enhanced charge reversal response that is clearly evident in the experimental characteristics of Fig. 6.18(i). The increase of the $|Q_2|/|Q_1|$ ratio for the State B Ti-target, which is in sharp contrast to the behaviour of the other materials can only be explained if it is assumed that the ion etching process has resulted in a significant increase in the Ti work function so that the tunnelling regime is altered from being "forward" to "reverse" biased: this effect is then assumed to predominate over the enhancement expected from the reduction of the oxide thickness. In support of this explanation, reference can be made to measurements which confirm that the necessary changes in the work function of Ti can occur following Ag-ion etching, the effect being attributed to ion impregnation [29,30]. As a final observation on the plots of Fig. 6.18(i) and (ii), it should be noted that the absence of charge reversal events at low fields can largely be explained by the fact that under such conditions particles invariably "stick" to the target surface [31]; a phenomenon that is thought to result from some form of particle-discharge welding process such as that proposed by Beukema [32] and described in section 4.5(ii), or that associated with electron scattering processes in the oxide layer of the MIM junction contact regime.

Referring now to Fig. 6.18(ii) and (iii), the significant lowering of the e-values for all three materials between their state A and state B surfaces can readily be explained in terms of the influences of the ambient surface oxide film which is generally known to be mechanically harder than its substrate metal. In addition, the reduction of the e-values with increasing impact velocity follows the behaviour associated with macro systems and has been discussed elsewhere by Latham et al. [17].

In considering the implication of these findings to the practical problem of the breakdown of commercially polished (state A) high voltage electrodes by microparticle impact following multiple bouncing discussed in section 4.8, it has to be assumed that particles will generally be of the same materials as their parent electrodes, so that $\phi_p = \phi_T$ and there will be no "forward" or "reverse" biassing effects: the charge reversal mechanism will therefore be controlled by the properties of the ambient oxide film [23]. If however the operational gap field exceeds $\sim 6 \times 10^6$ Vm^{-1}, which is frequently the case in practice, Fig. 6.18(i) indicates that all state A surfaces approach a common charge reversal response. Under these conditions any differences in the velocity enhancement from the bouncing mechanism must therefore arise from differences in the e-values. It would therefore appear that mechanically harder surfaces, such as would be provided by the refractory metals, would be more likely to promote the mechanism than the softer non-refractory metals.

Before concluding this discussion on microparticle bouncing phenomena, reference must be made to the investigations of Texier

[28,33,34] who, using a similar simulation technique, but with higher impact velocities (50-200ms^{-1}), has also studied the mechanical and electrical impact behaviour of micronyl iron microspheres on a comparable range of mechanically polished target materials (Al, Cu, Ni, Au). These measurements were however made under "commercial" vacuum conditions ($\sim 10^{-5}$mbar) without any in situ monitoring or treatment of the target surface state: also, they were restricted to an impact regime having a relatively low target field of $-2 \times 10^5 < E < +2 \times 10^5$ Vm^{-1}. The mechanical interaction was studied in terms of the coefficient of restitution and the dimensions of the associated indentation craters on the target surface, and shown to follow a semi-elastic type of impact behaviour as originally described by Tabor [35] for macrosystems. In common with the approach of Latham and Brah [23], the complementary electrical interaction between a particle and target was investigated by comparing the charge carried by an incident and reflected particle: however, the resulting data was interpreted using a simplified model based on the contact potential difference existing between the colliding surfaces.

6.7 References

1. Heard, H.G. and Laner, E.J., *UCLRL Report*, **2051**, (1953).
2. Olendzkaya, N.F., *Rad. Engng. Electron Phys.* **8**, 423-9, (1963).
3. Little, R.P. and Smith, T.S., *Proc.II-DEIV*, **41-49**, (1966).
4. Martynov, E.P. and Ivanov, V.A., *Rad. Engng. Electron Phys.* **14**, 1732-7, (1969).
5. Shelton, H., Hendricks, Jr. C.D. and Wuerker, R.F., *J.Appl. Phys.* **31**, 1243-7, (1960).
6. Friichtenicht, J.F., *Nucl. Instrum. Meth.* **28**, 70-8, (1964).
7. Brah, A.S. and Latham, R.V., *J.Phys.E: Sci.Instrum.* **9**, 119-23, (1976).
8. Brah, A.S., *Ph.D. Thesis*, University of Aston in Birmingham, (1978).
9. Hansen, D.O., *Appl. Phys. Lett.* **13**, 89-91, (1968).
10. Adams, N.G. and Smith, D., *Planet Space Sci.* **19**, 195-204, (1971).
11. Dietzel, H., Neakum, G. and Rauser, P., *J. Geophys. Res.* **77**, 1375-95, (1972).
12. Rudolph, V., *Z. Naturforsch.* **21a**, 1993-98, (1966).
13. Slattery, J.C., Friichtenicht, J.F. and Hansen, D.O., *Appl. Phys. Lett.* **7**, 23-28, (1965).
14. Chakrabarti, A.K. and Chatterton, P.A., *J. Appl. Phys.* **47**, 5320-28, (1976).
15. Auer, S., Grun, E., Rauser, P., Rudolph, V. and Sitte, K., *Space Research VIII*, North Holland, Amsterdam, 606-16, (1968).
16. Smith, D. and Adams, N.G., *J. Phys. D: Appl. Phys.* **6**, 700-719, (1973).

17. Latham, R.V., Brah, A.S., Fok, K. and Woods, M.O., *J. Phys. D: Appl. Phys.* **10**, 139-150 (1977).
18. Auer, S. and Sitte, K., *Earth Planet Sci. Lett.* **4**, 178-83, (1968).
19. Bandermann, L.W. and Singer, S.F., *Rev. Geophys.* **7**, 759-97, (1969).
20. Rudolph, V., *Z.Naturforsch.* **24a**, 326-331, (1969).
21. Cook, M.A., *In* "The Science of High Explosives", Reinhold, New York, (1958).
22. Brah, A.S. and Latham, R.V., *J. Phys.D: Appl. Phys.* **8**, L109-11, (1975).
23. Latham, R.V. and Brah, A.S., *J. Phys. D: Appl. Phys.* **10**, 151-67, (1977).
24. Fane, R.W., Neal, W.E.J. and Latham, R.V., *J. Appl. Phys*, **44**, 740-3, (1973).
25. Winterbottom, A.B., *J. Iron Steel Inst. Lond.* **156**, 9-21, (1950).
26. Archer, R.J., *J. Opt. Soc. Am.* **52**, 970-81, (1962).
27. Brah, A.S., Mohindra, S. and Latham, R.V., *Proc. VIII-DEIV*, **C6**. 1-9, (1978).
28. Texier, C., *Proc. VII-DEIV*, 92-96, (1976).
29. Smith, T., *Surface Sci.* **27**, 45-9, (1971).
30. Chang, Y.W., Lo, W.J. and Samorjai, G.A., *Surface Sci.* **64**, 588-94, (1977).
31. Cook, S. and Latham, R.V., *Proc. IX-DEIV, Physica,* **104c**, (1981), In press.
32. Beukema, G.P., *J. Phys.D: Appl. Phys.* **7**, 1740-55, (1974).
33. Texier, C., *Rev. Phys. Appl. (France)*, **13**, 13-22, (1978).
34. Texier, C., *Rev. Phys. Appl. (France)*, **13**, 165-70, (1978).
35. Tabor, D., *Proc. Roy. Soc.* **A192**, 247-74, (1948).

7 Diagnostic Studies of Electrode and Gap Phenomena

7.1 Electron emission orientated studies

(i) Emission imaging

(ii) Emission site location by "indirect" techniques

(iii) Emission site location by "direct" techniques

(iv) Gas desorption

(v) Optical emission spectra

(vi) Electron emission spectra

7.2. Microparticle orientated studies

(i) Particle detection by "indirect" techniques

(ii) Particle detection by "direct" in-flight techniques

7.3 References

In parallel with the development of the electron emission and microparticle based theoretical models for breakdown initiation and their associated laboratory simulation studies, there has been an on-going effort to devise increasingly sophisticated experimental techniques for identifying and studying the fundamental physical processes associated with these models in "real gap" situations. Wherever possible, the emphasis has been to link a diagnostic facility directly with an operational HV gap so that "dynamic" in situ measurements of a particular phenomenon can be made.

The aim of the present chapter is therefore to provide a review of those investigations that have led to an important insight into the processes occurring on both electrode surfaces and in the gap between them. It must however be added that in most instances it will only be possible to give an outline description of the experimental principles involved, leaving the reader to refer to the relevant source publication for further details of the instrumental complexities and ancilliary procedures.

7.1 Electron emission based phenomena

The most widely studied phenomenon resulting from electron emission processes is the finite prebreakdown conductivity of a high voltage gap as represented by the F-N plot of its current-voltage characteristic. This topic was extensively discussed in Chapter 2 where it was shown how such plots can provide "indirect" information about the microscopic properties of the emitting regime, including its geometry, work function and emitting area. In the present section, we shall be concentrating on describing specialised experimental techniques that have been developed for making "direct" quantitative measurements of the physical parameters of these emission sites.

7.1(i) Emission imaging

The basic concept behind this type of experiment is to use some sort of anode electrode that is capable of recording the spatial distribution of any impinging electrons. An obvious first approach would therefore be to replace the conventional anode of a high voltage gap by a phosphor screen. It is found however that such a technique is unsatisfactory, particularly with millimeter gap regimes, since the electro-mechanical forces associated with the high interelectrode fields tend to strip the phosphor particles from their glass substrate and precipitate the premature breakdown of such a gap, presumably by microparticle-based mechanisms. A better approach would be to use an anode that is faced with an electron sensitive chemical medium such as a silver iodide crystal or a film of photographic emulsion, although here again the use of such surfaces is not entirely satisfactory since, apart from also being prone to damage by the high gap fields, they can

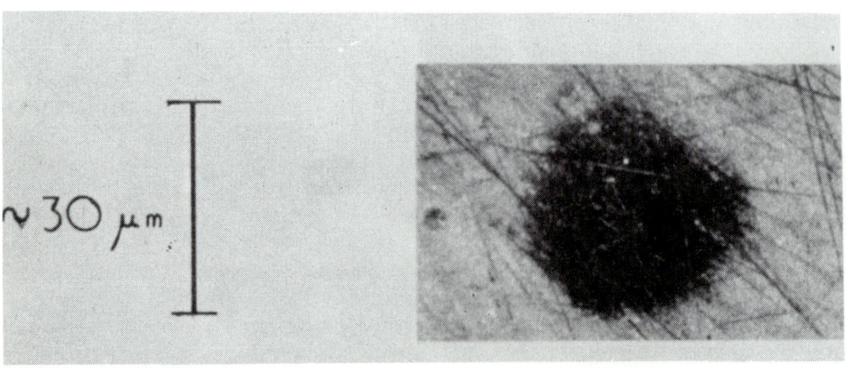

Fig. 7.1 An optical micrograph of a "burn mark" on a diamond polished copper anode.
(From Latham and Braun [1], with permission).

hardly be said to faithfully simulate the conditions existing in a normal vacuum gap. It happens however, that the earliest satisfactory evidence of the discrete nature of emission sites was obtained fortuitously as a consequence of the poor vacuum conditions ($\lesssim 10^{-5}$mbar) available at that time. Under such conditions, high-energy bombarding electrons will "crack" the large organic pumping oil molecules that are inevitably present on electrode surfaces so that any local region that is subjected to continuous electron bombardment will be "marked" by a build-up of carbon. Such surface features, of which Fig. 7.1 is a typical example [1], have come to be known as "burn marks" and can be used to measure the diameter $2R_a$ of the electron impact zone referred to in Section 3.2(ii). For millimeter gaps, $2R_a$ is typically

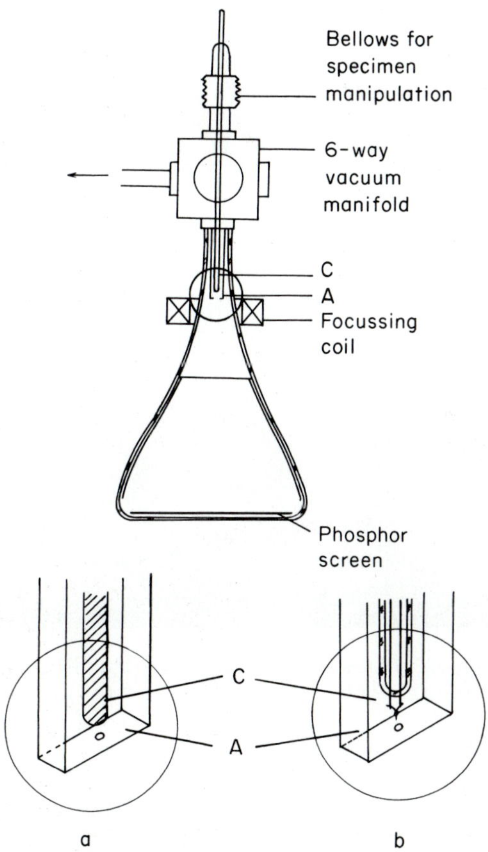

Fig. 7.2 A field emission microscope facility for studying the electron emission from small-area electrodes. Inserts (a) and (b) show respectively the specimen assemblies for "rounded" and "micropoint" cathodes.
(From Juttner [6], with permission).

∿ 5-10μm, which, when substituted into the electron trajectory equations 3.31 to 3.35, confirm that the associated emitters have microscopic dimensions.

A more versatile approach to emission imaging is to use a transparent grid anode with a phosphor screen placed behind this in the field-free space [2-6]. This type of technique has not only provided further positive identification of the discrete nature of emitting sites, but has also been used to identify the spatial location of individual breakdown events [5]. With small-area cathodes, Tomaschke et al. [4] and later Jüttner [6] were able to use a projection technique based on a modified field emission microscopic regime. The system used by Jüttner [6] is illustrated in Fig. 7.2, where an image of the emission sites on a 5mm diameter rounded molybdenum cathode C (insert a), or on tungsten microtips of radius ∿ 250nm (insert b), can be projected onto a phosphor screen. In this arrangement, the apertured anode A acts as an electron "extracting" electrode such as used in field emission electron guns [7]; i.e. it provides the necessary cathode field but allows a large percentage of the resulting emission to be projected onto the screen. Fig. 7.3 is an example of the type of image obtained from emission sites found on these rounded cathodes, and is seen to be characterised by a random distribution of sub-emission centres, each having emission

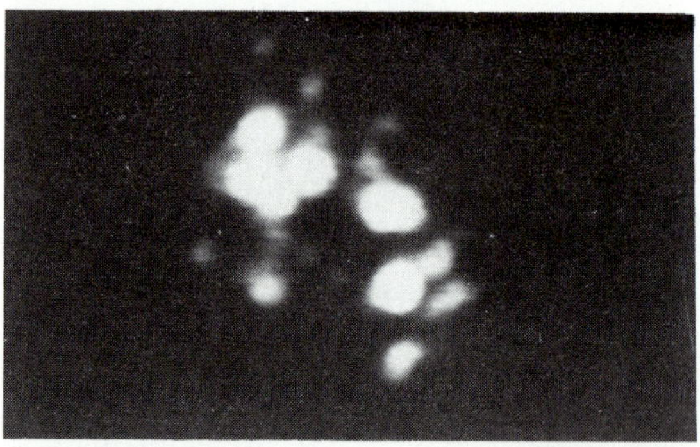

Fig. 7.3 A typical projection image of the electron emission processes that occur with the "rounded" type of cathode shown in Fig. 7.2.
(From Juttner [6], with permission).

areas with linear dimensions of ∿ 5nm. Another important characteristic of these images is that they appear to "flicker", which is caused by individual sub-emission centres randomly switching on and off; not surprisingly, this phenomenon also gives rise to a complementary "pulsing" of the total emission current. It is particularly significant that Tomaschke et al. [4] found that this instability persisted even down to liquid helium temperature since such behaviour is quite contrary to normal experience with metallic micropoint field emitters: in fact, this observation will be referred to again in Chapter 8 when discussing a non-metallic type of electron emission mechanism.

The immediate visual response of this type of technique also makes it a particularly valuable tool for studying the influence of physi and chemi-sorption processes on the emission properties of the sites found on such semi broad-area electrodes. For example, Jüttner et al. [8] have conducted a detailed investigation into how the corrosive action of such gases as CO, CO_2 and H_2O in the pressure range 10^{-10}-10^{-7}mbar affects the long-term spatial distribution and stability of the electron emission drawn from these types of cathode. These studies showed that such corrosion processes resulted in an initially bright and well defined emission image from an atomically clean surface becoming progressively "granulated" by the creation of numerous secondary sub-microscopic emission centres thought to be whisker-like structures having emitting area dimensions of $\sim$ 5-10nm. Accompanying this change, which occurs at a constant gap voltage, it was also found that there is a dramatic decrease in the total emission current level which was attributed to an increase in work function following the initial corrosive action of these gases. There is however a partial recovery of both the emission image and the total current level over a period of 2-3 hrs, due apparently to the partial removal of these corrosive layers by the sputtering action of positive ions formed by the impact of those electrons that are trimmed by the anode; an explanation that was also supported by Auger spectroscopy studies. These corrosion processes could also be important in the understanding of the electron emission mechanisms operating at the microscopic sites on broad-area electrodes and will therefore be referred to again in Chapter 8, when discussing the interpretation of the electron energy spectra of the emission from such sites.

An alternative approach to identifying the emission sites on broad-area electrodes is to employ the type of manual scanning technique developed by Cox and Wort [9]. This is illustrated schematically in Fig. 7.4(i), and shows how the cathode C is effectively scanned in a raster pattern in front of an anode A having a fine probe hole of 0.1mm diameter behind which there is a Faraday cage collector FC and picoammeter detecting facility to record any current passing through the anode probe hole. The type of current contour map obtained with this arrangement is shown in Fig. 7.4(ii). However, as discussed later (see Fig. 7.11) it is possible to refine such a system to obtain more detailed contour plots that resolve the spatial distribution of the electron current density associated with individual emitting sites.

7.1(ii) Emission site location - indirect techniques

With the recognition that the emitting sites on broad-area electrodes had sub-micron dimensions, it also became clear that the resolution of optical microscopy was too low for obtaining

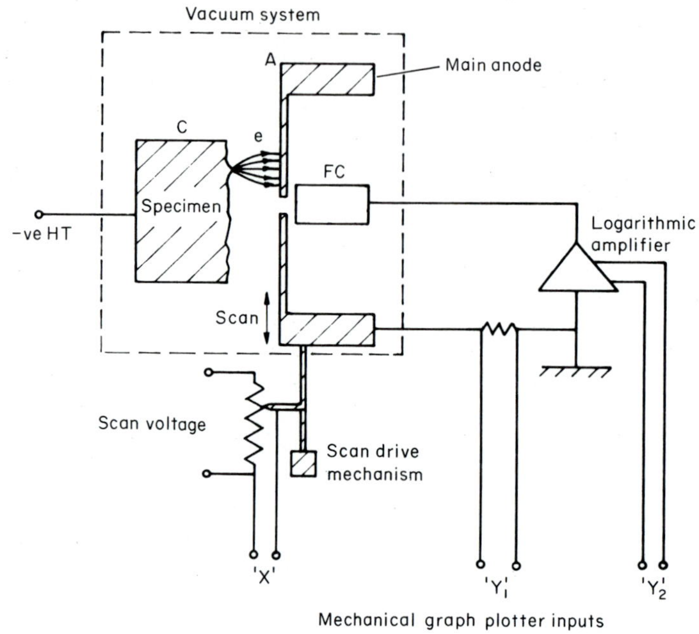

(i)

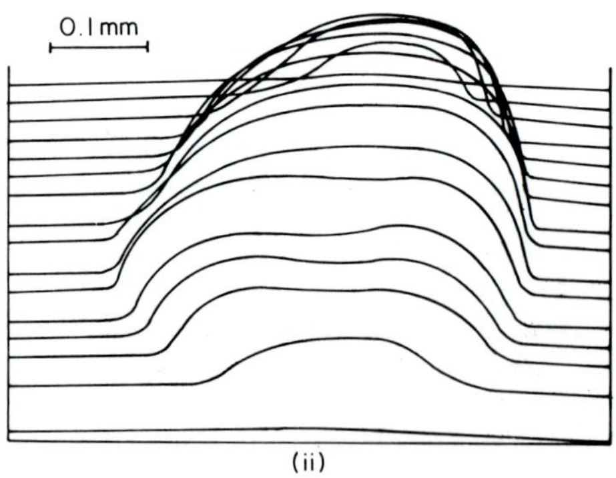

(ii)

Fig. 7.4 (i) The mechanical and electrical systems of a mechanically-scanned anode probe hole technique for locating the isolated electron emission sites found on broad-area electrodes (ii) A typical set of current traces obtained with this facility as a site is scanned across a 0.1mm diameter probe hole. (From Cox and Wort [9], with permission).

any detailed information about their microtopography. Accordingly ingly, attention was directed towards the application of electron optical techniques for looking at electrode surfaces. However, in the late 50's and early 60's when this work was being pioneered, the scanning electron microscope had not yet become a commercially available instrument, so it was therefore only possible to use the conventional transmission microscope for studying the profile of electrode surfaces. An early report of the application of this technique was by Bogdanovskii [10] in 1959 who was studying the growth of dendritic structures on microelectrodes. However, Little and Smith [11] and Jedynak [12] were the first to study the profiles of HV electrodes, with follow-up developments of the technique by Latham and his co-workers [1,13]. An essential requirement for this type of measurement is to choose a cathode electrode geometry that permits the imaging of the surface structures contained in a single plane that is orthogonal to the electrode surface, i.e. a geometry that offers an "edge" rather than a planar surface to the imaging electron beam. In the system of Latham and Braun [1] illustrated in Fig. 7.5, the high voltage electrode assembly, consisting of a filamentary hairpin cathode C separated by a 0.5mm gap from a planar anode A, was mounted in situ in the specimen chamber of an electron microscope so that the high voltage cycling (up to 10-15 kV) could be interrupted at any stage to observe the cathode profile.

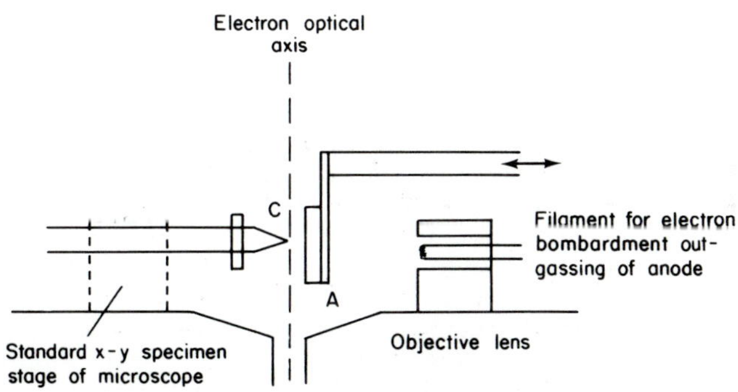

Fig. 7.5 The specimen stage of an EM3A electron microscope, as modified for studying the surface profile of a filamentary high voltage electrode.
(After Latham and Braun [1]).

The important conclusion to emerge from this type of investigation is that before any voltage is applied between a pair of "test" HV electrodes, the cathode surface appears smooth within the resolution of the imaging system (∿ 50Å) as shown in Fig. 7.6(i), and that it is only after the occurrence of a microdischarge or breakdown event that the surface becomes "decorated" with the type of microprotrusions shown in the micrograph of Fig.

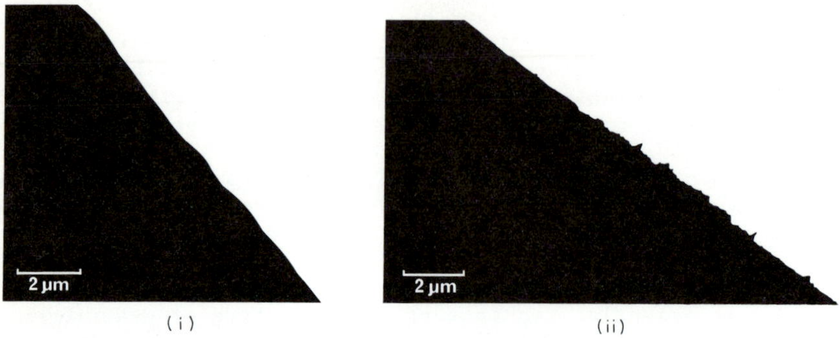

Fig. 7.6 Electron micrographs of (i) the smoothly undulating profile of a virgin electrode, and (ii) the damaged surface of an electrode that has suffered a breakdown or microdischarge event. (From Latham and Braun [1], with permission).

7.6(ii). Also, that the occurrences of such microprotrusions is accompanied by an increase in the slope of the F-N plot of the gap, typically corresponding to a reduction in the β-factor from an initially high value of ∿ 200-300, for which there is apparently no complementary surface microfeatures, to a much lower value of ∿ 50-100 which can then be realistically correlated with the dimensions of the observed microprotrusions (see Section 3.2(ii)). In support of the proposition that such features can subsequently act as microemitters, there is the type of evidence shown in the micrograph of Fig. 7.7, where it is assumed that the tip of an initially sharp protrusion has become blunted as a result of local melting caused by the resistive heating of an excessive electron emission current. Whilst attractive, this interpretation cannot however be regarded as conclusive, since it was subsequently shown that such features are also commonly observed following the sparking or arcing of say vacuum switch contacts, where they are normally attributed to droplets of molten metal which have solidified as they rebound from a metal substrate [14, 15].

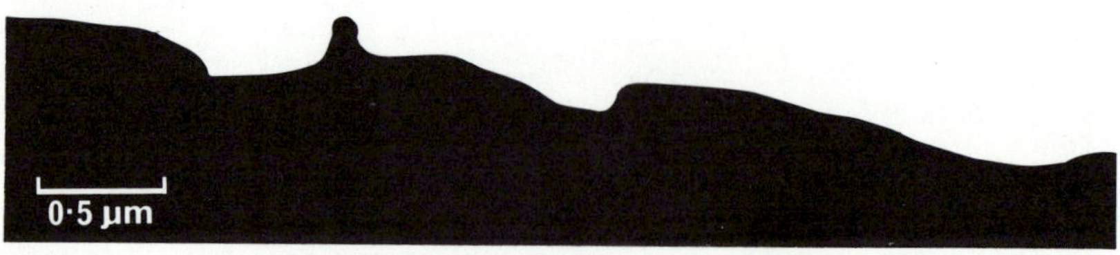

Fig. 7.7 A fusion-induced microfeature commonly found on arced electrodes.

To gain further insight into the time-scale of the physical mechanism responsible for the formation of these protrusions, Latham and Chapman [13] extended the in situ technique illustrated in Fig. 7.5 to the use of single-shot HV pulses in the micro-millisecond range. With this development, it was possible to obtain a sequence of micrographs such as shown in Fig. 7.8 which illustrate how the microtopography of the cathode surface is progressively degraded between successive pulses from its initially smooth profile of Fig. 7.6(i). This evidence therefore clearly shows that "groups" of these microfeatures form in times that are less than $\sim$ 20μs, which was the minimum pulse width available for the experiments.

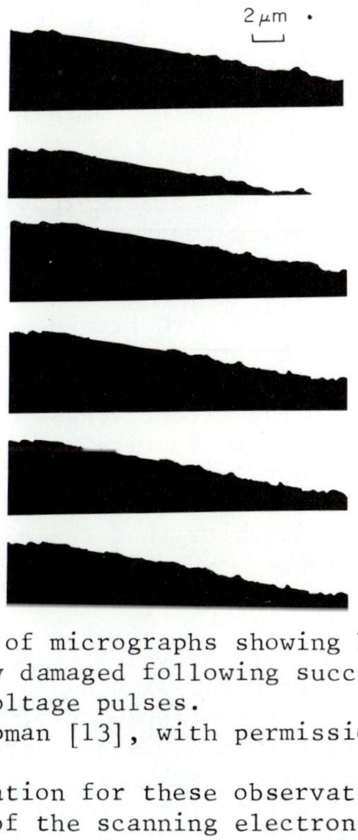

Fig. 7.8 A sequence of micrographs showing how an electrode surface is progressively damaged following successive 20μs, breakdown-inducing high voltage pulses.
(From Latham and Chapman [13], with permission).

A complete explanation for these observations had however to wait for the advent of the scanning electron microscope, which provided a complementary high-resolution means of studying the 3-dimensional nature of the microtopography on electrode surfaces. With such a facility, it was readily established [16] that these groups of electrode microprotrusions are associated with the microcratering of an electrode surface following some form of local fusion process. Thus, referring to Fig. 7.9, which is the complementary scanning electron micrograph of the same cathode surface imaged in profile in Fig. 7.6, it is clearly seen that the microprotrusions are in fact the "frozen" tongues of molten

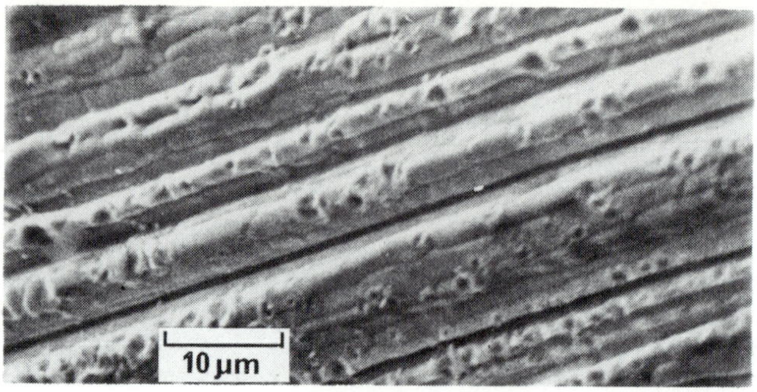

Fig. 7.9 A complementary scanning electron micrograph revealing the topographical nature of the electrode damage previously shown in profile in Figs. 7.6 to 7.8.
(From Latham and Braun [16], with permission).

metal projecting from the rim of these "splash" microcraters. On the basis therefore of the cathode-initiated microprotrusion breakdown model described in Chapter 3, it would appear that the presence of these features on the surface of an electrode would represent a serious hazard to the subsequent stability of the gap. However, whilst an isolated breakdown event does in practice frequently lead to a serious initial deterioration in the insulating performance of a gap, this need not be a permanent change, as evidenced by the effectiveness of the "spark" conditioning procedure described in Section 2.3(iv): in this connection, it would be relevant to cite several other investigations that have led to a similar conclusion [17-22]. This important observation therefore indicates that the presence of metallic microprotrusions and loosely adhering microparticles may not be the only important factors determining the voltage hold-off capability of a gap.

The physical origin of this type of damage has been plausibly attributed to both electron emission and microparticle based mechanisms. In support of the former explanation it will be noted from Fig. 7.9 that these cathode microcraters are predominantly located along the field enhancing ridges created during the initial extrusion of the tungsten filament. This observation therefore strongly suggests that they stem from microscopically localised electron emission processes that have degenerated into the "explosive emission" mode discussed in Section 5.3, possibly also involving the type of cathode-spot migration phenomenon discussed by Jüttner [23]. Since however there is no evidence from these studies to suggest that such a profusion of potential emission sites are initially present on an undamaged cathode, it has to be concluded that they are probably created as a result of some "primary" initiating event that, by its explosive action, sprays the electrode surface with sub-micron molten metal droplets that are immediately extruded by the field to form efficient microemitters, i.e. by a similar mechanism to that operating in mercury arc devices. The alternative microparticle explanation of this cratering will be delayed until Section 7.2(i).

7.1(iii) Emission site location - direct techniques

The location of electron emission sites by either the profile or topographical electron optical techniques described so far suffers from the obvious limitation that it is not possible to positively identify a particular microfeature as being the dominant electron emitter responsible for the prebreakdown current measured in the external circuit. Indeed, it could be said that none of the previous "indirect" evidence is representative of the important class of "high-β" emitting sites that are characteristic of undamaged electrodes whose surfaces appear to be free of any sharp microprotrusions. This deficiency was however largely overcome by a "direct" in situ electron optical technique developed by Cox [24] in which the specially designed "test" high voltage electrode assembly shown in Fig. 7.2 is mounted in the specimen chamber of a scanning electron microscope whose operating pressure is $\sim 10^{-8}$mbar. With this system it was possible to

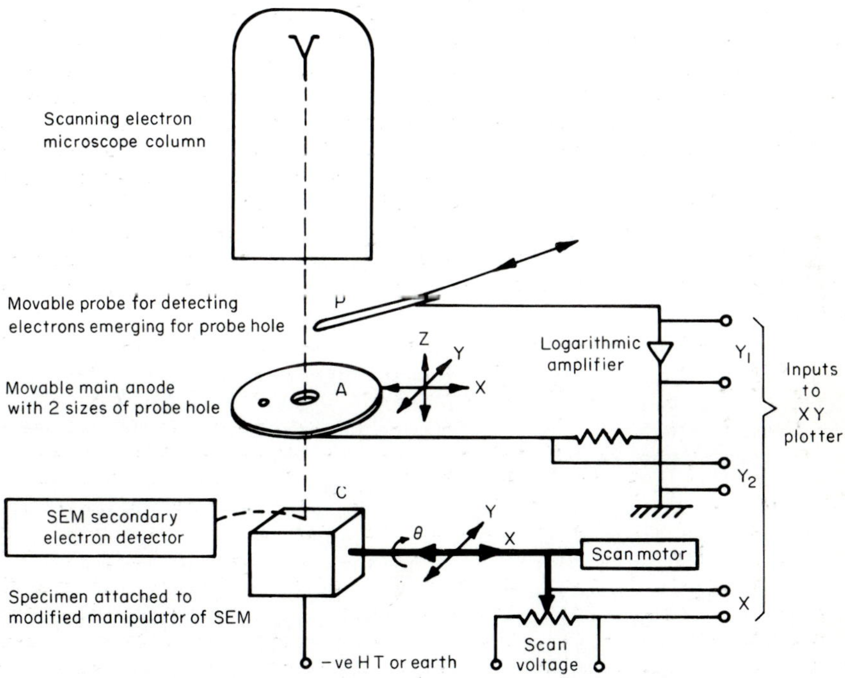

Fig. 7.10 An anode probe facility for the dynamic study of field emission sites on broad-area electrodes in situ in a SEM. (From Cox [24], with permission).

firstly locate and measure the electron emission characteristics of a given isolated site, and then to study its microtopography using the built-in SEM facility.

Referring to Fig. 7.10, a plane-parallel "test" gap is formed between a specimen cathode C and a stainless steel anode A with 500μm and 5μm diameter probe holes that can alternatively be accurately located on the axis of the SEM. Having thoroughly out-gassed both electrodes with an ancilliary electron bombardment facility (not shown), the subsequent experimental procedure is to use the micrometer controlled specimen stage to mechanically scan the cathode in a raster pattern in front of the coarse 500μm probe hole until a reading is obtained on the retractable current-sensor P; i.e. indicating that an emission site has been located approximately on the axis of the SEM. At this stage, the current-voltage characteristic of the site is recorded by varying the voltage across the test gap and noting the corresponding collected current which, with the larger probe hole, represents practically all the emission from the site: subsequently, this data can be used to construct a F-N plot of the emitter. The site may then be more accurately located on the SEM axis by firstly transferring to the 5μm probe hole and then progressively reducing the d-spacing of the electrode gap to $\sim$ 0.05mm: at this stage, the main anode and current sensor are removed and the microtopography of the on-axis region of the electrode is examined by the SEM facility. By using an electron trajectory technique that involves recording how the specimen coordinates corresponding to maximum collected current vary as the d-spacing is reduced, it is possible to locate the position of an emitting site with a spatial resolution that can approach $\sim$ 10μm. A typical example of the evidence obtained from this technique is illustrated by the micrograph of Fig. 7.11(i) in which the "circled" area represents the localised region of the arced surface of a copper-chrome alloy vacuum switch contact electrode that includes an emitting site. The most important conclusion to be drawn from this and similar observations on other sites, is that the identified region contains no field-enhancing microfeatures corresponding in "sharpness" to the β-factor of $\sim$ 200-300 measured indirectly from the F-N plot of the site. Unfortunately, the resolution of the technique is too low to identify which of the microfeatures within this region is giving rise to the emission; however, the presence of a grain boundary could well be significant, since similar types of site location were found in more recent studies [25,26]. Although a detailed consideration of the physical implications of this important observation will be delayed until the following chapter, when other more recent complementary data can also be taken into account, it can be stated at this stage that the evidence of Fig. 7.11 strongly suggests that there are other emission mechanisms apart from the metallic microprotrusion model for explaining the origin of prebreakdown currents. In addition to this microtopography information, it is also pos-

(i)

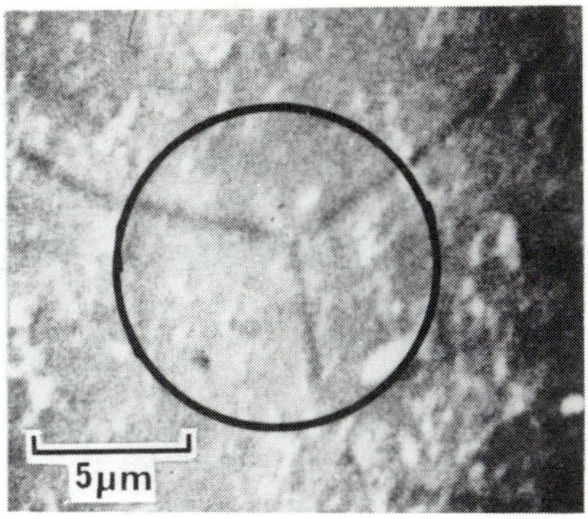

(ii)

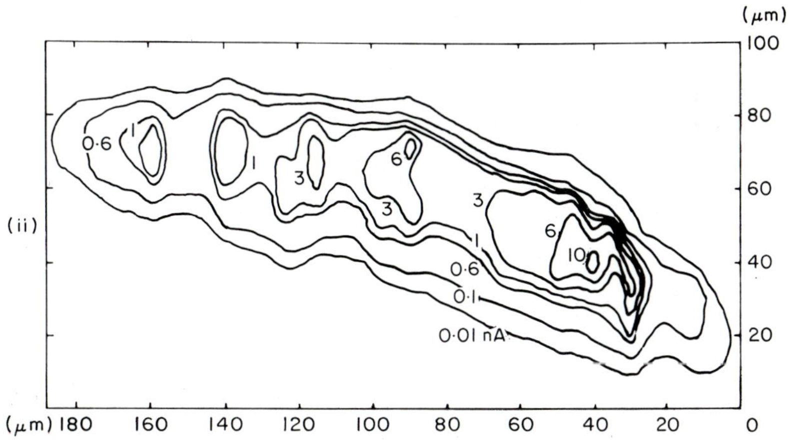

Fig. 7.11 (i) A scanning electron micrograph showing the region of an electrode surface (circled) that has been identified as containing an emission site, and (ii) the complementary distribution map of the field emission current associated with this site. (From Cox [24], with permission).

sible to use the specimen scan facility in conjunction with the fine probe hole current detection regime for obtaining a contour map of the current density from a given site as it appears in the plane of the anode; i.e. using the system of Fig. 7.2 described earlier in this chapter. Thus, Fig. 7.11(ii) is the complementary distribution of the emission obtained from the site imaged in Fig. 7.11(i), and is seen to consist of at least two sub emission centres which is a typical characteristic of the emission sites studied with this technique. It will be recalled that the direct projection imaging technique of Jüttner et al. [6,8], described earlier in this chapter, also indicated that the emission sites found on extended surfaces are composed of "clusters" of sub-centres (see Fig. 7.4).

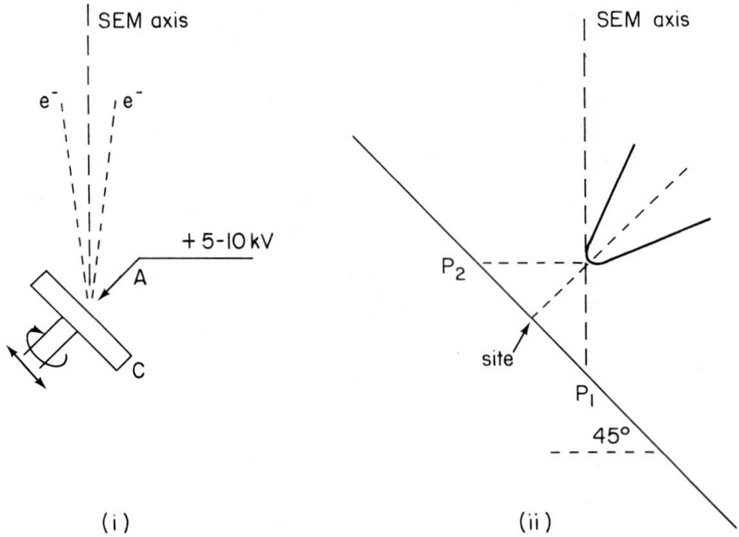

Fig. 7.12 (i) The experimental regime of an anode microprobe technique for locating electron emission sites on broad-area electrodes in situ in a SEM, (ii) The electrode geometry in the vicinity of an emission site.
(From Athwal and Latham [27], with permission).

In a more recent approach aimed at improving the resolution of emission site location, Athwal and Latham [27,28] have adapted the anode microprobe technique of Hurley [29] for direct use in a scanning electron microscope as illustrated in Fig. 7.12(i). Here, a standard electrolytically etched tungsten microtip (see Fig. 5.2), having a typical radius of 20-50nm, is located on the axis of the SEM by means of a bellows-operated adjustable mounting that has an insulated feed-through to the tip capable of supporting a positive potential of 5-10 kV. The specimen cathode C, which is orientated normally to the probe anode A and at 45° to the SEM axis, is mounted on the goniometer stage of the instrument such that its surface can be scanned in a spiral pattern in front of the fixed probe. By arranging for the specimen to be electrically insulated from the earthed mechanical stage, it is possible to use a series picoammeter (electrometer) to monitor any emission current drawn from the specimen. With the probe-to-specimen distance initially set to ∿ 0.5mm and the probe potential to the higher value of ∿ 8-10 kV, the first stage of the experimental procedure is to systematically scan the specimen until an emission site is roughly located as indicated by a specimen current of ∿ 10^{-8}amp. The second stage is to intermittently use the SEM facility for gradually reducing the probe-to-specimen distance to ∿ 5-10μm, ensuring that throughout this sequence of

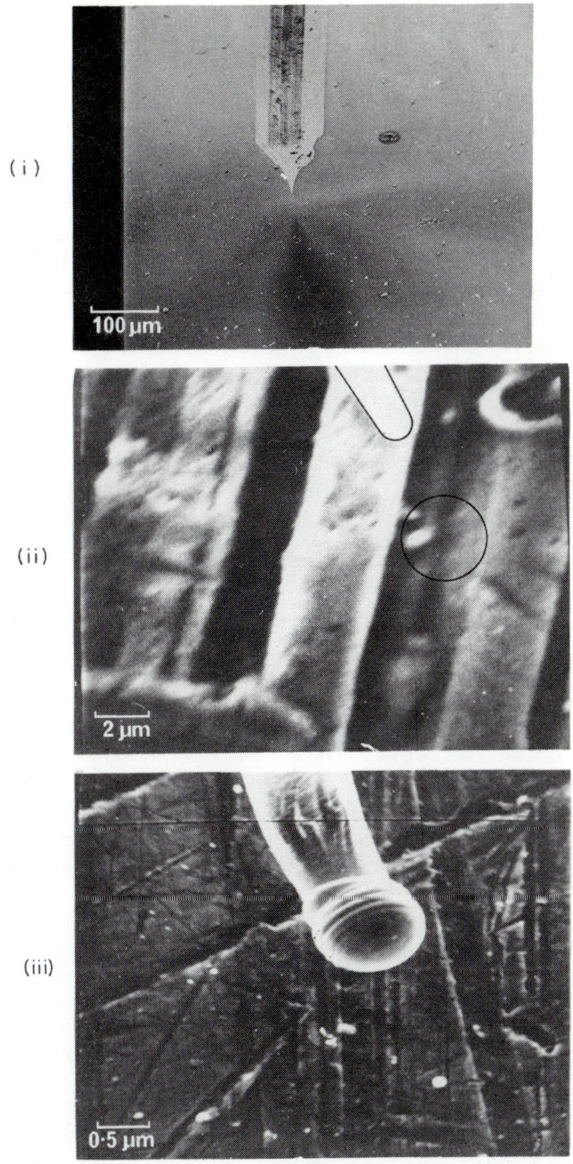

Fig. 7.13 Scanning electron micrographs showing (i) the anode microprobe electrode regime of Fig. 7.12, (ii) the tip of the probe immediately above the localised microregion of the cathode surface (circled) containing an emission site, and (iii) a probe that has suffered thermal instability as a result of collecting a high emission current.
(From Athwal and Latham [27], with permission).

operations the probe potential is progressively reduced to keep the specimen current approximately constant: at this final stage of adjustment, the probe/specimen micro-regime will be as shown in Fig. 7.12(ii). The emission site can then be assumed to be mid-way between the points P_1 and P_2, which can be respectively located in the centre of the field of view by (i) focussing through the tip onto the specimen and (ii) focussing on the tip profile, then, without altering the lens conditions, removing the tip and translating the specimen laterally until the surface is again in focus. With this technique it is possible to improve the resolution of site location to better than ±2μm. To provide the reader with a perspective of the point-plane electrode regime of this facility, the low-magnification scanning electron micrograph of Fig. 7.13(i) shows the microprobe anode (etched from a 0.1mm diameter tungsten wire) superimposed against the planar cathode. In contrast, the high resolution micrograph of Fig. 7.13(ii) illustrates the final stage of the technique where the site being studied has been localised to within the superimposed 2μm diameter circle. Typically, this is seen to contain a sub-micron insulating inclusion which strongly points to such features being the source of the electron emission. Although the resolution of the technique is still not good enough to precisely identify the emission site, this type of result even more strongly confirms the earlier findings of Cox and co-workers [24-26] that these emission processes are evidently not associated with a field enhancing surface microfeature having a β-value in the range 200-300, such as typically predicted from the corresponding F-N plot of the emitter. This conclusion will be further supported by the optical and electron spectrometry studies to be described respectively in Sections 7.1(v) and (vi).

Two further significant observations should be briefly mentioned. Firstly, with the aid of a Kevex X-ray analysis facility, it is frequently possible to identify a "foreign" element within the site region: thus in Fig. 7.13(ii) the insulating particle was shown to contain silver, probably in the form of an oxide. A similar finding had been reported earlier by Allen, Cox and Latham [26] using the anode probe hole technique to identify a site, although in this case the impurity element was aluminium. The second interesting observation involves the identification of an alternative type of emission site that apparently requires a minimum threshold field to "switch" it on, after which it emits copiously without a further increase in field. Such sites manifest themselves experimentally by the sudden blunting of the probe anode during its systematic scanning of a localised region of the cathode surface under gradually increasing field conditions. The typical outcome of such an event is shown in the micrograph of Fig. 7.13(iii), which clearly shows how the tip of the probe has been thermally blunted as a result of the excessive heat generated by the sudden collection of a high electron current. It will be recalled from Chapter 5 that a similar modification of a tip profile occurs when an excess current is drawn from such an emitter in a point-plane configuration.

7.1(iv) Gas desorption

From the discussion in Chapters 3 and 4 of the "active" physical phenomena that can occur in a high voltage gap, it could be anticipated that there will be essentially two processes that can give rise to an increase in the vapour pressure of a gap. Firstly, during the prebreakdown phase, there will be the thermally activated desorption of occluded gas that will occur principally at the anode "hot-spot" formed by electron bombardment, and secondly at a breakdown or microdischarge event (electron emission or microparticle initiated), there will be a transient increase in the electrode metal vapour pressure indicative of some form of thermal instability at either the cathode or anode. To verify the existence of the first of these two processes, mass spectrometry techniques have been used to monitor the partial pressure of the residual gas species present in an interelectrode gap as the applied voltage is gradually increased towards breakdown. The detection of transient changes in metal ion concentration requires very much more sophisticated techniques that will be described in Section 7.2(ii).

From measurements made during the prebreakdown phase [30-34], it has been established that, irrespective of the electrode material, there is a characteristic increase in the total pressure during the initial application of a voltage to a gap; i.e. during its "current" conditioning. The magnitude of this increase is dependent on the prebreakdown current, but can typically reach half an order of magnitude at an ambient pressure of $\sim 10^{-8}$mbar with a gap current of $\sim 10^{-6}$A. However, if the gap voltage, and hence mean current, is maintained at a constant value, any such pressure increases will very gradually decay away over a period of several hours. It is then found that during any subsequent voltage application to this value, there is no further significant evidence of gas desorption: from this observation it follows that a fully "conditioned" gap is similarly free of desorption processes. There is also some evidence [32] to suggest that, for a given electrode material, there is a characteristic "voltage threshold" or electron impact energy at which desorption is activated; e.g. 10-12 kV for Al and Bi, 14-17 kV for Cu and 19-20 kV for Ni and Zr. One possible explanation for this effect is that the gas is released from several atomic layers beneath the anode surface so that differing electron energies are required to penetrate to a given depth among the various electrode materials. Alternatively, the effect may have a simple thermal explanation in terms of a characteristic electron power loading required to raise the anode surface temperature above the value reached by the system during the original UHV bake-out procedure.

When the composition of this desorbed gas is analysed by mass spectrometry techniques [30-34], it is found to consist predominantly of CO and CO_2 for all electrode materials, with the partial pressure of CO_2 being typically twice that of CO. The selective desorption of these particular gases is a well known phenomenon in UHV technology and can be explained both in terms of the high solubility of these species in most metals, and the thermal oxidation of the carbon that is a common residual impurity.

7.1(v) Optical emission spectra

Anode spots: If a pair of operational (i.e. conditioned) high voltage electrodes are viewed in a darkened environment, it is common to observe the presence of several stable pin-points of light on the surface of the anode [35-39] such as illustrated in Fig. 7.14. These *anode spots* as they are termed, also occur on unconditioned electrodes, except that here the "spots" are more numerous and unstable; however, as conditioning procedes, many of the initial population are extinguished whilst the dominant ones that remain become progressively more stable. Their origin has generally been associated with the anode "hot spots" discussed in Section 3.3(ii) which are caused by the impact of the fine pencils of high energy electrons emitted from microscopically localised cathode sites. However, it has also been reported by Jüttner [38] that there is another type of anode spot that has a fixed location on the anode surface and is not spatially related to the electron emission sites on the cathode surface; accordingly, these were tentatively attributed to some form of electroluminescent process at thermally stable microinclusions. From studies of the former type of anode spot, it has been confirmed that a breakdown or microdischarge event is frequently associated with the disappearance of a specific spot; i.e. indicating a cathode-initiated process in which a particular emitter has been thermally eliminated [36]. The light from these spots was

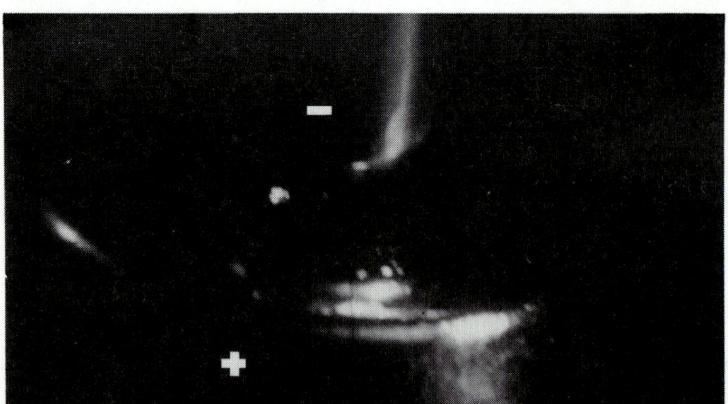

Fig. 7.14 Distribution of anode spots on an electrically stressed planar electrode, as viewed with an image intensifier. (From Young [39], with permission).

initially thought to be high temperature black body radiation until measurements revealed that the short wavelength composition of its spectrum was incompatible with the maximum temperatures likely to be attained at the anode surface due to electron heating [40,41]. Subsequently, its origin was correctly identified as transition radiation resulting from atomic excitation processes in the surface layers of the target following the scattering of the high velocity bombarding electrons [40]. It should also be noted that anode spots have an associated X-ray spectrum; in fact, Zeitoun-Fakiris [41] has used a pin-hole camera technique to obtain an X-ray image of anode spots. The transition radiation phenomena has been analysed theoretically by Boersch et al. [42] who showed that the angular dependence of the spectral power in the emitted radiation $W_\theta(\lambda)$ is given by

$$W_\theta(\lambda) = (3.6 \times 10^{-11} P_o/\lambda^2)\left\{(\varepsilon' - 1)^2 \sin^2\theta\cos^2\theta / [\varepsilon' \cos\theta + (\varepsilon' - \sin^2\theta)^{\frac{1}{2}}]^2\right\} \quad (7.1)$$

where P_o is the power in the incident electron beam, λ is the wavelength being considered and ε' [= $f(\lambda)$] is the complex dielectric constant of the anode surface. Thus, for intensity measurements at a given angle and wavelength, one has

$$W_\theta(\lambda) \propto P_o \quad (7.2)$$

This latter proportionality was used by Young [39] as the basis of an elegant experimental technique for studying the behaviour of individual broad area electron emission sites in which the optical intensity of a given anode spot could be directly related to its associated electron current; i.e. it provided a "visual" method of measuring the current-voltage characteristic of the individual electron emission site associated with any of the anode spots shown in Fig. 7.14. In the experimental system of Young illustrated schematically in Fig. 7.15, an optical detecting system OD (consisting of a telescopic focussing element, an image intensifier and a photomultiplier as shown in Fig. 7.16), records the intensity of the light emitted at a wavelength λ and at a fixed angle θ from a given anode spot in terms of the photomultiplier current i_p (dark current corrected). Thus if the gap voltage is V and i_n is the electron current flowing to the n'th spot, it follows that

$$i_p(n) \propto V\, i_n = KVi_n \quad (7.3)$$

where K is a constant that can be determined from a calibration measurement in which the photomultiplier current $i_p(T)$ corresponding to the total intensity from all the anode spots is compared with the total prebreakdown current flowing across the gap. Recalling that the F-N representation of the I-V characteristic of an emission process is a plot of $\log(I/V^2)$ against $(1/V)$, it

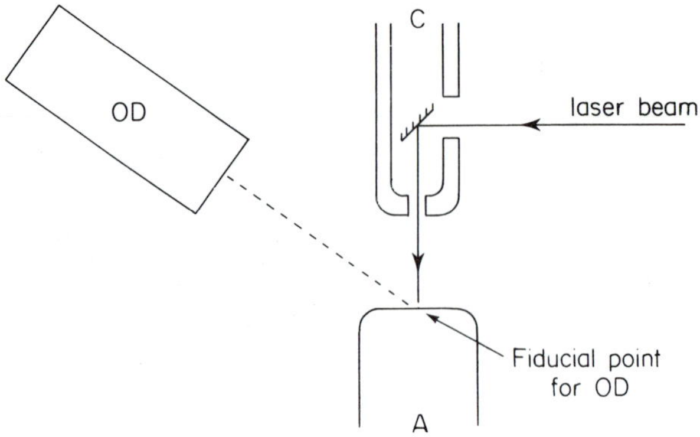

Fig. 7.15 The experimental regime used for recording the anode spots shown in Fig. 7.14.
(After Young [39]).

will be seen from equation 7.3 that for the present regime, the F-N characteristic of the n'th site will be given by a plot of $\log(i_p/V^3)$ against $(1/V)$. After correcting for the non-uniformity of the gap field, Young found that the β_n-values for individual sites typically ranged between 150-250; the 'total' β-factor of the gap, as measured from either $\log(I/V^2)$ versus $(1/V)$ or $\log(i_{pT}/V^3)$ versus $(1/V)$ F-N plots, would be $\sim$ 220. From such information, it is possible to identify the sites that are potentially most vulnerable to instability; i.e. those having the highest β-values (see analysis of Chapter 3). It is then possible to visually confirm that it is one or more of these that are destroyed with the first breakdown event. The technique also offers a powerful tool for studying how the choice of electrode material and surface preparation determines the incidence of emission sites and how such sites are affected during electrode conditioning procedures.

Cathode or k-spots: In the course of a follow-up investigation to the work of Young on anode spots, Hurley and Dooley [43] established the existence of complementary *cathode or k-spots*, as they are named to distinguish them from the well known phenomenon associated with the vacuum arc. Since this was a surprising finding, not to be anticipated from the metallic microprotrusion model for electron emission, these authors subsequently re-arranged the experimental chamber for a more detailed study of the optical properties of this new cathode phenomenon [44]. Their system, which is illustrated in Fig. 7.16, used a plane-parallel electrode geometry inclined at an angle to the axis of the optical detecting system previously used by Young [22], thus providing a line-of-sight to all parts of the cathode surface. To gain an insight into the physical mechanism responsible for the phenomenon, it was arranged to record a spectrum of the emission

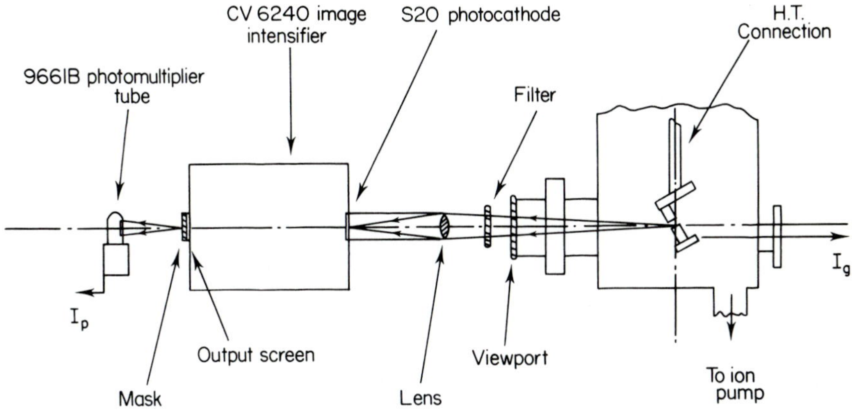

Fig. 7.16 Image intensifier and electrode regime used for studying k-spots.
(From Hurley and Dooley [43], with permission).

by using a series of high-pass sharp cut-off filters. This technique was then used to study a range of electrode materials (OFHC copper, stainless-steel, dural, gold and molybdenum) and in all cases k-spots were observed that had characteristic emission spectra [44,45]. As an example, that obtained from copper is reproduced in Fig. 7.17(i) and is seen to have two dominant lines at 650 and 700nm, which Hurley tentatively attributed to an accumulation of cuprous oxide, probably at a grain boundary. For comparison, the spectrum of the complementary anode spot is shown in Fig. 7.17(ii) and is seen to be characteristically shifted to shorter wavelengths. From these studies, it was also noted that breakdown events generally resulted in the disappearance of one or more spots, and that discharges originated from within light emitting regions; i.e. strongly suggesting that k-spots were associated with electron emission processes.

To confirm this latter possibility, Hurley [15] subsequently replaced the planar electrode geometry of Fig. 7.16 with the point-plane arrangement of Fig. 7.18, in which a micropoint probe anode is mechanically scanned in front of a planar test cathode until an emission site is accurately located on its surface, as evidenced by a finite specimen current recorded by the electrometer in the low-voltage cathode line. If the same image intensifier viewing system shown in Fig. 7.16 is then focussed on the cathode surface immediately below the micropoint probe, it is possible to observe luminous k-spots on all occasions that electron emission is detected. It should be added that a complementary anode spot is also invariably observed on the probe anode, although, as already pointed out, its emission spectrum of Fig. 7.17(ii) is characteristic of transition radiation and therefore

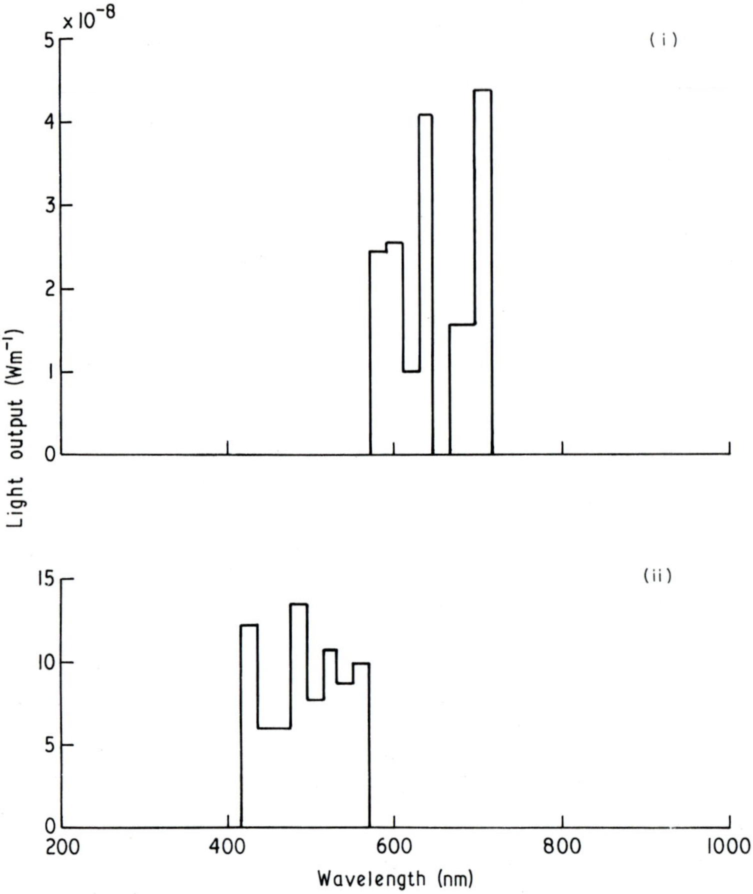

Fig. 7.17 The spectra of light emitted from (i) k-spots and (ii) anode spots.
(From Hurley [45], with permission).

readily discriminated from the cathode emission. Another important finding of these probe measurements was that there are two sorts of emission site [46]: type (a) that are characterised by high-β factors ($\gtrsim$ 200) and give rise to breakdown events at a critical current of $\sim 5 \times 10^{-5}$amp, and type (b) that have low β-factors at low-fields, but become current-limiting through a negative resistance effect at high fields and consequently do not give rise to breakdown events.

In seeking a physical explanation for the k-spot phenomenon, it would be logical to consider first the only apparent mechanism by which the established metallic microprotrusion model for electron emission discussed in Chapter 3 might give rise to the

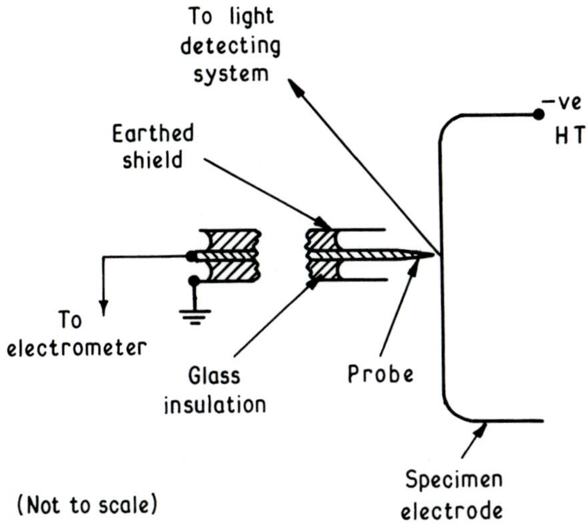

Fig. 7.18 An anode probe technique for correlating the electron and optical emission characteristics of individual k-spots. (From Hurley [45], with permission).

observed optical effects, viz. by thermal radiation from a sub-critically heated emitter. Such an explanation must however be discounted since as in the case of anode spots, it would require a black-body type of emission spectrum which is clearly not supported by the experimental evidence of Fig. 7.17(i). The alternative explanation proposed by Hurley and Dooley [44] is that the k-spot emission arises from an electroluminescent effect. This interpretation was strongly supported by measurements of the brightness dependence of a given emission line (as measured by the photomultiplier current i_p) on the applied voltage V which were shown to obey the anticipated Alfrey-Taylor relation [47] by giving a linear plot of log i_p versus $V^{-\frac{1}{2}}$. Since electroluminescence is a "non-metallic" phenomenon, it is clear that this interpretation is incompatible with the simple metallic protrusion model for electron emission. Instead, these authors attributed the emission to a more complex emitting mechanism involving some sort of metal/semiconductor micro-regime at highly localised sites on an electrode surface, possibly associated with impurity inclusions, i.e. similar to the type of regime proposed earlier by Walters et al. [48], Cox and Williams [25] and Farrall et al. [49] from qualitative reasoning based on indirect experimental evidence. The same conclusions emerged independently from the direct evidence obtained from electron spectrometry studies of these emission processes by Latham and his co-workers, to be described in the following section.

7.1(vi) Electron emission spectra

It has been a long held conviction of the present author [1, 48] and others [24,25,49,50], that the traditional metallic microprotrusion model for explaining the localised electron emission processes that occur on broad-area electrodes does not provide a satisfactory explanation for much of the experimental data. In particular, it is difficult to justify the unrealistically high β-factor ($\gtrsim 250$) and widely varying values of emitting areas predicted from the F-N plots of the I-V characteristic of a gap; also, there is an absence of any direct electron optical evidence of microprotrusions of the appropriate dimension on the surface of virgin electrodes [1]. The possibility of there being an alternative emission mechanism has therefore been gaining acceptance over recent years, particularly following the work of Cox [24], Hurley and Dooley [44] and that are to be described in the present section. Early speculative suggestions as to what form such a mechanism might take [1,48,49] were centred on the concept of a Malter emission process [51] which involved the presence of insulating inclusions in the cathode surface that could become positively charged by some form of electron emission or positive ion capture mechanism and so create an internal field sufficient to "heat" electrons injected from the Fermi level of the metal substrate by a further 4-5 eV so that they could escape into the vacuum. However, without any direct experimental evidence to support the existence of such a mechanism, there has been a reluctance to make a radical departure from the accepted microprotrusion interpretation of prebreakdown currents. Other mechanisms that have been considered as providing possible alternative explanations of "high-β" emission include resonance tunnelling effects [52,53] such as might occur at islands of alkali impurities created by surface diffusion [54],and a lowering of the surface potential barrier by either induced depth layers [55] or the interaction of charged dislocations at the electrode-vacuum surface, such as discussed by Shockley [56] in the case of semiconductors. However, all such suggestions lack conclusive experimental evidence to confirm that they indeed play an important role in the vacuum gap. A particularly powerful experimental technique for resolving this uncertainty is suggested by the extensive literature on the application of electron spectroscopy for studying the various forms of electron emission, where it is well established that the electrons emitted by any given mechanism have a characteristic energy spectrum. Accordingly, if such spectral measurements could be made on the emission from the isolated sites on high voltage electrodes, it would be possible to positively identify, for example, whether it stems from a metallic microemitter or some sort of semiconductor/insulator regime.

Following this reasoning, Latham and his co-workers [57-60] developed the sophisticated UHV ($p \lesssim 10^{-10}$mbar) analytical facility illustrated schematically in Fig. 7.19, consisting of a high-

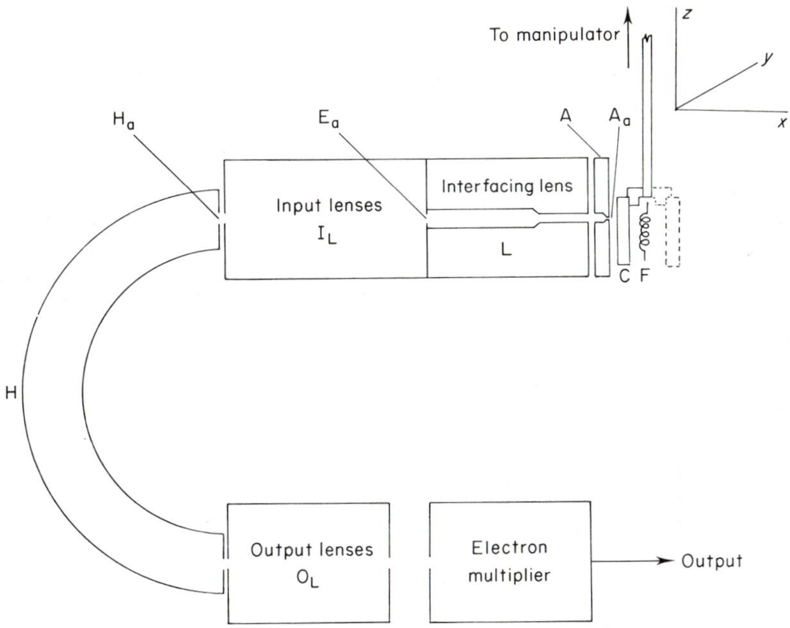

Fig. 7.19 The experimental regime used for recording the energy spectra of individual electron emission sites on broad-area electrodes.
(From Allen and Latham [58], with permission).

resolution electron spectrometer interfaced with a "test" high voltage gap. The latter has a plane parallel geometry consisting of the specimen cathode C and a highly polished stainless steel anode A having an axial 1.0mm diameter probe aperture A_a. A mechanical scan facility allows the specimen to be moved parallel to the anode in the y-z plane, whilst maintaining a known constant gap between the two electrodes. The specimens used in this work are discs 14mm in diameter with a suitably rounded edge profile, and are mounted in a specimen holder that is insulated for applying negative voltages of up to $\sim$ 15 kV. A 50 watt electron bombardment facility, provided by a low voltage heated filament F, is used for outgassing either the specimen or the front anode. The anode aperture A_a in conjunction with electrode L form an electrostatic lens which has been specially designed as an interfacing element between the test gap and the analyser. It has the two-fold action of (a) focussing the diverging beams of electrons leaving the anode aperture A_a into a parallel beam, and (b) decelerating the electrons from a typical energy of $\sim$ 5 keV at A_a to the $\sim$ 2 keV requirements at the entrance aperture E_a of the analyser. The spectrometer, with a resolution of $\lesssim$ 30 meV, is based upon a 180° hemispherical electrostatic deflecting element H with associated input and output lenses I_L and O_L respectively. The function of the input lens assembly is to decelerate the electrons to the analysing energy of ~ 2 eV and focus them onto the entrance aperture H_a of the hemispherical deflecting element H. Those electrons which have the correct energy to be transmitted by the deflecting element are then re-accelerated by the output lenses and focussed onto an electron multiplier. Full details of the construction, operation and performance of this instrument can be found elsewhere [57-60].

The experimental procedure is initiated by applying a gradually increasing voltage of ~ 5-10 kV across the test gap between C and A to confirm that there is a finite pre-breakdown current and hence the presence of an emitting site(s) on the specimen cathode C. To position a site opposite the probe hole A_a, the specimen is mechanically scanned in a raster pattern in front of A_a until a current is registered at L. Microadjustments are then made to maximise this current when the site will not only be centralised with respect to the probe hole, but its total emission will be collected by L: at this stage, a current-voltage characteristic, and hence a F-N plot of the site, can be recorded. By applying a suitable positive voltage to L, the electron beam can then be focussed to pass into the analyser input lens I_L, after which, adjustments can be made to the focussing of the analyser in order to obtain the energy spectrum of the electrons emitted from the site.

The initial measurements were made on copper specimens [58] since HV gaps made from this material are generally known to have high pre-breakdown current levels (and consequently poor voltage hold-off characteristics), indicating the presence of suitably "strong" emitting sites for commissioning the technique. Thus Fig. 7.20 compares a typical energy spectrum previously obtained from a reference tungsten emitter at room temperature and a pressure of $\lesssim 10^{-10}$mbar using this instrument [57], with that obtained under identical temperature and pressure conditions from a site situated near the centre of one of the copper samples used in the investigation.(N.B.electron energy is decreasing from left to right). In both cases, the spectra are stable with time and are reproducible from specimen to specimen. As seen from Fig. 7.20, it is also possible to use another important feature of this type of spectrometer to identify the position of the Fermi level FL of the substrate cathode of each emitting regime on their respective spectra; a measurement that is based on a previous calibration of the instrument [57]. The corresponding Fowler-Nordheim plot of the copper site obtained as described above, predicts a β-value of ~ 750 if a work function of 4.5 eV is assumed for the emitter. From a comparison of the two spectra of Fig. 7.20, three important differences in the emission characteristics can immediately be identified: (i) unlike the reference tungsten emitter, all electrons from the site on the copper electrode are emitted from states well below the Fermi level, (ii) the half-widths of the copper distribution (~ 360 mV) is

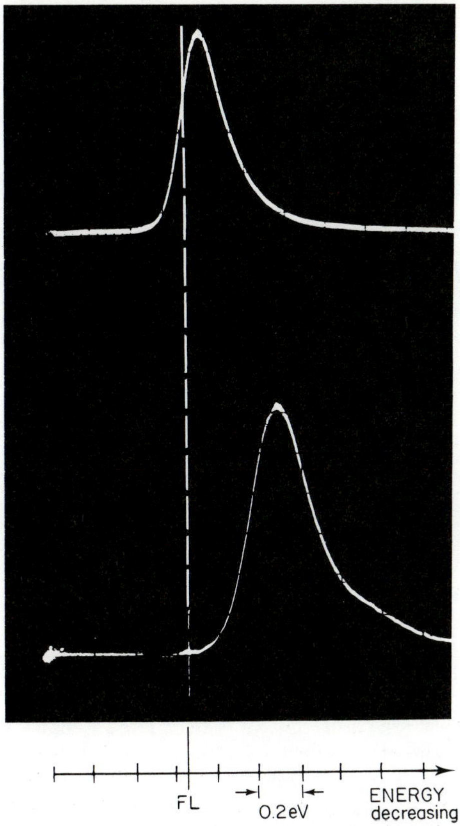

Fig. 7.20 Electron energy spectra obtained from (i) a reference tungsten micropoint emitter, and (ii) an emission site on a broad-area copper electrode: in both cases, the spectra are referred to the Fermi level FL of the substrate cathode. (From Allen and Latham [58], with permission).

broader than that of the tungsten emitter (∿ 240 mV) and (iii) the shape of the copper spectrum is almost symmetrical, i.e. lacking the characteristic sharp high energy slope found for tungsten.

Measurements were subsequently extended to the sites found on stainless steel and titanium specimens [59,61], i.e. materials that are widely used commercially for HV electrodes and, in contrast to copper, are characterised by generally having stable, low-level prebreakdown currents. The typical spectra obtained from sites on these materials are shown in Fig. 7.21 and are seen to share most of the characteristics noted above for copper. It will be seen however, that the spectrum from the site on the titanium specimen has a broader double peak structure extending further into the low-energy range. This phenomenon has also been

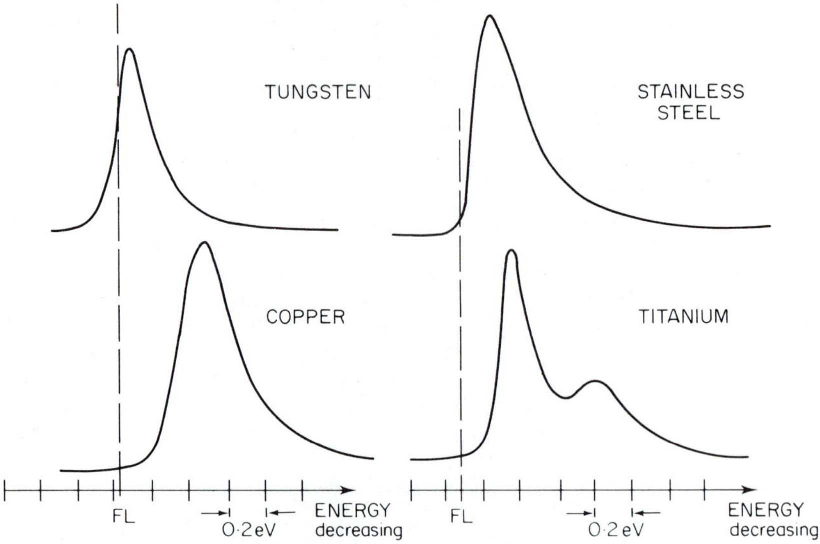

Fig. 7.21 A comparison of the electron spectrum of a reference tungsten emitter with those obtained from sites on copper, stainless steel and titanium electrodes.
(From Allen and Latham [61], with permission).

observed for copper-chrome alloy electrodes [26] and sometimes with copper when the specimen has not been thoroughly out-gassed [59]. As with copper, complementary F-N plots for the stainless steel and titanium sites again predicted high β-factors of 400 and 500 respectively. For the convenience of the reader, the emission characteristics of the sites found on these three materials have been collated in the following table, and also contrasted, where appropriate, with those of a reference micropoint tungsten emitter. Following the accepted convention of Young [62], spectra have been characterised in terms of (i) their full width at half maximum (FWHM), normally referred to simply as their "half-width", (ii) the steepness of their high energy slopes, quantified as the energy spread between the 10% and 90% points and (iii) the shift of the 78% point up the high energy slope from the Fermi level of the substrate cathode.

Material	Half-width (FWHM) (eV)	Energy Slope Width (eV)	Spectral Shift (eV)	β-value
Tungsten	0.23	0.11	NIL	-
Copper	0.35	0.16	0.30	700
Stainless Steel	0.25	0.14	0.10	400
Titanium	-	0.14	0.25	500

It can be concluded from these measurements that the general character of the electron energy spectra obtained from broad-area emission sites differs markedly from that to be expected from metallic emitters. Thus whilst the wide half-widths and symmetrical shape of the distributions could possibly be explained in terms of tip contamination [57],shifts of $\sim$ 0.1-0.3 eV in the position of spectrum relative to the Fermi level cannot be explained in terms of the Fowler-Nordheim free-electron model. In fact, such spectral shifts more closely resemble the behaviour of semiconducting emitters [63,64]. It is also significant that in all cases the β-factors predicted from the F-N plots are unrealistically high (400-700) for the metallic whisker model. These findings, taken in conjunction with the cathode spot electroluminescent measurements of Hurley and Dooley [44] described in the previous section, therefore strongly point to the existence of a more complicated electron emission mechanism, apparently involving semiconducting microinclusions. Clearly this conclusion has profound implications not only on the interpretation of prebreakdown current-voltage characteristics, but also on the technological approach to improving the voltage hold-off capability of vacuum gaps. Such considerations will be enlarged upon in the final chapter to this book when summarising the present state of the art. We shall also include in that discussion a review of possible alternative electron emission models that have very recently been proposed to explain this latest data.

7.2 Microparticle orientated studies

Since the early 50's, when Cranberg [65] formulated the first theory of microparticle initiated breakdown (see Chapter 4), there has been a sustained effort to devise experimental techniques for detecting the presence of the hypothesised high-velocity charged particles. In fact, this has proved to be a very challenging problem and it is only very recently that direct evidence of their existence has become available through the development of in-flight detecting systems. Prior to this, it was only possible to refer to indirect evidence which mostly took the form of observing changes in the microtopography of electrode surfaces that were attributable to the impact of such particles.

7.2(i) Particle detection by indirect techniques

The earliest experiments of this type were those aimed at obtaining positive evidence of material transfer between electrodes following breakdown events. Two techniques have been employed, although both share the common approach of using an electrode gap formed by disimilar electrode materials. In the first, such as used by Anderson [66], positive identification of the phenomenon has been obtained from an optical spectroscopy analysis of the elemental composition of electrode surfaces which revealed traces of "foreign" elements corresponding to the complementary electrode material. In the second approach, radioactive tracer techniques [67] were used to detect material transfer. Neutron activation analysis is another technique that has been used to obtain evidence of material transfer across a gap [16,68], whereby one of the electrodes is made artificially radioactive by the bombardment of fast neutrons so that any traces of it can subsequently be detected on the unradiated electrode. In the case of copper electrodes, for example [16], it is possible to use the β^+ activity ($T_{\frac{1}{2}}$ = 9.8 min) of ^{62}Cu produced by the reaction ^{63}Cu(n,2n)^{62}Cu. It must be added however, that the technique lacks spatial resolution and has a minimum mass detection limit of $\sim 10^{-13}$kg which probably corresponds to upwards of 50 microparticles. Nowadays, with the ready availability of the scanning X-ray microprobe surface analysis technique, it is a relatively routine experiment to confirm these earlier findings; also, with the high spatial resolution of these instruments ($\lesssim 1\mu m^2$), it is possible to establish that "foreign" species are highly localised on an electrode surface, as would be expected from the microparticle impact model.

The other major source of indirect evidence for microparticle phenomen also stems from the advent of scanning electron microscopy as a readily available analytical technique. With this facility it is possible to study the microtopography of electrode surfaces both before and after breakdown events and thereby respectively identify the characteristic structural changes resulting from microparticle impact processes. There have been several such reports in the literature [16,69] whose general findings can be typified by the micrographs previously shown in Fig. 7.9 together with that of Fig. 7.22 which shows the complementary

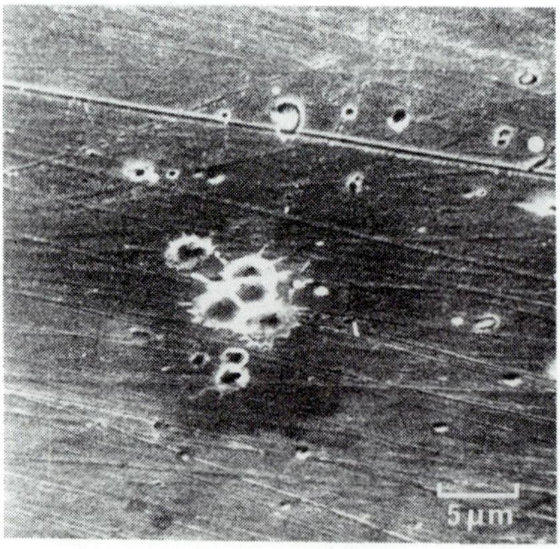

Fig. 7.22 A scanning electron micrograph of a ¼-micron diamond polished copper anode showing the type of microcratering damage that typically follows a breakdown event.
(From Latham and Braun [16], with permission).

localised "splash" microcratering damage on the planar anode used in conjunction with the hairpin cathode of the experimental system of Fig. 7.5. This latter micrograph of Fig. 7.22 is of particular significance to the present discussion since it is possible to identify embedded microparticles at the centre of these craters, i.e. strongly suggesting that they originated from either the high velocity impact or trigger discharge process discussed in Chapter 4. Both of these explanations are however open to some doubt, since on the one hand the estimated single-transit impact velocities of micron sized particles in the present regimes are too low ($\lesssim 300\ m.s^{-1}$) to cause the observed fusion cratering [16], and on the other hand, theory indicates that a trigger discharge is unlikely to occur with such small particles. Despite these doubts, it is nevertheless difficult to discount a microparticle-based explanation for at least some of this microcratering since, as discussed above, considerable evidence has been accrued from investigations using dissimilar electrodes suggesting that relatively large numbers of particles are in fact exchanged between electrodes. Another important feature of the micrographs of Figs. 7.8 and 7.22 is the distribution of loosely adhering "secondary" microparticles that have evidently been formed from molten droplets generated during the fusion process. On the basis therefore of the various microparticle mechanisms discussed in Chapters 4 and 6, it is reasonable to anticipate that such secondary microparticles could play an active role in the subsequent operation of the gap.

In another novel approach for obtaining indirect evidence of microparticle processes, Theophilus et al. [70] devised the experimental regime illustrated in Fig. 7.23 in which any particles generated between the high voltage electrode assembly L_1 and L_2 during a prebreakdown voltage cycling can escape from the gap through small perforations in L_2 to become attached to the collecting plate P. By examining this plate before and after an experiment in a SEM, these investigators were able to show that a large number of microparticles having dimensions that were typically $\sim 3\mu m$ had been active in the gap during the prebreakdown phase. However, since the experiment was conducted in poor vac-

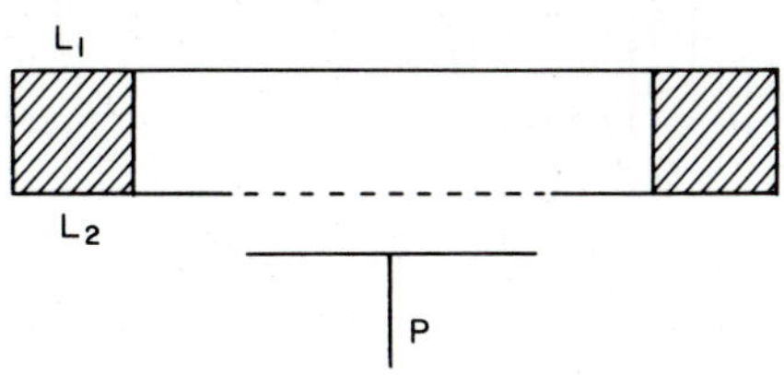

Fig. 7.23 An electrode regime used for collecting the naturally occurring microparticles that are active in a gap during the initial application of a high voltage (After Theophilus et al. [70]).

uum conditions ($\sim 10^{-5}$mbar) with a consequently greater likelihood of the occurrence of microdischarge events, some doubt must exist as to whether the collected sample of particles can be reliably assumed to be passively-launched "primary" microparticles. The interpretation of the findings was somewhat complicated by the presence of insulating ceramic particles among the collected sample; these could either have been derived from the alumina polishing medium, or have indicated that the insulating mounting of the electrodes was playing an active role in the experiment.

7.2(ii) Particle detection by direct techniques

The earliest attempts to record the actual transit of naturally occurring "primary" microparticles across a high voltage gap relied on the fact that they would be electrically charged and that it should therefore be possible to use fast electronic techniques to detect them as a charge transient superimposed upon any continuous prebreakdown current. Such a transient could then be used to directly characterise the microparticles in terms of their charge, mass and velocity. However, whilst this approach was conceptually very attractive, it had to be abandoned since no conclusive evidence was obtained, presumably due to the limitations of the electronic detecting systems which demanded the incompatible specifications of the highest charge sensitivity and the fastest response time.

Recently however, Texier [71] has developed an alternative *electrical* technique for the dynamic detection of charged microparticles. In this system, illustrated schematically in Fig. 7.24, one of the electrodes of a plane-parallel gap is replaced by a stainless steel grid and is followed by a capacitive drift tube detector system, similar to that described in Section 6.2,

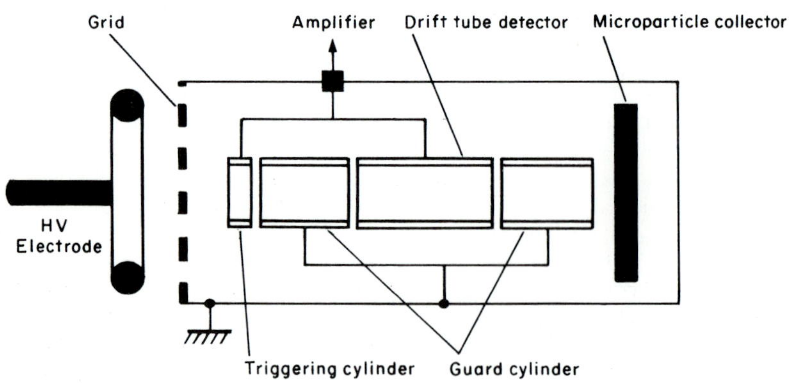

Fig. 7.24 An experimental regime for dynamically recording the charge and velocity of naturally occurring microparticles generated in a high voltage gap.
(From Texier [71], with permission).

for recording the charge and velocity of any microparticles that escape from the HV gap. In addition, there is a plate for collecting these particles so that their size and shape can be checked in a complementary SEM analysis. It was found that when a slowly increasing voltage is initially applied across the gap between the grid (cathode) and a freshly polished anode electrode A, large numbers of loosely adhering particles, typically ranging in size from 1-8μm, are extracted from the gap well before breakdown is approached, and that a further cycling of the gap voltage over this sub-breakdown range yielded no further particles; i.e. indicating that the initial voltage application had "electrostatically cleaned" the anode electrode of all loosely adhering "primary" microparticles.

A complementary elemental analysis of this sample of particles yielded the important but somewhat unexpected result that they were principally composed of the material used for the anode electrode A; unlike the findings of Theophilus et al. [70] described above, particles of the alumina polishing medium appeared to be of only secondary importance. Another interesting finding was that the size of the collected particles decreased with the applied voltage, which is in general agreement with Boulloud's theoretical reasoning as to the role played by Van der Waals adhesion forces [72]. As an extension of the technique, it was found, not surprisingly, that if the gap voltage is subsequently increased to breakdown, fresh bursts of "secondary" microparticles are detected whose characteristics appear to depend somewhat upon the target material. Whilst this technique undoubtedly represents an important new tool for the in situ study of microparticle phenomena, more reliance could be placed on the findings of any future application if it were (i) operated under UHV rather than the present "commercial" ($\sim 10^{-5}$mbar) vacuum conditions, (ii) incorporated some form of prebreakdown current/microdischarge monitoring facility to ensure that the apparent "primary" microparticles were not associated with electrical instabilities and (iii) reversed the polarity of the electrodes so that the field enhancing fine grid wires [73] could not play an active role as a source of electron emission.

An alternative approach to the dynamic detection of in-flight microparticles has been to use a laser-based *optical scattering* technique to detect the light scattered by microparticles as they cross an electrode gap. Here again however, the findings from early investigation [74,75] were inconclusive and it is only comparatively recently that Jenkins and Chatterton [76] have succeeded in obtaining reliable results from an improved experimental regime employing higher laser power and an improved detection efficiency. In the system used by these authors, illustrated schematically in Fig. 7.25, a 4W laser beam, with 1.6W in the 514.4nm line, is directed between the electrode gap to impinge on a suitable light dump so that only scattered radiation is collected by the lens and recorded by the photomultipler PM.

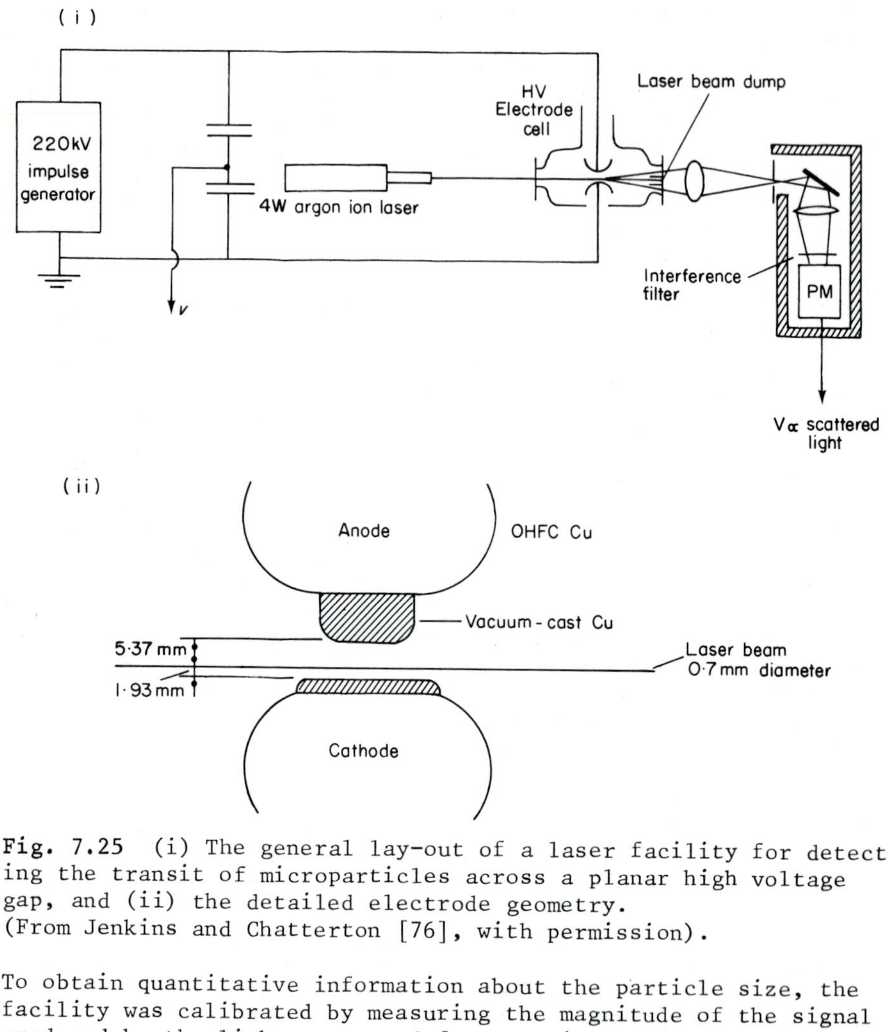

Fig. 7.25 (i) The general lay-out of a laser facility for detecting the transit of microparticles across a planar high voltage gap, and (ii) the detailed electrode geometry.
(From Jenkins and Chatterton [76], with permission).

To obtain quantitative information about the particle size, the facility was calibrated by measuring the magnitude of the signal produced by the light scattered from particles of known diameter, artificially introduced into the system: particle velocities were estimated from the duration of the light pulse, which corresponded to the time taken for a particle to cross the known diameter of the laser beam in the gap. The initial findings of this study showed that the first d-c voltage application to virgin electrodes is characterised by the passage of large numbers of "slow" particles having velocities in the range 15-30 $m.s^{-1}$, thus confirming the findings of Texier [71]. By using an impulse voltage technique, it was also demonstrated that a breakdown event is typically precursed by the detection of a microparticle crossing the gap $\sim$ 5μs before the voltage collapse; however, unlike the "slow" particles referred to above, this latter type have very much higher velocities (80-800 $m.s^{-1}$) and smaller diameters (0.1-0.2μm). Although not conclusive, this correlation between particle and breakdown events must be regarded as direct evidence in support of the general premise that breakdown can be microparticle initiated. This investigation also confirmed that as spark conditioning proceded, there was the expected rapid fall off in the number of particles crossing the gap. An unfortunate limitation of the present form of the technique is that it cannot discriminate between anode and cathode launched particles, or verify that they are electrically charged.

Finally, in this discussion of in-flight microparticle detection, it will be recalled from section 4.6(iii) that Davies and Biondi proposed a mechanism whereby microparticles can be vaporised by electron bombardment during their transit between electrodes and thereby induce breakdown. To obtain some experimental verification of this model, these same authors developed a *spectroscopic* technique for recording transient increases in the density of metal ions in a gap immediately prior to a breakdown [77]. Copper resonance radiation from an external source is focussed into a narrow beam to pass through the 1mm gap formed between a pair of plane-parallel copper electrodes. The transmitted light then enters a monochromator coupled to a photomultiplier so that it is possible to record rapid intensity variations in a given line of the copper resonance radiation. Such an "open shutter" system therefore provides a sensitive means of detecting transient increases in the vapour density of copper atoms in the inter-electrode gap, since the latter will constitute a strongly absorbing medium for the copper resonance radiation. To investigate the temporal correlation between the detection of metal vapour and the incidence of electrical discharge events as the gap voltage is gradually increased, the output signal from the photomultiplier, and that derived from a potentiometric resistor chain of 10kΩ and 50Ω carrying the total gap current in the low-voltage side of the circuit, are simultaneously monitored with a twin-beam oscilloscope. With this system it was established that a burst of neutral metal vapour is commonly liberated into the electrode gap ∿ 2-3 microseconds before a breakdown or microdischarge event. Since this relatively long time period is inconsistent with the anticipated delay time of ∿ nanoseconds for the avalanche growth of ionisation processes that would follow an "explosive" breakdown initiating event, Davies and Biondi were able to interpret these findings as strongly supporting their "heated-anode-particle" breakdown mechanism discussed in section 4.5(iii); i.e. in which a microparticle extruded from an anode "hot-spot" is vaporised by electron bombardment during its subsequent flight between the electrodes. Further evidence for the anodic origin of the initial vapour release was obtained from a development of this technique [78,79] illustrated in Fig. 7.26, in which dissimilar electrode materials

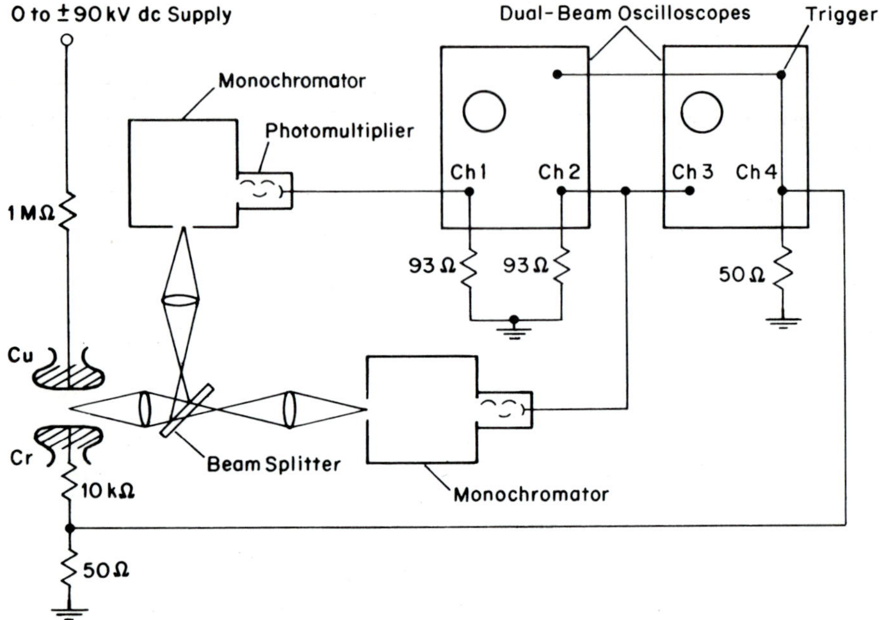

Fig. 7.26 An optical spectrometry facility for detecting and discriminating between the generation of anodic or cathodic metal vapour in a high voltage gap during a breakdown event. (From Davies and Biondi [78,79], with permission).

(copper and chromium) were used in conjunction with twin monochromator detecting systems tuned respectively to the resonance lines of Cu and Cr. With this system these authors were able to establish that, although both anode and cathode vapour are liberated at a breakdown, the anode species consistantly appears in the gap ∿ 30-150 nanoseconds before cathode vapour; i.e. consistent with the model of breakdown being initiated in the vapour medium generated from the anode particle, followed by erosion of the cathode by the ensuing discharge.

7.3 References

1. Latham, R.V. and Braun, E., *J. Phys. D: Appl. Phys.*, **1**, 1731-5, (1968).
2. Little, R.P. and Whitney, W.T., *J. Appl. Phys.* **34**, 2430-2, (1963).
3. Brodie, I. and Weissman, I., *Vacuum*, **14**, 299-301, (1964).
4. Tomaschke, H.E., Alpert, D., Lee, D.A. and Lyman, L.M., *Proc. II-DEIV*, 13-21, (1966).
5. Farrall, G.A., *J. Appl. Phys.*, **42**, 2284-93, (1971).
6. Jüttner, B., *Proc. VI-DEIV*, 101-6, (1974).

7. Crewe, A.V., Eggenberger, E.N., Wall, J. and Welter, L.M., *Rev. Sci. Inst.* **39**, 576-83, (1968).
8. Jüttner, B., Wolff, H. and Altrichter, B., *Phys. Stat. Sol.*, **27a**, 403-12, (1975).
9. Cox, B.M. and Wort, D.E.J., *Vacuum*, **22**, 453-55, (1972).
10. Bogdanovskii, G.A., *Sov. Phys.-Solid State*, **1**, 1171-6, (1959).
11. Little R.P. and Smith, S.T., *J. Appl. Phys.*, **36**, 1502-4, (1965).
12. Jedynak, L., *J. Appl. Phys.*, **36**, 2587-9, (1965).
13. Latham, R.V. and Chapman, C.J.S., *J. Phys. E: Sci. Instrum.* **3**, 732-4, (1970).
14. Udris, Y., 1st Int. Conf. on Gas Discharges, London, 108-12, (1970).
15. Cox, B.M., Jervis-Hunter, G. and Lloyd, O., *CEGB Lab. Rpt. RD/M/N593*, (1971).
16. Latham, R.V. and Braun, E., *J. Phys. D: Appl. Phys.*, **3**,1663-70, (1970).
17. Little, R.P. and Smith, S.T., *IEEE Trans. Electron Devices*, **ED-12**, 77-83, (1965).
18. Miller, H.C. and Farrall, G.A., *Gen. Elec. Rpt. No. 66-C-302*, (1966).
19. Cox, B.M. and Bloomer, R.N., *CEGB Lab. Rpt. RD/M/R91*, (1968).
20. Bouchard, K.G., *J. Vac. Sci. Technol.* **7**, 358-60, (1970).
21. Williams, D.W. and Williams, W.T., *J. Phys. D: Appl. Phys.* **6**, 734-43, (1973).
22. Cox, B.M., *J. Phys. D: Appl. Phys.* **7**, 143-50, (1974).
23. Jüttner, B., *Beitrage Plasmaphysik*, **19**, 25-48, (1979).
24. Cox, B.M., *J. Phys. D: Appl. Phys.* **8**, 2065-73, (1975).
25. Cox, B.M. and Williams, W.T., *J. Phys. D: Appl. Phys.* **10**, L5-9, (1977).
26. Allen, N.K., Cox, B.M. and Latham, R.V., *J. Phys. D: Appl. Phys.* **12**, 969-78, (1979).
27. Athwal, C.S. and Latham, R.V., *Proc. IX-DEIV, Physica DE*, **104c**, (1981), In press.
28. Athwal, C.S., Ph.D. Thesis, University of Aston, U.K. (1981).
29. Hurley, R., *J. Phys. D: Appl. Phys.*, **12**, 2247-54, (1979).
30. Cornish, J.C.L., Latham, R.V. and Braun, E., *Proc. IV-DEIV*, 28-32, (1970).
31. Jüttner, B., *Exper. Tech. Phys.*, **19**, 45-48, (1970).
32. Ghani, A., Ph.D. Thesis, University of Aston, U.K. (1971).
33. Panitz, J.A., *J. Appl. Phys.* **44**, 372-5, (1973).
34. Panitz, J.A., *J. Appl. Phys.* **45**, 1112-4, (1974).
35. DeGeeter, D.J., *J. Appl. Phys.* **34**, 919-20, (1963).
36. Alpert, D., Lee, D.A., Lyman, F.M. and Tomaschke, H.E., *J. Vac. Sci. Technol.* **1**, 35-50, (1964).
37. Bennette, C.J., Swanson, L.W. and Charbonnier, F.M., *J. Appl. Phys.* **38**, 634-40, (1967).
38. Jüttner, B., *Mber, Deut. Acad. Wiss. Berl.*, **11(2)**, 105-7, (1969).
39. Young, R.W., *Vacuum*, **24**, 167-172, (1973).

40. Chatterton, P.A., *Brit. J. Appl. Phys.*, **17**, 1108-10, (1966).
41. Zeitoun-Fakiris, A., *C.R. Acad. Sci. Paris*, **266**, 828-30, (1968).
42. Boersch, H., Radeloff, C. and Suerberg, L. , *Z. Phys.* **65**, 464- 9 , (1961).
43. Hurley, R.E. and Dooley, P.J., *Vacuum*, **28**, 147-149, (1977).
44. Hurley, R.E. and Dooley, P.J., *J. Phys. D: Appl. Phys.* **10**, L195-201, (1977).
45. Hurley, R.E., *J. Phys. D: Appl. Phys.* **12**, 2229-45, (1979).
46. Hurley, R.E., *J. Phys. D: Appl. Phys.* **13**, 1121-8, (1980).
47. Alfrey, G.F. and Taylor, J.B., *Brit. J. Appl. Phys.* **6**, Suppl. 4, 544-9, (1955).
48. Walters, C.S., Fox, M.W. and Latham, R.V., *J. Phys. D: Appl. Phys.* **7**, 911-19, (1974).
49. Farrall, G.A., Owens, M. and Hudda, F.G., *J. Appl. Phys.* **46**, 610-17, (1975).
50. Maskrey, J.T. and Dougdale, R.A., *Brit. J. Appl. Phys.* **17**, 1025-34, (1966).
51. Malter, L., *Phys. Rev.* **49**, 876-85, (1936).
52. Duke, C.B. and Alferieff, M.E., *J. Chem. Phys.* **46**, 923-37, (1967).
53. Kellog, G.L. and Tsong, T.T., *Surface Sci.* **62**, 343-60, (1977).
54. Todd, C.J. and Rhodin, T.N., *Surface Sci.* **42**, 109-38, (1974).
55. Schmidt, L.D. and Gomer, R., *J. Chem. Phys.* **45**, 1605-23, (1966).
56. Schockley, W., *Phys. Rev.* **91**, 228, (1953).
57. Braun, E., Forbes, R.G., Pearson, J., Pelmore, J.M. and Latham, R.V., *J. Phys. E: Sci. Instrum.* **11**, 222-8, (1978).
58. Allen, N.K. and Latham, R.V., *J. Phys. D: Appl. Phys.* **11**, L55-L57, (1978).
59. Allen, N.K., Ph.D. Thesis, University of Aston, U.K. (1979).
60. Allen, N.K., Athwal, C.S. and Latham, R.V., *Vacuum*, **32**, (1981), In press.
61. Allen, N.K. and Latham, R.V., *Proc. VIII-DEIV*, **C6 1-9**.(1978).
62. Young, R.D., *Phys. Rev.* **113**, 110-4, (1959).
63. Shepherd, W.B. and Peria, W.T., *Surface Sci.* **38**, 461-98, (1973).
64. Lewis, B.F. and Fischer, T.E., *Surface Sci.* **41**, 371-6, (19 (1974).
65. Cranberg, L., *J. Appl. Phys.* **23**, 518-22, (1952).
66. Anderson, H.W., *Elec. Eng.* **54**, 1315-1320, (1935).
67. Browne, P.F., *Proc. Phys. Soc.* **B68**, 564-6, (1955).
68. Tarasova, L.V. and Razin, A.A., *Sov. Phys.-Tech. Phys.* **4**, 879-85 (1959).
69. Chatterton, P.A. and Biradar, P.I., *Z. Ang. Phys.* **30**, 163-70, (1970).
70. Theophilus, G.D., Srivastava, K.D. and Van Heeswijk, R.G., *J. Appl. Phys.* **47**, 897-9, (1976).
71. Texier, C., *J. Phys. D: Appl. Phys.* **10**, 1693-1702, (1977).

72. Boulloud, A., *Le Vide*, **99**, 240-3, (1962).
73. Feynman, R.P., Leighton, R.B. and Sands, M., Feynman Lectures on Physics, Addison Wesley: Massachusetts, **2**, 710-714, (1970).
74. Piuz, F., *CERN Report TC-L/Int*. 72-8, (1972).
75. Smalley, J., *J. Phys. D: Appl.Phys*. **9**, 2397-401, (1976).
76. Jenkins, J.E. and Chatterton, P.A., *J. Phys. D: Appl. Phys*. **10**, L17-23, (1977).
77. Davies, D.K. and Biondi, M.A., *J. Appl. Phys*. **41**, 88-93, (1970).
78. Davies, D.K. and Biondi, M.A., *Proc. VI-DEIV*, 45-50, (1974).
79. Davies, D.K. and Biondi, M.A., *J. Appl. Phys*. **48**, 4229-33, (1977).

8 Recent Advances in the understanding of Prebreakdown Electron Emission

8.1 A non-metallic field emitting microregime
8.2 Band theory interpretation
8.3 Filamentary interpretation
8.4 Insulator "switching" model
8.5 References

8.1 A non-metallic field emitting microregime

The picture to emerge from the recent experimental studies described in Chapter 7 on the origin of the prebreakdown electron emission currents associated with small gap ($d \lesssim 1$mm) virgin electrodes, is that they appear to stem invariably from microscopically localised "non-metallic" emission sites that are characterised by having (i) linear high-β Fowler-Nordheim current-voltage characteristics, (ii) no significant field-enhancing surface structure (see Fig. 7.11), (iii) associated electroluminescent effects (see Fig. 7.18), and (iv) semiconductor-like electron emission spectra (see Fig. 7.20). These studies also showed that a similar predominance of "non-metallic" sites occurs on arced electrodes: however, with this type of regime, it is known that there are also large numbers of metallic microprotrusions (see Figs. 7.6, 7.9 and 7.22) which occasionally may be sharp enough to provide the necessary field enhancement for a "metallic" field emission process. The question as to whether breakdown results from a "cathode" or "anode" process is now a more complex issue than that discussed in Chapter 3. Clearly, if the prebreakdown current stems solely from a traditional "metallic" emitter, this earlier detailed analysis will still hold: however, if it originates from a "non-metallic" electron source, it must be assumed that, although the critical "anode" condition will remain unchanged, there will be a different set of critical conditions for a "cathode" initiated event, and consequently, new criteria for "cathode" versus "anode" initiation.

The model originally proposed by Latham and his co-workers [1,2] was developed from the electron spectrometry measurements described in the previous chapter and is based on the physical regime of a semiconducting/insulating micro-impurity that is in intimate contact with the substrate metallic cathode; i.e. perhaps partially embedded as illustrated in Fig. 8.1.

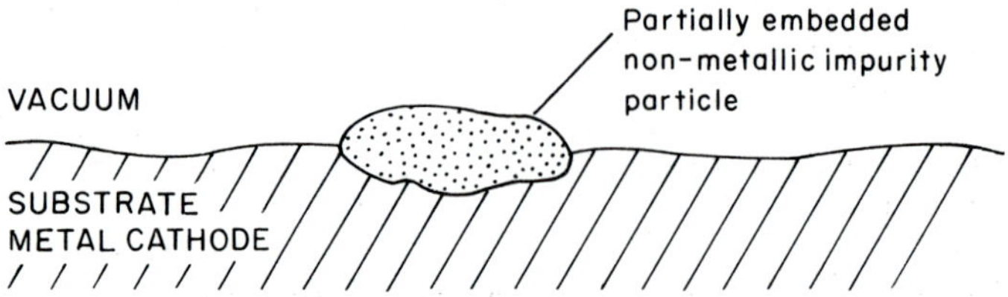

Fig. 8.1 The microregime proposed by Latham and his co-workers [1,2] as being responsible for the electron emission processes on broad-area high voltage electrodes.

8.2 Band theory interpretation

Very little is known about the possible composition of such impurities, although there is a suggestion from follow-up X-ray microprobe measurements that they may frequently contain elements that are alien to the substrate electrode: in one study, for example, aluminium, possibly in its insulating oxide form, was found to be associated with an emitting site on a copper electrode [2]. In the absence of an applied field, the idealised energy band representation of such a composite surface would appear as shown in Fig. 8.2, where ϕ_1 is the work function of the substrate metal and ϕ_2 that of the overlaying semiconducting/ insulating impurity: the band bending at the metal/non-metal and non-metal/vacuum interfaces is a well known effect arising from work function differences and the presence of surface states as discussed for example in [3] and [4]. If now a high

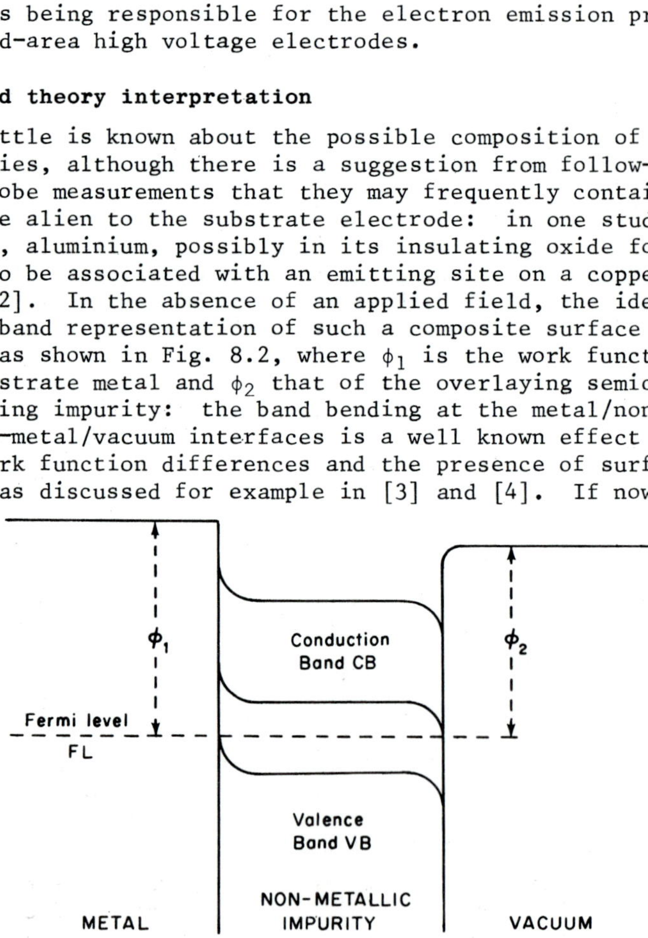

Fig. 8.2 The zero-field energy band configuration of the composite microregime shown in Fig. 8.1.

external field is applied to this regime, the dielectric properties of the non-metallic impurity will allow the field to penetrate into its surface, so that the band structure and potential barrier of Fig. 8.2 will be modified to that shown in Fig. 8.3(i) and (ii) for the extreme cases of a small band-gap semiconductor and a wide band-gap insulating material, where both are assumed to have a similar thickness s. In the former case, the presence of a high density of free electron carriers or surface states will screen the bulk of the semiconductor from the applied field and hence limit its penetration to a thin surface region as shown in Fig. 8.3(i). As the conductivity of the semiconductor decreases the field penetration correspondingly increases until,

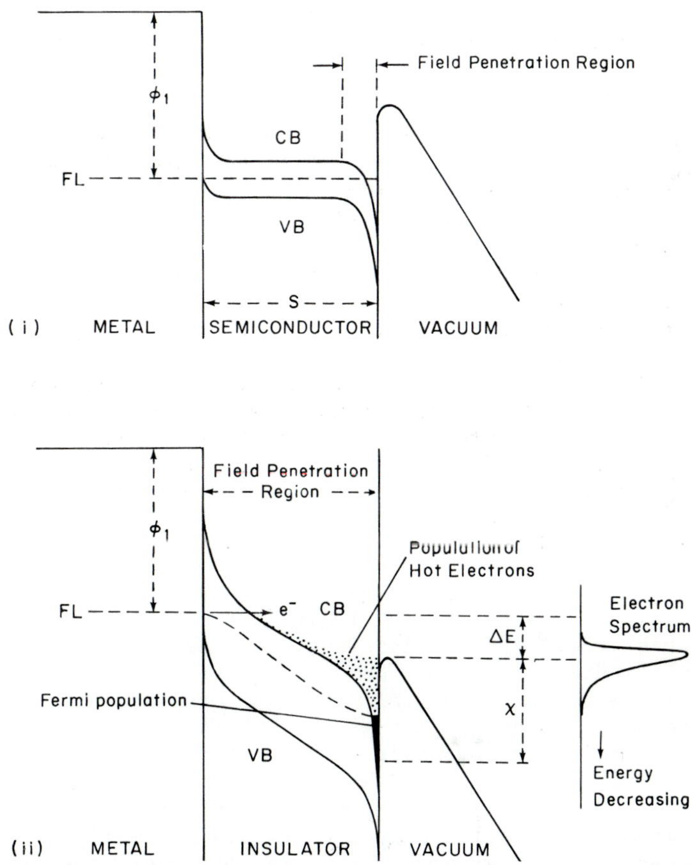

Fig. 8.3 The high-field energy band configuration of the composite microregime when the impurity has (i) semiconductor and (ii) insulator like properties. For case (ii), an electron emission mechanism has also been illustrated that gives rise to an energy spectrum that is displaced from the Fermi level of the substrate metal cathode.

for the limiting case of an insulator, complete penetration to the substrate metal occurs producing the highly distorted band structure shown in Fig. 8.3(ii).

From the point of view of promoting a continuous field electron emission process, the latter regime has several favourable features. Firstly, and most important, the field penetration can create the necessary condition for *initiating* such a process; viz. by tilting the energy bands to a point where electrons can tunnel from the Fermi level in the metal into the bottom of the conduction band of the insulator. Secondly, such electrons will then be accelerated or "heated" by the internal field so that they can acquire sufficient energy to escape over the low electron affinity barrier χ at the insulator/vacuum surface that is characteristic of good insulators. Thus, such an "internal" electron heating mechanism avoids the need to invoke the concept of geometric field enhancement at surface microprotrusions. It also follows from Fig. 8.3(ii) that the spectrum of these heated electrons will be displaced by some energy ΔE from the Fermi level as is indeed found experimentally (see Fig. 7.20). Associated with this electron heating there will inevitably be electron-phonon scattering tending to thermalise the electron population. However, some electrons will presumably acquire energies approaching the total potential dropped across the insulator, and hence be capable of ionising deep-lying trapped states and exciting inter-band electron-hole pairs. The existence of such processes is strongly supported by the electroluminescent effects described in section 7.1(v) that are associated with these emission processes. In fact, their spectra, which typically lie in the range 500-750nm [5], also confirm that the band gap of the emitting regime must be $\gtrsim 2.5$ eV; i.e. indicating that an insulating rather than a semiconducting type of material is involved. If it is also assumed that such an insulating material has the most favourable dielectric properties for supporting the maximum initial internal field, viz. that it should have a low dielectric constant with $\varepsilon_r \to 1$, the necessary thickness of such an impurity to drop ~ 2.5 V in a field of $\sim 10^7 Vm^{-1}$ is $\gtrsim 0.25\mu m$. Significantly, this order of dimension is typical of the surface features identified by the direct SEM techniques described in section 7.1(ii) as being responsible for the localised emission sites. It must be added however, that since the assumption of such a low value of ε_r is questionable for low vapour pressure inorganic surface impurities that can withstand vacuum processing (e.g. baking to $\sim 300^oC$), the alternative possibility cannot be ruled out that impurities having higher ε_r values could also provide emission centres if they occurred in regions where the field was locally enhanced by surface roughness, e.g. at cracks or grain boundaries as suggested by the findings of Cox [6] and Allen, Cox and Latham [2]. Finally, and in general support of this proposed emitting regime, there are the experimental findings of Cox [6], Farrall et al. [7,8], and Pokrovskaya-Soboleva et al.

[9] which directly confirm that micron-sized insulating particles, both superficially adhering to an electrode surface or embedded in it, frequently promote strong electron emission.

As an early approach to explaining the second low-energy peak that is sometimes present in the spectra of these sites (see Fig. 7.21), Latham and his co-workers [1,2] attributed it to an unstable surface effect, and suggested that the model of Fig. 8.3(ii) could be modified to take account of the possibility of ad-atom resonance tunnelling as described by the models of Duke and Alferieff [10] and Gadzuk [11]. Thus referring to Fig. 8.4, it is assumed that under certain conditions, an ad-atom can provide a favourable resonance tunnelling state relative to the population of hot electrons so that those within the appropriate narrow energy band will have a high probability of escaping to the vacuum by this additional mechanism. In the early discussion of the basic model of Fig. 8.3(ii), consideration was also given to the possible role played by inter-band impurity states. This followed from the recognition that the least plausible aspect of the model was the requirement that there should be sufficient band bending to allow the initial tunnelling of electrons from the Fermi level in the metal into the bottom of the conduction band of the insulator. To alleviate this difficulty, it was suggested that the model could be further modified as shown in Fig. 8.4 to include a level of inter-band impurity

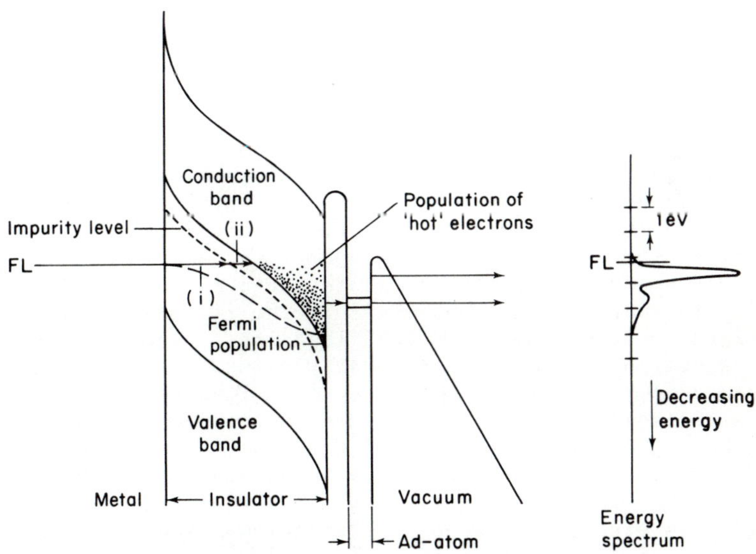

Fig. 8.4 The high-field electron emission regime of Fig. 8.3(ii) as it is modified by the presence of interband impurity levels and ad-atom surface states. (From Allen, Cox and Latham [2], with permission).

states near the bottom of the conduction band in the insulator that would provide an intermediate "resting place" for an electron undergoing a two-stage tunnelling process (i) + (ii).

8.3 Filamentary interpretation

In a recent detailed discussion of the cathode or k-spot electroluminescent measurements described in section 7.5, Hurley [5, 12] has proposed an alternative explanation of the electron emission that can stem from the type of microregime shown in Fig. 8.1. This is based on a well known phenomenon exhibited by nanometer to micron thick films of certain semiconducting and insulating materials, particularly oxides, nitrides, fluorides and amorphous semiconducting glasses, whereby the application of a high electric field (10-100 $MV.m^{-1}$) via surface electrodes can lead to the device "switching" from a non-conducting "off" state to a conducting "on" state in which the externally measured conductivity of the film can be increased by as much as a factor of 10^8. Such a switching event is also accompanied by the simultaneous appearance of two further "external" phenomena that are of particular significance to the present discussion, viz. microscopically localised electroluminescent and electron emission processes. For a full discussion of the early work on the switching and associated properties of these devices, the reader is referred to the review articles of Dearnaley et al. [13] and Boer and Ovshinsky [14]. The underlying physical mechanism thought to be responsible for the phenomenon involves the establishment of a thin conducting channel or filament in the dielectric between the two metal electrodes. Estimates of the initial cross sectional dimensions of these filaments show that they depend on the film thickness, varying from $\sim$ 1nm to 50μm for 40nm - 500μm thick films [13,15]: once established in a given film, however, a filament section will also depend on the current it is conducting. Another important feature of this phenomenon is that if the field is applied for a sufficient length of time, a filament may become "electroformed" through the permanent or semi-permanent rearrangement of the atoms or molecules within the filament: electroforming times are typically in the millisecond to second range, whereas switching times are generally $\lesssim$ 1μs.

According to the model of Hurley [5], impurity inclusions, such as illustrated in Fig. 8.1, are distributed at random throughout the surface. A few of these occur in regions where the field is locally intensified at cracks and grain boundaries by a factor β above average values. The field throughout the impurity is given, to a good approximation, by $\beta E/\varepsilon_r$ where E is the average field, so that if both β and ε_r are of the order of 5 to 10, then electroforming of filaments is possible when $E \approx 10^5$V/cm. This situation will be as illustrated in Fig. 8.5, from which it follows that such a filament will behave as a metallic-like whisker and hence give rise to a local field

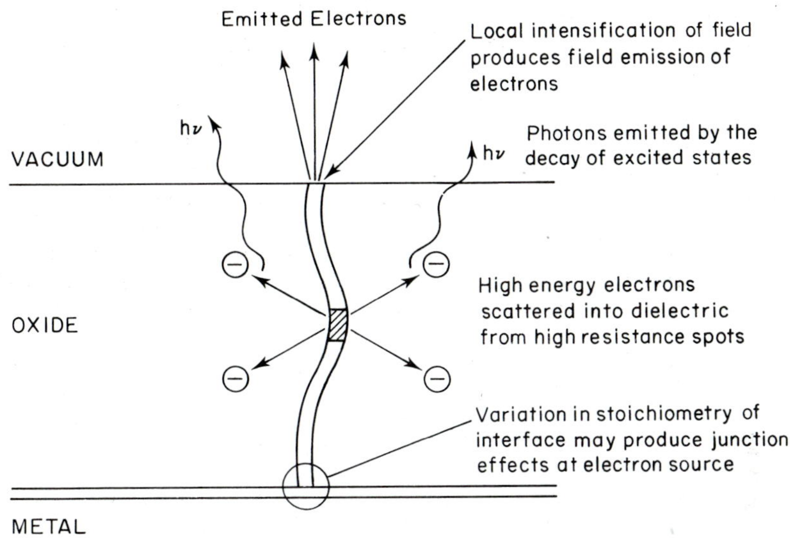

Fig. 8.5 The simultaneous production of electroluminescence and electron emission from an electroformed conducting filament in an oxide microimpurity.
(From Hurley [12], with permission).

enhancement that could be sufficient to promote field electron emission at its intersection with the vacuum interface. Extending the anology with the Dearnaley filamentary model [16], it can be assumed there are likely to be high resistance spots in the electroformed filament where the enhanced electric field will give rise to a population of "hot" carriers that will subsequently be scattered by the surrounding oxide to give rise to electroluminescence effects through some form of impact ionisation or recombination process such as discussed by Hickmott [17]. The injection of electrons from the metal substrate into the filament is assumed to arise from complex semiconductor/metal junction effects. To evaluate this model, Hurley [12] made reference to his measurements on the electron and optical emission sites on copper electrodes. By assuming that the microimpurity involved in this case was Cu_2O, he was able to show that most of the observed phenomena were strikingly similar to those observed in independent measurements made on switching devices of this oxide by Cook [15] and Morgan and Howes [18]. Here, particular mention should be made of the threshold switching field and the breakdown delay time associated with over-voltage pulse experiments. The actual breakdown mechanism envisaged for this filamentary regime is based on the thermal instability model of Cook [15], whereby at a certain current level, the conducting filament becomes thermally unstable and "explodes" so that a molten impurity particle is ejected from the electrode surface as illustrated in Fig. 8.6. Vivid support for such a mechanism is provided by the type of open-shutter photograph shown in Fig. 8.7, which not only records the track of such a particle, but also establishes a positive correlation between a breakdown event and a previous electroluminescent centre [19].

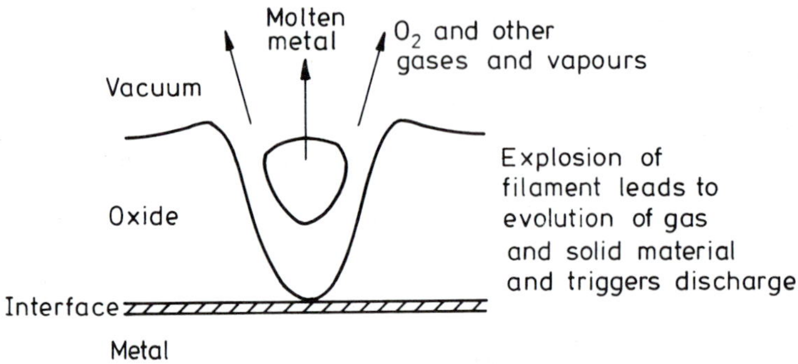

Fig. 8.6 An illustration of the breakdown mechanism associated with the conducting filament model of Fig. 8.5.
(From Hurley [5], with permission).

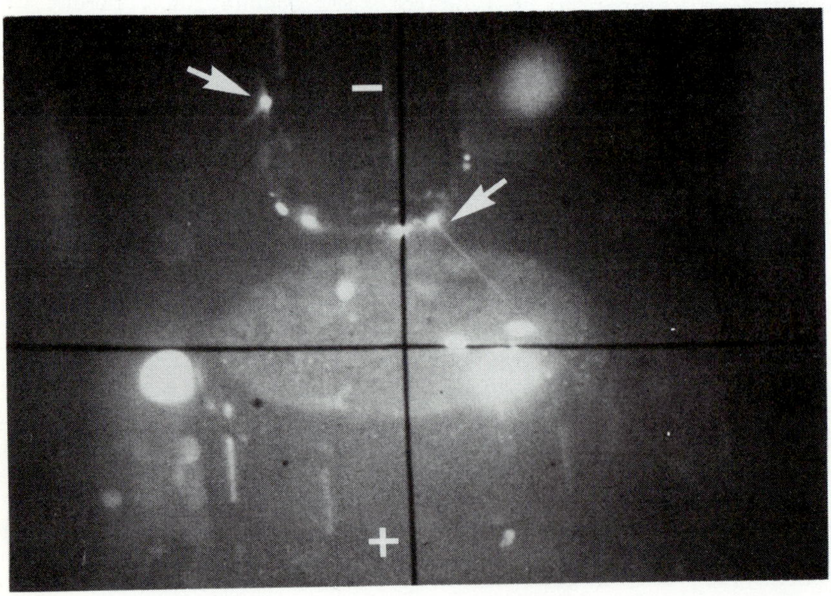

Fig. 8.7 An open-shutter photograph of an electrically stressed planar high voltage gap showing both anode and cathode spots. Also shown arrowed are flares and discharge tracks emanating from cathode-spots.
(From Hurley and Dooley [19], with permission).

There are several other important phenomena that can satisfactorarily be explained on the basis of this type of model [5,12]. Firstly, discontinuities in the current-voltage characteristic of a broad-area gap can be attributed to either the thermal rupture and possible reforming of the filaments that are contributing to the total emission, or the "switching-on" of new filaments as the gap field is raised. In support of this latter concept, there have recently been reports [20,21] that the prebreakdown current can exhibit just such a "switching-on" effect, presumably associated with the formation of the first conducting filament. Secondly, this new model offers not only an alternative and very plausible interpretation of the experiments of Juttner et al. [22,23] described in section 7.1(i), which demonstrate how electron emission is selectively suppressed by such "active" gases as O_2, CO and N_2, but also explains the more recent observation of Hurley [5] that the associated electroluminescence is also suppressed by increasing the ambient pressure. Thus, these effects can now be attributed to the "poisoning" mechanism discussed by Dearnaley [16], in which absorbed gases such as oxygen or nitrogen will fill up the oxygen vacancies that are thought to characterise a conducting filament. It follows from this reasoning that oxygen should have a more marked influence than say nitrogen, which is indeed borne out by the measurements of

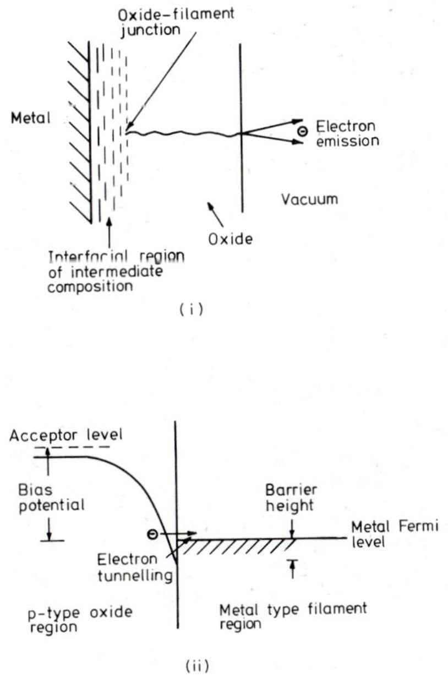

Fig. 8.8 (i) A conducting filament penetrating from the oxide-vacuum boundary into a p-type impurity, (ii) The energy band diagram of the filament-oxide junction regime.
(From Hurley [24], with permission).

Juttner et al. [22,23]. Lastly, attention must be drawn to the recent finding of Cox [20] and Hurley [24] that there are two types of emitting site, termed a- and b-sites by Hurley. The a-sites are the more common and give rise to the familiar linear F-N plots and breakdown events, whilst the b-sites are distinguished by being current-controlled through a negative resistance characteristic, and hence do not give rise to breakdown events.

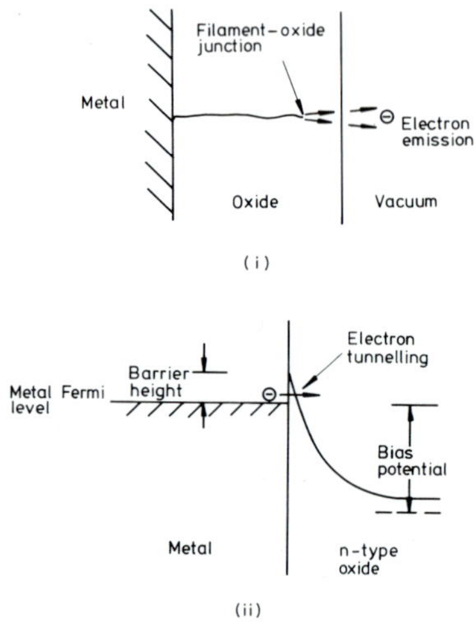

Fig. 8.9 (i) A conducting filament penetrating from the base-metal into an n-type oxide impurity, (ii) The energy band diagram of the filament-oxide junction region.
(From Hurley [24], with permission).

In terms of the present discussion,the b-sites are particularly interesting since their behaviour bears a striking resemblance to the current-controlled switching states in electroformed oxide filaments. Hurley [24] has suggested two possible models that could account for the observed current-voltage characteristic of b-sites. Both involve filaments that only partly penetrate the surface impurity and give rise to the emission of hot electrons that are produced at distances no greater than $\sim$ 100Å from the surface. In one interpretation, (Fig. 8.8) a conducting filament penetrates from the oxide surface and terminates in the dielectric, or within an oxide-metal interface region of intermediate composition. Electrons tunnel through this region into a metal type filament and are emitted from the point where the filament penetrates the surface by field enhanced tunnelling, or because they are hot relative to the Fermi level. In the other interpretation, (Fig. 8.9) a conducting filament penetrates from the base metal and terminates in the oxide just below the surface: here hot electrons originate at the filament-oxide boundary and are emitted from the oxide-vacuum surface. In each case, emission is controlled at a metal-oxide boundary located below the surface which may take the form of a reverse biased rectifier type junction and exhibit negative resistance characteristics if the bias voltage is increased beyond a certain point [25]. This effect is often attributed to junction heating but may also be attributed to the development of a semi-permanent space-charge distribution [26]. If positive holes migrate to the barrier interface then at higher fields electron-hole recombination will decrease because the holes are trapped in regions which only see high electron velocities. It should be pointed out that negative resistance (current controlled S-type curve) may also be attributed to impact ionisation, increasing mobility caused by decreasing cross-sections of certain scattering processes and phase changes or atomic re-arrangements (see for example Volkov and Kogan [27] or Dearnaley et al. [13]).

8.4 Insulator "switching" model

Although each of the emission models described so far have many attractive features, they also have evident limitations. For example, the energy band model of Figs. 8.3 and 8.4 does not readily explain how a significant number of the hot electrons will be able to cross the micron-dimension impurity without losing most or all of their energy through phonon scattering processes, whilst the filament model of Fig. 8.5 does not correctly account for the shift in electron spectra from the Fermi level: both models are also equally vague about the precise mechanism by which electrons tunnel from the metal into the impurity. In an attempt to overcome these limitations, and particularly to correlate the complementary optical and electron spectrometry data obtained from high-β sites, Athwal and Latham [21] have revised the earlier band models of Figs. 8.3 and 8.4. They now include the concept that the emission regime involves a substance that is capable of an Ovshinsky type "switching", through some electro-forming process, to an equilibrium high conductivity "on" state [14], in which the energy band structure of Fig. 8.3(ii) is altered to the configuration illustrated in Fig. 8.10; i.e. analogous to that assumed to occur in"metal-chalcogenide glass-metal" systems [28,29]. Such a switching event is envisaged as being associated with an avalanche process that is triggered by the onset of electrons tunnelling from the metal substrate into the insulating impurity which, at this stage, is experiencing a high penetrating field. Under these circumstances there will be a simultaneous production of positive and negative charge carriers, such as electron-hole pairs from impact ionisation by the hot electrons. Hole migration could then create a high field region at the metal-insulator boundary, whilst negative charge trapped in surface states could give rise to pronounced band bending at the insulator-vacuum boundary. A quantitative assessment of the effect of these processes on electron emission presents considerable difficulties in view of the unknown composition and micro-structure of the emitting region. For example, amorphous

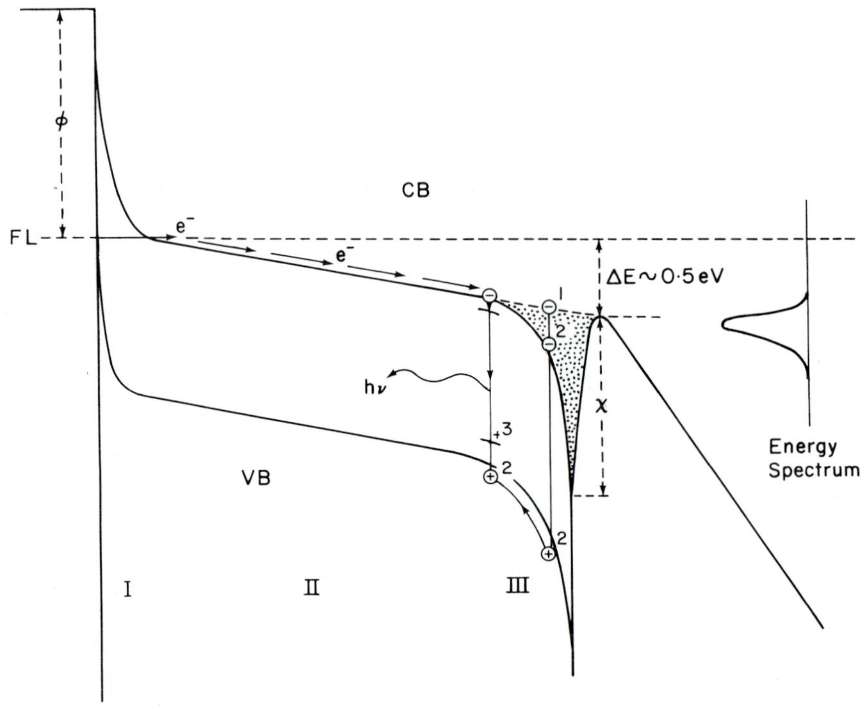

Fig. 8.10 The energy band configuration of the "on" state of an electron and photon emitting composite microregime. (From Athwal and Latham [21], with permission).

material would contain a profusion of trapping levels, and would require current densities of the order of $10^8 Am^{-2}$ to maintain the emitter in the switched 'ON' state, corresponding to Fig. 8.10 [28]. The estimated current density of known emitting sites is of the order of $5.10^5 Am^{-2}$ and hence the micro-channels involved may consist of relatively trap-free crystalline regions. In this respect, thermal effects during electro-forming [30], or even vacuum baking procedures may be important. It is worth noting that both baking and 'current-conditioning' described in section 2.3(i) have a stabilising effect on pre-breakdown electron currents.

Referring to Fig. 8.10, it will be seen that this emission regime is characterised by two very narrow high field regions I and III, located respectively at the metal/insulator and insulator/vacuum interfaces, with an extended intermediate low-field region II. According to this model, electrons will tunnel from the metal across the first high-field region and then be rapidly thermalised so that they are able to cross the extended low-field region in the bottom of the conduction band where their lifetime can be $\sim 10^{-8}$s [28]. They then enter the second narrow high-field region a few tens of nanometers thick where they are heated through the 2-3 eV necessary both for exciting the electron transitions required for producing the typical optical spectra shown in Fig. 7.17 and to escape over the depressed barrier at an energy that is experimentally found to be ∿ 0.2-0.5 eV below the substrate Fermi level as shown in Fig. 8.10. On the assumption that the optical spectra are associated with the emission of electrons, rather than just the presence of an applied field, their most likely physical origin involves an impact ionisation mechanism such as the sequence of events also illustrated in Fig. 8.10. Firstly, a hot electron $\ominus^1$ gives rise to an electron-hole pair $\ominus^2 + \oplus^2$. The hole then migrates towards the metal but soon relinquishes its energy to excite a luminescent centre $+^3$. Finally there is a recombination process with a conduction electron via an excited state in which an optical photon $h\nu$ is emitted. Another mechanism that may also contribute to the observed electroluminescent effects involves the production of an electron-hole pair by the field ionisation of a luminescent centre in one of the high field regions of Fig. 8.10. On either of these interpretations, the relative broad optical spectra spanning a typical wavelength range of 500-750 nm would indicate a complex distribution of interband states, i.e. such as might reasonably be expected to occur in impure microcrystalline regions.

According to the model of Fig. 8.10, Athwal and Latham [21] attribute the shift of the electron energy distribution from the Fermi level to be the sum of (i) the energy lost in thermalising into the conduction band minimum in region I, (ii) the ohmic energy loss in low field region II, and (iii) the energy lost due to electron-phonon scattering in region III. Since each of these losses may be expected to increase with increasing current, the total spectral shift should be strongly dependent on the applied field. It can also be observed that electrons which have thermalised in a parabolic conduction band minimum will have an energy distribution with a half-width of ∿ kT (∿ 0.04 eV at room temperature) before entering region III, so that if it is assumed that the electrons escape over the work function barrier, the half-width of the emitted distribution will be predominantly due to phonon scattering of hot electrons in region III: here again therefore, this spectral parameter could similarly be anticipated to increase with increasing current and hence applied field. These general conclusions have indeed been recently verified experimentally by Athwal and Latham [21] who extended the electron spectrometry studies described in section 7.1(vi) to a more detailed analysis of how the spectra of broad-area emission sites depend on the applied field and emission current. Thus, Fig. 8.11 contrasts the spectra obtained from a typical site on a copper electrode under (a) low-field and (b) high-field conditions, and clearly illustrates how this parameter influences their shape and position with respect to the Fermi-level of the cathode sub-

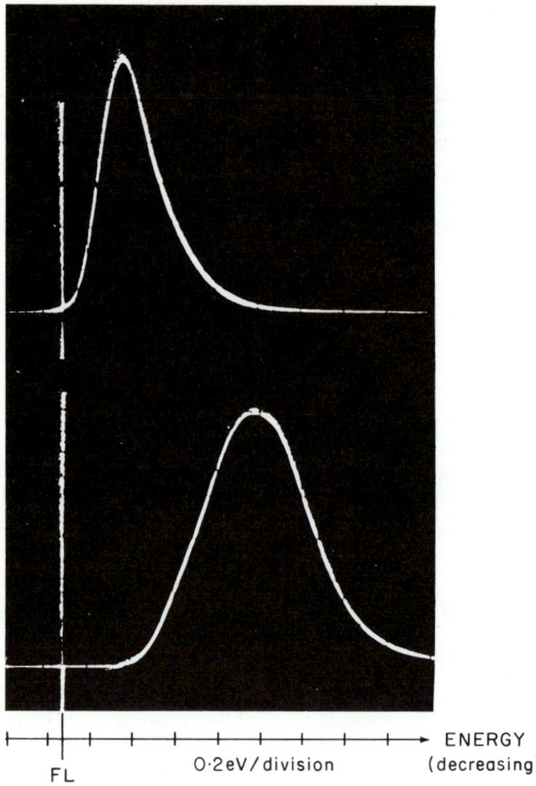

Fig. 8.11 Typical energy spectra of electrons emitted from the microregime illustrated in Fig. 8.10 under (i) low-field and (ii) high-field conditions.
(From Athwal and Latham [21], with permission).

strate. For this investigation such spectra were characterised in terms of (i) the shift of the maximum of the distribution from the Fermi level of the copper substrate, and (ii)the full width of half maximum (FWHM), and the variation of these parameters with total emission current for the same copper site is shown in Fig. 8.12. From these plots it is seen that both parameters are nearly constant at low current levels (i.e. $\lesssim 10^{-8}$A), but thereafter increase rapidly. This behaviour, particularly in the case of the FWHM, is therefore consistant with the concept that the dominant process controlling the emission spectrum is electron-phonon scattering in the final high field region III of Fig. 8.10.

There has been much discussion in the literature as to whether the electro-forming process implicit to this model is a thermal or electronic process. Thermal theories emphasise the constricted

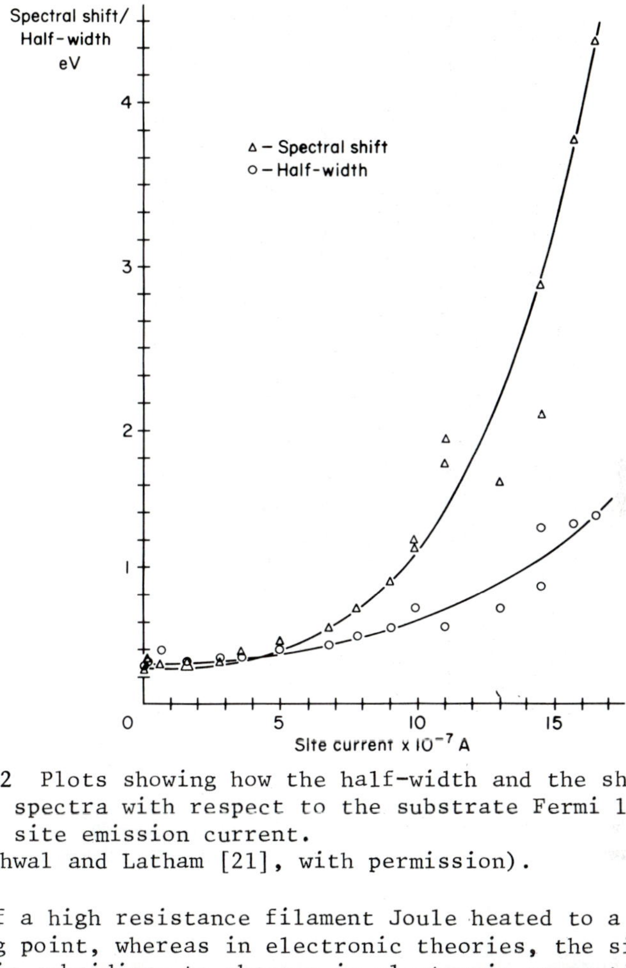

Fig. 8.12 Plots showing how the half-width and the shift of the electron spectra with respect to the substrate Fermi level vary with the site emission current.
(From Athwal and Latham [21], with permission).

nature of a high resistance filament Joule heated to a critical switching point, whereas in electronic theories, the size of the channel is subsidiary to changes in electronic properties, so that channel expansion is possible. This distinction is important to the present discussion, since in one case a constricted conducting filament in a dielectric medium produces field intensification as illustrated in Fig. 8.5, whilst distortions in band structure at the surface can produce hot electron emission such as suggested in the model illustrated in Fig. 8.10. Recent analyses of Chalcogenide alloy systems by Peterson and Adler [28] and Adler, Henisch and Mott [29] indicate that for these materials, the cross-sectional dimension of the conducting channel is a function of current. If this also applies to the impurities under consideration here, it then follows that the electron emission current could not be related to a fixed field enhancement factor β. Such an effect could therefore account for the high-field non-linearities in F-N plots that had previously been interpreted in section 3.1(iii) as a space charge effect associated with the metallic emitter model. If this concept of an expanding conducting channel is further related to the constraint imposed by the dimensions of the micro inclusion, Athwal and Latham [21] have pointed out that two extreme situations can be envisaged. For a small inclusion, the channel could occupy its whole cross-sectional dimension, so that there will be a constant β-factor with breakdown occurring when some critical current density is exceeded; for a large inclusion on the other hand, it may always be possible to accommodate the expanding channel so that the critical current density associated with breakdown is not exceeded. These alternative situations might therefore correspond respectively to the a- and b- sites referred to earlier.

Summarising the merits of this model, it can be said that it provides a qualitative explanation for most of the observed phenomena associated with the high-β emission sites. In addition it opens an alternative approach to the understanding of such well-known properties of high voltage vacuum gaps as the influence of the residual gas species, the physical significances of the "slope" and "intercept" of the traditional F-N plot of the current-voltage characteristic, the various conditioning procedures and the actual breakdown process itself. The concept of a potential emission regime undergoing a sub-microsecond "switching-on" process at some critical field also offers a very plausible explanation of the large-gap breakdown phenomenon; i.e. an alternative to the microparticle-based mechanism discussed in section 4.9(ii). However, this new model is based on a very complex phenomenon that is far from fully understood, even when studied under precisely controlled conditions, so it has to be anticipated that a great deal more fundamental investigation will be necessary before it will be possible to quantify the model and confidently prescribe a technological procedure for improving the insulating capability of vacuum that supersedes traditional "conditioning" techniques.

8.5 References

1. Allen, N.K. and Latham, R.V., *Proc. VIII-DEIV*, B3,1-13, (1978).
2. Allen, N.K., Cox, B.M. and Latham, R.V., *J.Phys.D: Appl. Phys*. **12**, 969-78, (1979).
3. Many, A., Golstein, Y. and Grover, N.B., *In* "Semiconductor Surfaces", p.131, North Holland Pub.Co., Amsterdam, (1965).
4. McKelvey, J.P., *In*"Solid State and Semiconductor Physics", p. 485, Harper & Row, New York and London, (1966).
5. Hurley, R.E., *J.Phys.D: Appl. Phys.*, **12**, 2229-45, (1979).
6. Cox, B.M., *J.Phys. D: Appl. Phys.*, **8**, 2065-73, (1975).
7. Farrall, G.A., Owens, M. and Hudda, F.G., *J. Appl. Phys.*, **46**, 610-7, (1975).
8. Farrall, G.A., *In* "Vacuum Arcs" (ed. J.M. Lafferty), John Wiley, New York and Chichester, (1980).

9. Pokrovskaya-Soboleva, A.S., Kraft, V.V., Borisova, T.S. and Mazurova, L.K., *Proc. V-DEIV*, 105-9, (1972).
10. Duke, C.B. and Alferieff, M.E., *J. Chem. Phys.* **46**, 923-37, (1967).
11. Gadzuk, J.W., *Phys. Rev.* **81**, 2110-29, (1970).
12. Hurley, R.E., *J. Phys. D: Appl. Phys.* **12**, 2247-52, (1979).
13. Dearnaley, G., Stoneham, A.M. and Morgan, D.V., *Rep. Prog. Phys.* **33**, 1129-91, (1970).
14. Boer, K.W. and Ovshinsky, S.R., *J. Appl. Phys.* **41**, 2675-81, (1970).
15. Cook, E.L., *J. Appl. Phys.* **41**, 551-4, (1970).
16. Dearnaley, G., *Thin Solid Films*, **3**, 161-74, (1969).
17. Hickmott, T.W., *J. Appl. Phys.* **37**, 4380-8, (1966).
18. Morgan, D.V. and Howes, M.J., *Phys. Stat. Solidi* **21**, 191-5, (1974).
19. Hurley, R.E. and Dooley, P.J., *Vacuum*, **28**, 147-9, (1978).
20. Cox, B.M., *CEGB Res. Rpt.* R/M/N1021 (1979).
21. Athwal, C.S. and Latham, R.V., *Proc. IX-DEIV, Physica*, **104c**, (1981), In press.
22. Juttner, B., Rohrbech, W. and Wolff, H., *Proc. V-DEIV*, 65-9, (1972).
23. Juttner, B., Wolff, H. and Altrichter, B., *Phys. Stat. Sol.* **27**, 403-12, (1975).
24. Hurley, R.E., *J. Phys. D: Appl. Phys.* **13**, 1121-8, (1980).
25. Benzer, S., *J. Appl. Phys.* **20**, 804-15, (1949).
26. Mott, N.F., *Contemp. Phys.* **10**, 125-38, (1969).
27. Volkov, A.F. and Kogan, S.M., *Usp. Sov. Phys.* **11**, 881-903, (1969).
28. Peterson, R.E. and Adler, D., *J. Appl. Phys.* **47**, 256-63, (1976).
29. Adler, D., Henisch, H.K. and Mott, S.N., *Rev. Mod. Phys.* **50**, 209-220, (1978).
30. Moridi, G.R. and Hogarth, C.A., *Int. J. Electron.* **44**, 297-304, (1978).

Appendix – Flashover across Solid Insulators in a Vacuum Environment

The mechanical design of any high voltage vacuum device must inevitably incorporate a glass or ceramic electrical insulating member for supporting the "high voltage" electrode, such as shown for example in Figs. 2.1 and 2.2. From the practical point of view it is therefore essential that the voltage hold-off capability of this "link" is at least as good as that offered by the operational vacuum gap. In fact, the actual performance of a solid insulator is generally poorer than that of a vacuum gap of similar dimensions, even though the *bulk* insulating properties of the material concerned would indicate a superior performance. The explanation of this anomaly centres on the role played by the *surface* of the insulator, which is highly susceptable to promoting an electrical flashover between the "high" and "low" voltage electrodes. One way of tackling this problem in a practical situation, is to arrange for the length of the solid insulator in the direction of the field to be considerably greater than the corresponding d-value of the vacuum gap. It is found however that this precaution alone is not sufficient to guarantee the performance of an insulator. Accordingly, there has been an on going research effort to understand the physical mechanisms responsible for this type of breakdown event, and to evolve design procedures for minimising the likelihood of its occurrence. An account of the early work in this field can be found in the review of Hawley [1] published in 1968, whilst for details of later developments there is for example the more recent review article of Cross [2].

From the early work of Boersch et al. [3], Smith [4], Bugaev and Mesyats [5,6], Watson [7], de Tourreil et al. [8], Sudarshan and Cross [9], Brainard and Jensen [10-12] and Anderson [13], it is now widely accepted that the surface flashover of a solid insulator is a direct consequence of secondary electron emission processes that lead to the positive charging of the insulator surface. Thus referring to Fig. A.1, the necessary conditions for initiating a breakdown event are assumed to stem from the field emission of electrons at the cathode "triple junction" formed at the metal/vacuum/insulator interface when the applied field exceeds some threshold value [10,13-15]. The first stage

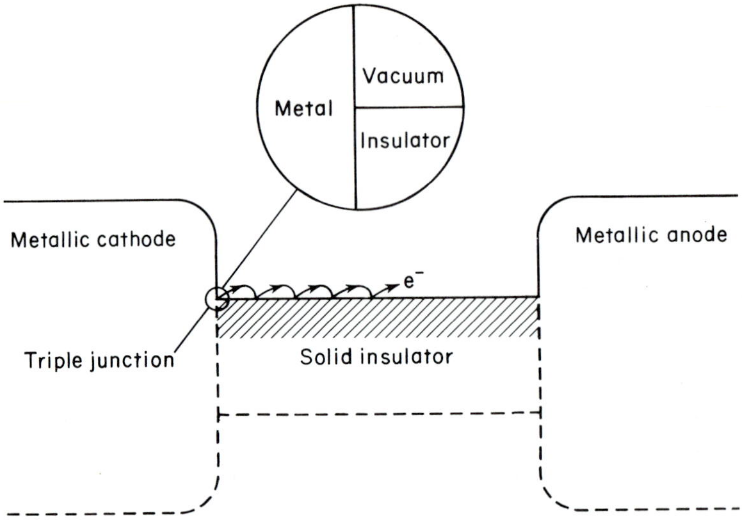

Fig. A.1 A schematic illustration of the physical regime associated with a "solid" high voltage insulator: also shown is the "hopping" mode by which electrons travel from cathode to anode.

of the process involves the insulator surface in the vicinity of the cathode acquiring an increasing positive charge as the result of a regenerative secondary electron emission mechanism that originates from the bombardment of the insulator by primary electrons field emitted from the triple junction. This leads to a growing cathode field, and hence the primary electron emission, until a point is reached where the region of regenerative charging can propagate rapidly across the surface of the insulator. The mechanism by which this is believed to occur is illustrated in Fig. A.1 where, under the influence of the applied field in the vacuum gap immediately above the surface of the insulator, electrons "hop" along the insulator towards the anode and so give rise to a pre-breakdown current [3]. However, since the dependence of the secondary electron yield δ_e on the primary energy U has the general form shown in Fig. A.2 for most insulating materials, where U_1 and U_2 are typically $\sim$ 20-100 eV and 1-5 keV respectively, with $(\delta_e)_{max}$ perhaps approaching 6, it follows that there is a wide range of primary energies for which δ_e is greater than unity. Hence, if the energy acquired by an electron during one of the "hops" illustrated in Fig. A.1 exceeds U_1, which is generally the case, the possibility exists for a progressive build-up of a positive charge distribution on the surface of the insulator as illustrated in Fig. A.3. However, the increasing field at the insulator surface now starts to return the "hopping" electrons more quickly to the surface until a point is reached where they only acquire an energy of $\sim$ 20 eV during any hop, keeping within

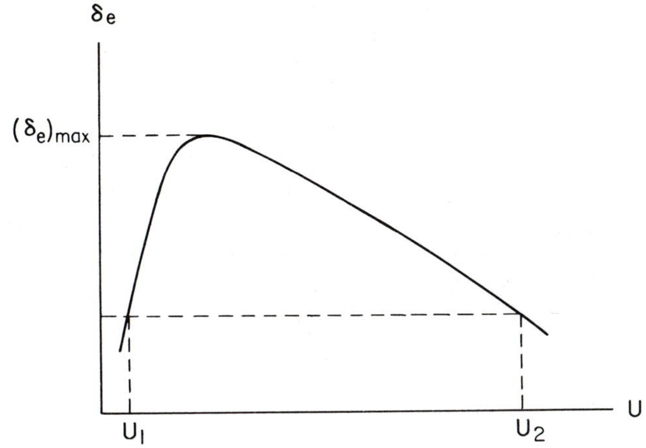

Fig. A.2 The typical dependence of the secondary electron yield δ_e on the energy of the primary electrons.

a few microns of the surface, so that from Fig. A.1, $\delta_e \to 1$ and there will no longer be any further charge multiplication by secondary emission. In practice, this charging of the insulator surface proceeds by an avalanche process [3,7,10-14] involving a high gain multiplication of secondary electrons over large areas of the insulator and hence large currents. On the other hand,the decay time of the surface charge distribution is typically several hours at a pressure of $\sim 10^{-9}$mbar, which is consistant with the bulk electronic relaxation times of insulating materials [10]. (In the context of this discussion, it should be noted that δ_e of Fig. A.2 is generally understood to refer to the "true" low-energy electron yield, i.e. excluding elastically and inelastically scattered primaries, whereas it is in fact the "total" secondary electron yield that governs the charging process. However, in practice, the contribution from reflected primaries is usually small, so that failure to recognise this distinction does not lead to large discrepancies).

To study the evolution of this secondary-emission avalanche, and hence obtain a better insight into the physical processes involved, single-shot pulse techniques have been employed; i.e. a similar approach to that used for studying the "cathode initiated" breakdown mechanism discussed in Chapters 3 and 5. From

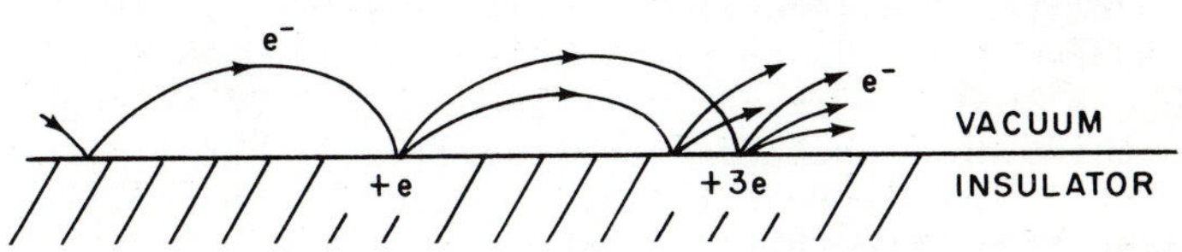

Fig. A.3 Illustrating how the "hopping" electrons can lead to the surface of an insulator becoming positively charged.

early microsecond pulse experiments of this kind by Brainard and Jensen [10,11], in which an avalanche was initiated by an auxiliary electron beam that bombarded a cylindrical alumina insulator in the vicinity of the triple junction (see Fig. A.1) to simulate real electron emission from this region, it was established that charging currents can reach several amperes in a few nanoseconds, and that the characteristic time for the charging process to reach a saturation state where $\delta_e \to 1$ was $\sim$ 50ns. For a given pulse rise-rate, the threshold voltage at which the avalanche was initiated was found to be strongly dependent on the magnitude of the simulated triple-junction electron emission current, with a minimum requirement of $\sim 10^{-9}$A. The total surface charge was also measured and found to be proportional to the pulse amplitude V_p for $V_p \gtrsim 25$ kV, which was in agreement with an earlier theoretical prediction of Boers [16] based on a solution of Laplace's equation. Finally, a delay-time was identified between switching on the simulated electron emission and the initiation of the avalanche, which was similarly dependent on the magnitude of the electron beam current for a given pulse rise rate: an effect that was attributed to the time required to build up the surface charge density to some critical value required for avalanche initiation.

The saturated surface charge distribution on an insulator has been investigated experimentally by a number of techniques including (a) measuring the deflection of an electron beam directed close to the charged surface [14,17], (b) measuring the charge induced on a static probe [3,8], static plate [12], or oscillating probe [18], all located in close proximity to the insulator surface, and (c) by use of the Kerr effect [19]. Where a technique has a good spatial resolution, such as that of Brainard and Jensen [18], it is found that the surface charge density rises and falls nearly symmetrically along the length of the insulator, reaching a maximum value in the centre which would typically be ~ 25nC.cm^{-2} for a 100 kV pulse applied across a 1cm insulator. This same research group also calculated the surface charge distribution from a numerical solution of Poisson's equation [18,20] and showed there to be good agreement with the experimental findings. The charging process has also been treated theoretically by Srivastava and his co-workers [21,22] using a numerical simulation technique. Although necessarily idealistic in its concept, good agreement was reported between the predictions of this model and the findings of the complementary diagnostic experiments of this group [8,17]: of particular interest, it predicted an irreversible discontinuity in the linear rate of increase of the triple junction field with applied voltage, such as would be expected to occur with the sudden onset of electron emission, insulator charging [10,11] and a resulting enhancement of the cathode field. Typically, the critical gap field associated with this phenomenon is $\simeq 0.8$ MV.m^{-1}.

Whilst the above model provides a well founded explanation of the prebreakdown behaviour of solid insulators, the mechanisms leading to a flashover and the development of an arc are less well understood. From the early measurements of Bugaev and Mesyats [5,6] and later Anderson [13,22,23] using fast-rise nanosecond pulses, it was established that the typical normalised voltage waveform associated with a breakdown event takes the form shown in Fig. A.4, where V is the voltage appearing across the gap at any instant and V_p is the pulse amplitude. The time t_d is defined as the breakdown delay time and can vary from less than a nanosecond to hundreds of nanoseconds in a reproducible manner depending on the applied field, whilst t_b is defined as the breakdown or voltage collapse time and tends to a nearly constant value of $\sim$ 1ns. Nanosecond pulse techniques have also featured in a variety of optical measurements of the velocity v_d with which a discharge is propagated across the surface of an insulator; these include for example the techniques of Smith [14], Condit and Pelliman [25], Anderson [13,23] and Cross and Sudarsham [26,27]. Although there was a considerable spread in the reported values of v_d, ranging from 0.8-3 x $10^7 ns^{-1}$ and virtually independent of field, it has to be noted, that not only were a variety of insulating materials employed having differing dielectric constants [23] and secondary electron yields [13], but the

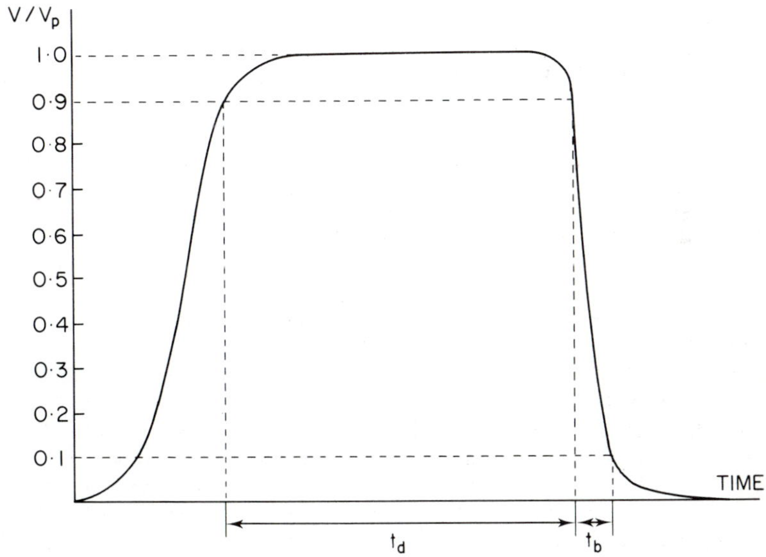

Fig. A.4 The typical form of the normalised voltage waveform V/V_p that appears across an insulator during a breakdown event, where V_p is the pulse amplitude: the breakdown delay time t_d and the voltage breakdown (or collapse) time t_b are defined in terms of the 10% and 90% points on the transient. (After Bugaev and Mesyats [5]).

measurements cover d-c, microsecond [26,27] and nanosecond [4,13, 23,25] pulsed field conditions. Also, v_d is sensitive to the shape of the insulator in so far as it affects the angle of the electric field relative to its surface [13]. Of the cited discharge velocity measurements, the higher 2 x $10^7 ms^{-1}$ value recently obtained by Anderson [23] using nanosecond pulse techniques is not only consistent with the widely accepted flash-over model of Boersch et al. [3], which required the previously discussed electron avalanche to precede breakdown, but is also in agreement with an earlier indirect measurement of v_d by a technique using crossed electric and magnetic fields [13]. On the basis of these measurements, the physical origin of the breakdown delay time is principally attributed to the initial threshold charging of the insulator in the vicinity of the cathode, since the flashover is thought to follow immediately upon the electron avalanche whose propagation velocity is comparably high.

The common feature of recent interpretations of the final flashover phase of a breakdown event, is the vital role played by the gas that is either thermally or electron-stimulated desorbed from the insulator surface. This is assumed to create an ionisable medium in the vicinity of the surface that can support regenerative ionisation processes and hence the development of an arc [28-32]. From early computations based on a thermal desorption model, Anderson [28] was able to show that, in the case of insulators having a low thermal conductivity, there could be a sufficiently large temperature rise within a few nanoseconds of the voltage application for there to be the necessary rapid desorption of gas. Further support for this type of mechanism is provided by indirect experimental evidence which confirms that the surface flashover voltage of certain insulators, such as polyethylene, does in fact exhibit the anticipated fall off with increasing temperature [29]. Recently, Anderson and Brainard [32] have developed a theoretical analysis of a more sophisticated version of this model based on the electron stimulated desorption of gas, and shown that the predicted dependence of the breakdown delay time on the length of the insulator and electric field are in good agreement with experimental observations. Referring to Fig. A.5 the sequence of events envisaged in their model are that (i) the insulator surface becomes positively charged by secondary electron emission until the unity-yield equilibrium situation described above is reached, (ii) in parallel with this process, there is an increasing electron stimulated desorption of neutral or positively ionised atoms and molecules from the surface of the insulator, (iii) further "neutrals" become ionised above the surface by electron impact, (iv) these positive ions drift towards the cathode and give rise to an enhanced field at the triple junction and hence an increased electron emission, (v) this then leads to a further increase in the rate of gas desorption and ionisation until finally, as this process continues and the cathode field rises, (vi) other regenerative proces-

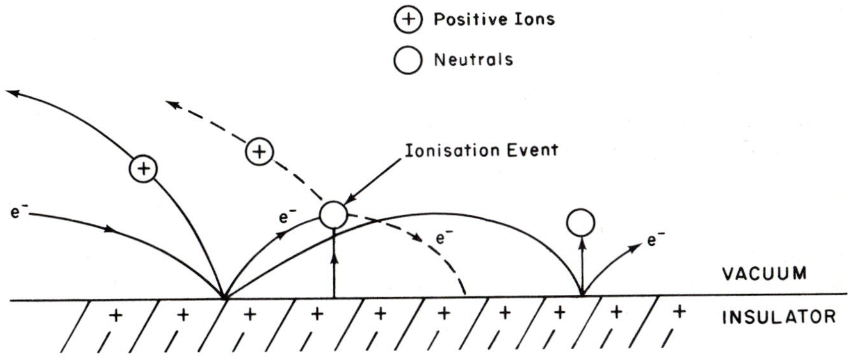

Fig. A.5 The mechanism by which gas molecules are desorbed from the surface of the insulator by electron-stimulation and subsequently ionised by electron impact.
(After Anderson and Brainard [32]).

ses, possibly involving photon emission, are initiated which result in the rapid breakdown of the insulator. A somewhat similar model of the breakdown mechanism has also been proposed by Cross [27], in that it too assumes an insulator charging process that is based on a secondary electron emission avalanche. However, the final flashover stage is now assumed to be initiated by a large burst of electron emission from the triple junction which, by a knock-on process, charges successive regions of the insulator negatively until the burst reaches the anode, thus leaving a channel of excited gas in its wake along which flashover finally takes place.

The general philosophy behind the technological procedures that have been developed for suppressing this type of breakdown mechanism is to inhibit the initiation of the above sequence of events by preventing the initial charging of the insulator. One of the earliest measures to be adopted, that consistently leads to an improved performance, involves electrically shielding the cathode triple junction to reduce the local field and associated electron emission processes [15]. There are also reports of an improved performance resulting from reducing the field at the triple junction by specially shaping the metal electrodes and insulator in this local region [7,33,34]. More generally, the shape of the insulator [1,7,35-40], and in particular the angle its surface makes with the metal electrodes [35,36], can be used to control the trajectories of the secondary electrons, and thereby significantly control the voltage hold-off capability of an insulator: in this connection, mention should be made of the use of a magnetic field to inhibit surface flashover [41]. The influence of the insulator material has also been extensively investigated [1,15,38,40,42-44]: however, whilst it has been conclusively demonstrated that this parameter plays a major role in determining the performance of an insulator, there is a considerable divergence among the published data as to the correct hierarchy of materials. Nevertheless, despite the evident difficulty in reproducing identical test regimes from laboratory to laboratory, it can be said that glass-like insulators exhibit a general trend towards providing better performances than those of comparable geometry fabricated from porous ceramic materials. Brief mention should also be made of an early finding [45] that an improvement in performance can be achieved by roughening the surface of the insulator near the cathode triple junction; an effect that presumably arises from a favourable redistribution of the charge on the insulator surface that leads a reduced cathode field.

Another approach that has received considerable attention in recent years is to coat the surface of an insulator with a material having a low secondary electron yield, ideally with $\delta_e \lesssim 1$, so as to inhibit the initial build-up of positive charge. This requirement therefore points to the use of a metallic or semiconducting based treatment since insulating materials generally have high values of δ_e. An important secondary consequence of using such coatings is that the surface conductivity of the insulator will be raised, so that any residual charging effects will also be minimised. The successful application of this technique was first demonstrated by Fryszman et al. [46] who, by depositing a thin layer of semiconducting Fe_2O_3 on a cylindrical ceramic insulator, obtained a significant improvement in its voltage hold-off capability: these workers also showed that this treatment is most effective when applied at the cathode end of the insulator. More recently, Cross and Sudarshan have reported on their detailed investigation into the performance of alumina insulators that have been coated with cuprous oxide [47] and chrome oxide [48], whilst Miller and Furno [49] have made a similar study of the influence of a manganese/titanium coating on alumina, and later chrome on alumina [50], using a quasi-metalising process,in an attempt to develop insulators that can survive breakdown events. In the case of the Cu_2O treatment, where $\delta_e \simeq 1.25$, Cross and Sudarshan [47] found that whilst there was a considerable improvement in performance for μs pulsed field operation, the dc and low frequency behaviour was only comparable with a fully conditioned uncoated insulator: it should be noted however that this latter observation still points to important practical advantages. In contrast, these authors showed that with a Cr_2O_3 coating [48], where $\delta_e \sim 0.98$, the dc insulating performance is now improved by a factor of 2-3, whilst that obtained with μs pulses is less marked. The findings from both of these investigations were however shown to be in good agreement with the predictions of an associated computer simulation model [51]. With Mn/Ti coated insulators Miller and Furno [49] found that the voltage hold-off capability for both d-c and μs pulsed operation could be consistently raised by about 25% above that of uncoated control insulators. Apart from lowering δ_e and decreasing the surface resistivity, these authors also attributed the improved performance in part to the more uniform dielectric properties of a coated insulator. It should however also be noted in connection with this discussion of the control of secondary electron yield, that care has to be taken when quoting δ_e-values to specify the angle of incidence of the primary electrons, since δ_e can show large increases at glancing angles such as are involved in an avalanche [52]. The possibility must also be recognised that the effects associated with using different insulator coatings may also, at least in part, be due to changes in the efficiency of the electron-stimulated desorption process, as could be anticipated from recent breakdown models [24,32,53].

Whatever the physical origin of the observed changes in insulaator performance, it is apparent that because both mechanisms would be very sensitive to surface contamination, such as might follow a flashover event, the hold-off voltage of a device will depend very much upon its operational history. This phenomena has been systematically investigated by Chatterton and Davies [54] for Macor, Lucalox and Plexiglas insulators. To simulate the conditions that are likely to exist on the contaminated surface of an insulator following a large number of flashovers, they also studied Plexiglas insulators that had been coated with thin layers of Ti and C. By using the electron probe technique of Sorensen [55] for measuring δ_e in situ both before and after flashover events, these authors were able to show that, for all the uncoated samples, there is a general lowering of δ_e following flashover conditioning; i.e. they established a dynamic correlation between the voltage hold-off capability and the secondary electron yield coefficient. However, they were unable to establish a similar correlation for the more complex surface regime existing on the coated insulators: one suggested reason for this is that the surface contaminants cause drastic changes in the emitting properties of the cathode field emitting sites, and that this effect masks that resulting from small changes in δ_e.

Before concluding this discussion of electrical flashover across solid insulators, mention must be made of three other physical mechanisms that could also play a significant role in initiating some breakdown events. Firstly, it follows indirectly from the experiments described in Section 7.2, and also from the direct measurements of Cross and Srivastava [56], that there is an abundance of microparticles in the size range 0.5-2μm present in a high voltage gap. This therefore means that the possibility exists for any of the microparticle breakdown initiating mechanisms described in Chapter 4 to operate in the present regime: in particular, microscopic damage to the insulator surface, with the consequent local change in δ_e, would seem to be a strong possibility. The second mechanism is thought to be associated with the modification of the cathode field following the injection of charges into the insulator. This effect shows itself as a sensitivity of the hold-off voltage to the history of the field sequences applied to the insulator. For example, it has been found that the impulse flashover voltage can be significantly influenced by a d-c pre-stress treatement where, depending on whether or not it has the same polarity as the following impulse voltage, the insulating strength will be respectively increased or reduced [56]. Although the phenomenon has many features in common with a similar effect exhibited with bulk dielectrics [57], there is a discrepancy of two orders of magnitude in the value of the applied field required for observing the phenomenon in the two cases: for bulk breakdown it is $\simeq 5 \times 10^8 Vm^{-1}$ whilst for surface flashover it is only $\simeq 5 \times 10^6 Vm^{-1}$. This therefore suggests that a direct analogy between the bulk and surface processes is unlikely to represent the true physical situation. Finally, it has been reported by Anderson [35,58] that breakdown can also take place by an anode-initiated mechanism where the flashover propagates from anode to cathode. The mechanism is extremely fast ($\sim$ nanoseconds), electronic in origin, is particularly associated with conical insulators having angles between 40° and 70°, and is also characterised by producing a tree-like or dendritic form of damage to the insulator surface. This type of breakdown has tentatively been attributed to a mechanism involving a small area of plasma on the insulator surface that causes a local breakdown of the bulk dielectric and hence the formation of new plasma to carry forward the discharge.

References

1. Hawley, R., *Vacuum*, **18**, 383-90, (1968).
2. Cross, J.D., *Proc. VII-DEIV*, 24-37, (1976).
3. Boersch, H., Hamisch, H. and Erlich, W., *Z. Angew Phys.* **15**, 518-25, (1963).
4. Smith, I.D., *Proc. I-DEIV*, 261-80, (1964).
5. Bugaev, S.P. and Mesyats, G.A., *Sov. Phys-Tech. Phys.* **10**, 930-2, (1966).
6. Bugaev, S.P., Iskol'dsky, A.M. and Mesyats, G.A., *Sov. Phys-Tech. Phys.* **12**, 1358-62, (1968).
7. Watson, A., *J. Appl. Phys.* **38**, 2019-23, (1967).
8. de Tourreil, C.H., Srivastava, K.D. and Woelke, V., *IEEE Trans. Elec. Insul.* **EI-7**, 176-9, (1972).
9. Sudarshan, T.S. and Cross, J.D., *IEEE Trans. Elec. Insul.* **EI-8**, 122-8, (1973).
10. Brainard, J.P. and Jensen, D., *1972 Ann. Rpt. CEIDP*, 298-303, (1973).
11. Brainard, J.P. and Jensen, D., *1973 Ann. Rpt. CEIDP*, 250-7, (1974).
12. Brainard, J.P. and Jensen, D., *J. Appl. Phys.* **45**, 3260-5, (1974).
13. Anderson, R.A., *Appl. Phys. Lett.* **24**, 54-6, (1974).
14. de Tourreil, C.H. and Srivastava, K.D., *Proc. V-DEIV*, 295-99, (1972).

15. Kofoid, M.J., *Trans. AIEE (USA), Pt. III* **79**, 991-1004, (1960).
16. Boers, J.E., *Proc. 11th Symp. on Electron, Ion and Laser Beam Tech., San Francisco Press Inc.*, pp. 167-72, (1971).
17. de Tourreil, C.H., Ph.D. Thesis, Univ. Waterloo,Ont.Can(1971).
18. Brainard, J.P. and Jensen, D., *1974 Ann. Rpt. CEIDP*, 442-50, (1975).
19. Brainard, J.P., *Proc. VI-DEIV*, 198-203, (1974).
20. Anderson, R.A. and Brainard, J.P., *1977 Ann. Rpt. CEIDP*,128-35, (1979).
21. de Tourreil, C.H. and Srivastava, K.D., *IEEE Trans. Elec. Insul.* **EI-8**, 17-21, (1973).
22. Sudarshan, T.S., Cross, J.D. and Srivastava, K.D., *IEEE Trans. Elec. Insul.* **EI-12**, 200-8, (1977).
23. Anderson, R.A., *J. Appl. Phys.* **48**, 4210-5, (1977).
24. Anderson, R.A. and Brainard, J.P., *Proc. VIII-DEIV*, **D4**, 1-15, (1978).
25. Condit, W.C. and Pellinen, D., *Phys. Rev. Lett.* **29**, 263-5, (1972).
26. Cross, J.D. and Sudarshan, T.S., *IEEE Trans. Elec. Insul.* **EI-11**, 63-6, (1976).
27. Cross, J.D., *IEEE Trans. Elec. Insul.*, **EI-13**, 145-8, (1978).
28. Anderson, R.A., *1974 Ann. Rpt. CEIDP*, 435-41, (1975).
29. Ohki, Y. and Yahagi, K., *J. Appl. Phys.* **46**, 3695-6, (1975).
30. Avdienko, A.A. and Malev, M.D., *Sov. Phys-Tech. Phys.* **22**, 986-92, (1977).
31. Avdienko, A.A. and Malev, M.D., *Vacuum*, **27**, 643-8, (1977).
32. Anderson, R.A. and Brainard, J.P., *J. Appl. Phys.* **51**, 1414-21, (1980).
33. Shannon, J.P., Philp, S.F. and Trump, J.G., *J. Vac. Sci. Technol.* **2**, 234-9, (1965).
34. Brainard, J.P., *1975 Ann. Rpt. CEIDP*, 482-8, (1978).
35. Anderson, R.A., *1975 Ann. Rpt. CEIDP*, 475-81, (1978).
36. Anderson, R.A., *Proc. VII-DEIV*, 252-6, (1976).
37. Mazurek, B. and Tyman, A., *Proc. VII-DEIV*, 265-9, (1976).
38. Hamidov, N., Aritov, V.A., Isamuhamedov, S.D., Kelman, M.C. and Agsamov, A., *Proc. VII-DEIV*, 282-5, (1976).
39. Golden, J. and Kapetanakos, C.A., *J. Appl. Phys.* **48**, 1756-8, (1977).
40. Svinjin, M.P., Sivkova, A.V., Smirnov, L.V. and Ershov, V.V., *Proc. V-DEIV*, 301-5, (1972).
41. Bergeron, K.D. and McDaniel, D.H., *Appl. Phys. Lett.* **29**, 534-6, (1976).
42. Kondsatosv, O.I., *Proc. V-DEIV*, 289-94, (1972).
43. Akahane, M., Kanda, K. and Yahagi, K. *J. Appl. Phys.* **44**, 2927-32, (1973).
44. Suzuki, T., *Japan J. Appl. Phys.* **13**, 1541-6, (1974).
45. Gleichauf, P.M., *J. Appl. Phys.* **22**, 766-71, (1951).
46. Fryszman, A., Strzyz, T. and Wasinski, M., *Bull. Acad. Polon. Sci. Ser. Sci. Tech.* **8**, 379-83, (1960).
47. Cross, J.D. and Sudarshan, T.S., *IEEE Trans. Elec. Insul.* **EI-9**, 146-50, (1974).

48. Sudarshan, T.S. and Cross, T.D., *IEEE Trans. Elec. Insul.* **EI-11**, 32-5, (1976).
49. Miller, H.C. and Furno, E.J., *J. Appl. Phys.* **49**, 416-20, (1978).
50. Miller, H.C., *IEEE Trans. Elec. Insul.* **EI-15**, (1981), In press.
51. Sudarshan, T.S., Ph.D. Thesis, University of Waterloo, Ontario, Canada, (1975).
52. Brainard, J.P. and Anderson, R.A., *1977 Ann. Rpt. CEIDP*, 136-41, (1979).
53. Bergeron, K.D., *J. Appl. Phys.* **48**, 3073-80, (1977).
54. Chatterton, P.A. and Davies, D.K., *Proc. VIII-DEIV*, D2.1-11, (1978).
55. Sorensen, H., *J. Appl. Phys.* **48**, 2244-50, (1977).
56. Cross, J.D. and Srivastava, K.D., *IEEE Trans. Elec. Insul.* **EI-9**, 97-102, (1974).
57. Bradwell, A., Cooper, R. and Varlow, B., *Proc. IEEE*, **118**, 247-52, (1971).
58. Anderson, R.A., *1978 Ann. Rpt. CEIDP*, 173-8, (1979).

Subject Index

Accelerators (*see* particle accelerators,
Anode flares, 70
Anode "hot-spots"
  burn mark evidence, 172-3
  critical power loading, 77
  dimensions, 65-6
  microparticle source, 96-7, 205-6
  optical emission (*see* electroluminescence)
  steady-state temperature distribution, 66-9
  thermal stability, 5,76-9
  transient temperature distribution, 74-6
  transition radiation, 188-90
  X-ray emission, 189

β-factor (*see* microprotrusions)
Bibliographies, 8,10
Breakdown
  anode initiated, 3,5,60,76-9
  cathode initiated, 4,5,60-5, 70,76-9,217-8
  cathode versus anode initiation, 76-9
  critical field, 2,5,77,125
  commutation time, 70-2
  delay time, 70-2, 73
  electrode damage, 177-81
  in-flight particle vaporisation, 96-100
  large gaps, 3,4,7,22,38,226
  microparticle initiated, 4, 84-6,93-6,96-100,110-3, 205-6
  practical implications, 1,6-8
  residual gas pressure (*see* pressure "effect")
  residual gas species, 34
  small gaps, 4,7,22,38
  suppression (*see* conditioning, electrodes, external circuitry and pressure)
  total time, 70
  trigger discharge mechanisms, 27, 91-6,112-3,149
  voltage waveform (*see* plane-parallel gap)
Broad-area emission sites
  electron spectra, 194-9
  emission imaging, 172-4,190-1
  location, 175-6,181-6,193-6
  optical spectra, 190-3
  physical properties, 56,174-5, 182-3,186,192-3,199,211-26

Cathode
  flares, 70,131-2
  flare velocity, 71,131-3
  microprotrusions (*see* microprotrusions)
  thermal response time, 73
Clumps (*see* microparticles and breakdown, microparticle initiated)
Coefficient of restitution (*see* microsphere simulation studies)
Conditioning
  "current", 3,7,25-7,222
  "gas", 28
  gas desorption, 187-8
  "glow-discharge", 27
  "spark", 7,28-30

Drift tube (*see* microparticle detection and microsphere charge and velocity measurement)

Electrochemical polishing (*see* electrode surface preparation)
Electrode
  conditioning (*see* conditioning)
  damage, 156-8,177-81
  gap (*see* electrode separation)
  geometry, 36-8
  "high-voltage", 14-5,22
  insulating inclusions, 186,192-3,211-26
  "low-voltage", 14-15,22
  material, 7,34,39-40,44,98-101,103,158-9,167-9,187-8,198
  microtopography, 177-81
  profile, 7,16
  separation, 38-9 (*see also* plane-parallel gap)
  surface coatings, 42
  surface field, 37-8
  surface state, 162-3
  surface preparation, 7,40-2,166-9
  work function, 20,33-4,53,167,175
  yield strength, 87-9, 101
Electroforming (*see* FEE, "non-metallic" mechanisms)
Electroluminescence
  anode spots, 188-90
  cathode or k-spots, 190-3,214,216-21
  experimental observation, 188-93
Electron bombardment (*see* anode "hot-spots")
Electron emission (*see* field electron emission)
Electron "heating" (*see* FEE, "non-metallic" mechanisms)
Electron spectra
  experimental measurement, 194-6
  "metallic" microemitters, 196-7
  "non-metallic" emission sites, 197-9,223-6
Ellipsometry, 162-3
Emission sites (*see* broad-area emission sites)
Explosive emission
  broad-area electrodes, 70-1
  point-plane diodes, 132-5
External circuitry, 42,131-3

Field electron emission
  high-temperature "metallic" mechanism, 54-5,73
  low-temperature "metallic" mechanism, 51-4
  "non-metallic" mechanisms, 186,192-3,211-26
  sites (*see* broad-area emission sites)
  space charge effects, 55-6,71
Field enhancement factor (*see* microprotrusions, β-factor)
Field penetration (*see* FEE, "non-metallic" mechanisms)
Flashover (*see* breakdown and solid insulators)
Fowler-Nordheim
  plots (*see* plane-parallel gap and micropoint cathodes)
  theory (*see* FEE, low-temperature "metallic" emission)

Gas
  adsorption, 33-4,175
  electron stimulated desorption, 234
  field desorption, 18,27,33
  thermal desorption, 18,37,187-8
  voltage-dependent desorption, 187

Historical, 2-6

Ignition phenomenon, 34-5
Impulse voltages (*see* plane-parallel gap)
Insulators (*see* solid insulators)

Ion-etching, 166-9 (*see also* "gas" and "glow discharge" conditioning)
Ion-exchange processes, 18,19, 25-7

Joulian heating (*see* microprotrusions, temperature response)

k-spots (*see* electroluminescence)

Light emission (*see* anode and cathode flares and electroluminescence)

Mass spectrometry techniques, 149-56,205-6
Mechanical polishing (*see* electrode surface preparation)
Microcratering (*see* electrode damage)
Microdischarges, 18-9,25-7
Microparticles, naturally occurring (*see also* microsphere simulation studies)
  bouncing, 26,104-110
  bouncing impact charge exchange, 106-110
  bouncing impact contact time, 107
  charge acquisition, 88
  charge to mass characteristics, 89,202-6
  critical inelastic impact velocity, 100-3
  detachment criteria, 26,87-91
  idealised geometries, 87-8
  impact cratering, 107
  impact vaporisation, 102-3
  impact welding, 95-6
  impact velocities, 100-3
  indirect detection, 199-202
  in-flight detection, 143-4, 202-6
  in-flight electron emission, 91-6,112-3
  in-flight vaporisation, 96-100, 205-6
  kinetic energy enhancement, 104-5
  microscopic surface field, 93-5, 112
  origin, 4,83,199-202
  "primary" and "secondary", 87,90
  velocity measurement, 143-4, 202-6
Micropoint cathodes
  d-c emission characteristics, 121-6
  d-c experimental regime, 119-21
  emission image, 118-20,122
  "explosive" emission regime, 132-8
  fabrication, 118
  material vaporisation, 135-6
  oscillatory emission regime, 136-8
  profile, 119,122,125
  pulsed field emission characteristics, 128-38
  pulsed field experimental regime, 126-7
  space charge effects, 124-5, 128-9
  surface fields, 120,123-4,133
  thermally assisted emission, 129-30
Microprotrusions, (*see also* broad-area emission sites)
  β-factors, 19-21,56-8,78
  blunting, 26,28
  direct observations, 5,177-81
  emission characteristics, 59-60
  field enhancement (*see* β-factors)
  field sharpening (*see* surface diffusion)
  geometries, 58
  growth (*see* surface diffusion)
  removal, 26-8
  steady-state temperature response, 62-5
  thermal stability, 76-9
  transient temperature response, 72-3
Microsphere simulation studies
  bouncing impact charge exchange,

160,165-8
breakdown initiation, 141-2, 146-9
charge and velocity measurement, 144-5,150,160-5
coefficient of restitution, 161,166-9
gun sources, 142-6,161-2
impact damage, 156-9
impact ionisation, 149-56
inelastic impact, 157-9
kinetic energy enhancement, 164-5
microcrater dimensions, 157-8
particle bouncing, 159-69

Negative resistance characteristic (*see* FEE, "non-metallic" mechanisms)
Neutron activation analysis, 200 (*see also* microparticle, indirect detection)
Nottingham effect
experimental investigation, 64-5
inversion temperature, 64
theoretical basis, 61-5

Optical phenomena (*see* electroluminescence, anode and cathode flares)

Particle accelerators, 19
Plane-parallel gap
a-c voltages, 43-5
breakdown characteristics, 38-9 (*see also* breakdown)
electrode material, 7,29,32-4
electrode polarity, 22-4
electrode separation, 21-2
electrode temperature, 24
experimental regime, 14-7, 42-3
F-N plots, 19-21,54
impulse voltages, 45-6,110-2
I-V characteristics, 17-24,35, 220
pulse voltages, 46
residual gas pressure, 34,219
Plasmas (*see also* cathode flares)
analysis of ion species, 153-6
charge separation, 131-2,138
oscillations, 136-8
particle impact (*see* microsphere impact ionisation)
Point-plane diode (*see* micropoint cathodes)
Polishing (*see* electrode surface preparation)
Prebreakdown currents (*see also* plane-parallel gap)
field dependence, 3,17-24,35,54
origin, 3,19-21,192-3,211-26
Pressure
"effect", 2-3,28-34,44
residual gas, 28-34,219
residual gas species, 27,187-8, 219
Protrusions (*see* microprotrusions)
Pulsed fields (*see* micropoint cathodes and plane-parallel gap)

References, 9-11,46-9,79-81,114-5, 139,169-70,206-9,226-7,238-40
Resonance tunnelling, 34-5,215
Reviews, 8,10

Simulation studies
using micropoint diodes, 5,55, 117-39 (*see also* micropoint cathodes)
using microspheres, 141-69, (*see also* microsphere simulation studies)
Solid Insulators
breakdown delay time, 233-4
breakdown time, 233
conditioning, 236-8
discharge velocity, 233-4
electrical shielding, 235
electron "hopping", 230
flashover mechanisms, 229-30,234-5,237-8
gas desorption, 234
insulating performance, 8,229-38

length, 229,234
material, 234-7
pulse breakdown, 232-4
secondary electron avalanche, 230-2,235
secondary electron yield, 230-1,234,237
shape, 234-5
surface charge distribution, 231-2
surface condition, 237
surface treatments, 236-7
thermal conductivity, 234
triple junction, 229-30,232-6
Space charge effects (*see* FEE, explosive emission and cathode flares)
Spectra
electron (*see* electron spectra)
optical (*see* electroluminescence)
Spot-knocking (*see* "spark" conditioning)
Sputtering phenomena, 22,27-8, 32-3
Surface diffusion, 6,22-4,33,72 125
Surface states (*see* FEE, "non-metallic" mechanisms)
Switching phenomena (*see* FEE, "non-metallic" mechanisms)

"Total-voltage" effect, 22
Transition radiation (*see* anode "hot-spots" and electroluminescence)
Trigger discharges (*see also* microparticle in-flight electron emission)
particle detachment, 112-3
particle impact, 27,91-6,149
Triple junction (*see* solid insulators)

Vacuum
pumping systems, 16
switches, 29,43
Van der Waals force, 90-1 (*see also* microparticle detachment)

Work function (*see* electrodes)
Work hardening, 41

X-rays
anode "hot-spot" emission, 189
flash tubes, 70
surface analysis, 186,200

Yield strength (*see* electrodes)